Clinical
Dermatology
for Students and Practitioners

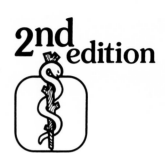

Clinical Dermatology

for Students and Practitioners

2nd edition

Joseph W. Burnett, MD
Professor and Head of Dermatology
University of Maryland

Harry M. Robinson, Jr, MD
Professor of Dermatology
University of Maryland

YORKE MEDICAL BOOKS
666 FIFTH AVENUE, NEW YORK, NEW YORK

To
Kitsie and Betty

FOREWORD

Dermatology at the University of Maryland has a rich heritage. This school, the fifth oldest in the United States, established the first formal teaching program for students in 1876. I.E. Atkinson, the first professor, and two of his Maryland schoolmates, Brown and Yandell, were three of the fourteen founders of the American Dermatological Association. G.H. Rohé, one of their contemporaries, and another Maryland graduate, wrote one of the first texts on dermatology to be published in the United States. Later, Rohé and T.C. Gilchrist published several revised editions of the book. R.B. Morison (University of Maryland, 1874) established the first teaching program in dermatology at the Johns Hopkins Hospital in 1887. Atkinson, the first professor at the University of Maryland, was successively followed by T.C. Gilchrist, M. Rosenthal, H.M. Robinson, Sr, H.M. Robinson, Jr, and J.W. Burnett (who assumed the position of chairman in 1977).

Atkinson and his successors stressed the importance of observing the minutiae, so helpful in making a clinical diagnosis. He taught, as we do today, that the clinical diagnosis should lead to the selection of the laboratory tests necessary for confirmation.

The original text by Harry M. Robinson, Jr, and Raymond C.V. Robinson, published in 1959, proved to be a good instrument with which to teach dermatology to medical students, and served as a practical reference for the primary care practitioner.

With the passage of time and the development of newer, more efficient diagnostic and therapeutic modalities, revision has become mandatory. In rewriting this book, we have preserved the original format but have deleted obsolete material. In an effort to present a modern, up-to-date text, we have consulted Butterworth's ''Syndromes'' and the latest editions of the major dermatology texts.

Joseph W. Burnett, MD
Harry M. Robinson, Jr, MD

PREFACE

The skin is a protective covering and a functioning organ which has nervous, vascular and hormonal communications with the viscera, the nervous system and the vascular system. The skin is the largest organ in the body and frequently reflects disturbances in normal physiologic functions or pathologic changes initiated elsewhere in the body.

The art of diagnosis applied to dermatology requires careful and thorough inspection of the entire cutaneous surface, regardless of the presenting complaint. The physician must compile a detailed record of the clinical manifestations and attempt to correlate them with the laboratory findings.

We have not attempted a comprehensive text; therefore, the clinical descriptions are concise. This monograph has been designed for practical use by students and practitioners. For more detailed information it will be desirable, at times, to consult a larger text.

In the first part of the book, general topics are introduced and discussed. In Part II, the dermatoses are classified by their morphological appearance so that the student may use this text as a diagnostic aid and as a tool to compile a differential diagnosis.

For simplification, the diagnostic terms have been anglicized as much as possible. Where feasible, the old names have been included as synonyms. In keeping with modern times, the heading "Venereal Diseases" has been replaced with "Sexually Transmitted Diseases". Every effort has been made to modernize without sacrificing content.

The authors gratefully acknowledge the contributions made by Drs. Ronald Goldner, William M. Gould, Irving D. Wolfe and Andrew G. Smith in revision of the chapters on Allergy, Mycology, Therapy, and Sexually Transmitted Diseases.

Joseph W. Burnett, MD
Harry M. Robinson, Jr, MD

CONTENTS

PART ONE
General Principles

Anatomy of Skin

The skin is the largest organ in the human body and completely envelops all other anatomic structures. At the mucocutaneous orifices it becomes continuous with mucous membranes through transitional epithelium. Its complicated structure contains blood and lymph vessels, nerves and specialized dermal appendages. It is thickest on the palms and soles and thinnest on the eyelids. Dermal appendages are specially distributed to meet the needs of the area. The palms and soles contain eccrine sweat glands but no sebaceous glands, whereas the apocrine glands predominate in the axillae and genital area. The face, scalp and upper back are rich in sebaceous gland.

Histologically the skin is divided into three layers: the epidermis (the outmost layer); the corium (true skin); and the subcutaneous tissue (fatty layer).

Epidermis. The epidermis consists of four strata:

The Basal Layer or Stratum Germinativum. This is the innermost layer of the epidermis and consists of a single layer of columnar cells, arranged perpendicularly to the surface. All of the other layers of the epidermis are formed from these cells which undergo morphologic and nuclear changes as they progress toward the most superficial layer. As long as this layer of cells remains intact, the epidermis will regenerate without scar formation. Mitoses are restricted to this layer or the immediately supra-adjacent cells.

The Stratum Granulosum. The cells of this layer are named for their histidine-rich cytoplasmic granules (keratohyalin) which are thought to be important in keratin formation.

The Stratum Lucidum. This layer is only present on the palms and soles.

The Stratum Corneum. This is the outmost layer of the epidermis and is formed of keratinized cells in which the nuclei are not normally present. The keratin present in those cells is a proteinaceous substance which has a high sulfur content.

Dermis. The dermis or corium is collagenous tissue which contains some elastic fibers. It is divided into the papillary portion (closest to the epidermis) and the reticular portion which lies between the papillary portion and the subcutaneous tissue. The capillary loops in the papillary bodies (ridges of the dermis in apposition to the basal layer of the epidermis) join the larger blood vessels in the reticular portion, and these larger blood vessels become large arteries and veins in the subcutaneous tissue. Nerves, sweat glands and sebaceous glands are found in the dermis.

Subcutaneous Tissue. This layer of the skin consists of fat cells in a fibrous tissue stroma. Large arteries, veins, lymphatics and nerve trunks are found in this layer. Some sweat glands also extend into the subcutaneous tissue. The subcutaneous tissue varies in thickness in

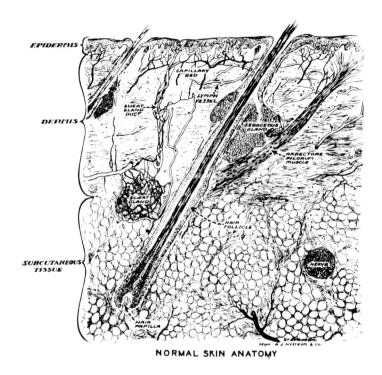

NORMAL SKIN ANATOMY

different parts of the body.

Appendages. The appendages of the skin are nails, hair, sebaceous glands, sweat glands and mammary glands.

Nails. The nail plate arises from the proximal nail fold and is adherent to the nail bed. It normally grows continuously at the rate of approximately 1 mm a week, and is composed of hard keratin.

Hair. The hair arises from a papilla located in the lowermost portion of the hair follicle. The portion of the hair contained within the follicle is known as the root. The lowermost portion of the hair root arising from the papilla is known as the hair bulb. The shaft is the portion of hair extending from the opening of the follicle. It grows at the rate of about 3 mm a week. There are two general types of hair: the fine, lightly pigmented type (lanugo), and the coarse, pigmented terminal hairs.

Sebaceous Glands. Sebaceous glands, classified as holocrine glands, arise from follicle walls. These structures produce sebum, a substance responsible for lubrication of the skin surface. This oily material is emptied onto the skin through the follicular orifice. Each gland has a rich vascular supply.

Sweat Glands. Sweat glands (coil glands) are of two types: apocrine and eccrine. Apocrine sweat glands are located in the axillae, the areolae of the nipples, about the umbilicus, the perianal region and the genital region. These glands are hormone-dependent and do not function until puberty. Eccrine sweat glands are primarily important in thermoregulation. They secrete a hypotonic salt solution which contains some nitrogenous materials. Each gland is surrounded by a plexus of capillaries, lymphatics and nerves.

Skin Muscles. Arrectores pilorum muscles are bundles of smooth muscle fibers attached to hair follicles. When these contract, the skin has a "gooseflesh" (cutis anserina) appearance. Striated muscles in the skin are limited to the face and neck (platysma).

CHAPTER 2

Physiological and Chemical Functions of the Skin

The skin accounts for 6-16% of total body weight. The surface area of an adult's skin, which approximates two square yards, is increased by invagination of the hair follicles. This large surface offers a passage for percutaneous absorption of many topically applied substances and is important in pharmacology. The skin is the external protective sheath which enables man to perceive pain, touch, temperature changes and other signals.

Principal Functions of the Skin

Protection. The skin is the elastic, resistant, covering organ which protects man from his complex environment. It prevents the influx of harmful physical and chemical agents and inhibits the excessive loss of water and essential electrolytes.

Thermoregulatory Function. Heat is lost from the body by conduction, convection, radiation and evaporation. The relative importance of these mechanisms varies with external conditions such as temperature, humidity, clothing and air movement.

Conduction. The poorest conducting layers of the skin are the horny layer and the adipose tissue. The dermis lying between these layers is a better heat conductor and tends to equalize any temperature differences.

Convection. This process is a constant source of heat loss. The thin layer of air in direct contact with the skin warms up rapidly and is replaced by cool and dry air. At air temperatures higher than 34.5°C, the heat loss by convection is negligible. Heat loss by convection increases with movement of the air.

Evaporation. Water loss from the skin has been divided into two categories: insensible, and visible or sensible water loss. The active secretion of the eccrine sweat glands, commonly referred to as sweat or perspiration is an example of visible water loss.

Radiation Heat Loss. The amount of heat loss by radiation varies with different individuals and with different postures.

Sensation. The four basic sensations of pain, temperature, touch and pressure are perceived in the skin. The ability to discriminate between sensations is a result of the stimulating pattern presented to the cerebral cortex as well as the type of receptor.

Secretory Mechanism. The skin has many active secretory cells. Sebum, secreted by the sebaceous glands, has some antifungal and antibacterial properties and aids in maintaining the texture of the skin.

Sweat is a true secretion. It is a hypotonic solution containing nitrogen, trace metals, lactate and potassium.

Percutaneous Absorption. The skin is the armor protecting the deeper tissues from trauma and desiccation. The oily surface film makes the skin water-repellent, and the constant desquamation of the horny layer retards the inward movement of materials which come in contact with the skin. The skin is permeable, however, and penetration occurs across the epidermal cells and through the follicular orifices. The stratum corneum plays a major role as a barrier to absorption, and hyperkeratosis does not greatly retard transfer rates. The epidermis is not supplied with blood vessels but the upper dermis has both a rich capillary bed and lymphatic drainage; therefore, materials which penetrate into the corium are absorbed.

All substances which pass through normal human skin are soluble in fat or water, but substances soluble in both solvent systems penetrate the skin best. Vehicles such as ointments or solvents may act as transport systems or simply bring the active ingredient in contact with skin.

Experimental evidence indicates that normal intact human skin is usually impermeable to water, electrolytes, carbohydrates, fats and proteins; however, all true gases and many vaporized or volatile substances will pass through the epidermis.

Mercury, lead, copper, arsenic and bismuth penetrate the skin under certain conditions, and sex hormones are readily absorbed when applied in a solvent vehicle.

Keratinization Process. Keratinization is the most important function of epidermal cells. It is the process of transformation of living epithelial cells into a horny substance called keratin. During this change there is a loss of cellular structure and cell death.

Hair growth is also a part of the keratinization process, and it varies in different regions of the body. It is most rapid on the chin (0.38 mm a day), less on the scalp (0.35 mm a day), axilla (0.30 mm a day), thigh (0.20 mm a day), and eyebrow (0.16 mm a day). The growth is more rapid in summer than in winter. After the third decade, the rate of hair growth declines slightly.

Pigmentation. Normal pigmentation is genetically controlled. Hyperpigmentation is produced by trauma, irradiation, exposure to the elements or inflammation.

The formation of pigment is believed to begin with tyrosine, which itself is probably formed from the essential amino acid, phenylalanine. Tyrosine is first oxidized to dopa (3,4-dihydroxyphenylalanine) by the enzyme tyrosinase. This enzyme also aids in transforming dopa through a series of oxidation and reduction reactions to an indole compound, which then polymerizes to form melanin. Melanin is packaged inside cytoplasmic granules. These granules are initially manufactured in the Golgi apparatus or endoplasmic reticulum. They appear to possess tyrosinase and become melanized as they move to the cell periphery. Some granules are "injected" into the cytoplasm of keratinocytes. It is primarily the clustering of these granules within their vacuoles that explains the dark pigmentation of blacks. The black's granules are larger and therefore can be packaged singly, thereby being better dispersed in the melanocyte's cytoplasm.

Pigmentation and Hormones. *Pituitary Gland.* The hypophysis influences pigmentation by its control over other endocrine glands, and through the production by the intermediary lobe of the melanocyte-stimulating hormone (MSH).

Thyroid. The thyroid has a "permissive" role in the production or control of pigmentation in the mammal.

Adrenal Glands. The adrenal glands are the most important endocrine glands in the control of pigmentation in the mammal because of their "feedback" effect on the production of MSH from the pituitary. If the adrenals are hypoactive or nonfunctioning, as in Addison's disease, MSH is produced in large quantities and abnormal pigmentation results.

Sexual Glands. Gonadal secretions promote pigment formation in specialized sites of the skin.

Sebaceous Secretion

The substance which forms the "surface film" of the body is derived from sweat, sebum and desquamating epidermal cells. The amount of sebum secreted is usually 1-2 gm a day for the entire body.

Distribution. The sebaceous glands are holocrine glands which usually develop by the fifth fetal month. They are distributed over the entire skin surface except the palms and soles. These glands are most numerous on the scalp, forehead, nose, cheeks and chin, and are also abundant on the chest and shoulders. Modified sebaceous glands on the penis produce smegma and in the ear canals produce wax. The meibomian glands of the eyelids are also variants of these glands. The mammary glands are variants of apocrine glands, not sebaceous glands.

Factors Influencing Sebum Production. The two most important factors controlling the production of sebum are the atmospheric temperature and hormonal factors. There is no direct nerve control.

Sebum is a fluid or semisolid oily material which is deposited on the skin surface. When the external temperature increases, the viscosity of sebum de-creases and the rate of flow is increased. Hormones play an important role in the production of sebum. Testosterone and progesterone are potent sebaceous gland stimulants.

Sebum is composed of waxes, triglycerides, cholesterol and squalene.

Chemistry of the Dermis

The dermis is composed of collagen, reticulum, elastin and ground substance. These substances, like keratin, are long chains of amino acids joined together by peptide linkages.

The most important and abundant amino acid in collagen is glycine. Collagen is attacked by pepsin but is resistant to trypsin. Collagen fibers, when heated, become rubbery and contract.

Reticulum. Reticulum is immature collagen formed by fibroblasts. Elastic fibers comprise only a small percentage of the corium and can be differentiated from collagen fibers by their resistance to pepsin, boiling water and boiling dilute acids. Elastic tissue is protein which lacks many of the essential amino acids.

Ground Substance. This is an organized network of protein molecules filled with hyaluronic acid, a mucopolysaccharide which contains hexosamine, glucosamine, uronic acid and acetyl groups. This material is important as a "filler" substance which allows rapid diffusion of needed nutrients but can impede the transmission of bacteria.

CHAPTER 3

Etiology of Dermatoses

Etiology is the science of investigation of the cause of disease. As the knowledge of pathologic physiology increases, it becomes more obvious that etiology and diagnosis are inseparable. The practitioner must make every effort to understand the nature of a condition, discover its cause, and thereby establish the correct diagnosis. When the cause of an eruption has been determined, some rational form of therapy may be devised, but when the etiologic agent is obscure, the physician must resort to the use of empirical measures.

A multiplicity of factors may combine to produce an eruption. Eczema (atopic dermatitis, lichenified dermatitis, lichen simplex chronicus, neurodermatitis) may have been originally caused by some endogenous or exogenous sensitizing substance. However, the ultimate picture is caused by a combination of endogenous factors and emotional stimuli. This syndrome may be complicated further by superimposed pyogenic infection produced by local inoculation (scratching).

The etiology of dermatoses is divided into predisposing causes (nonspecific factors which contribute to the development of an eruption) and precipitating causes (those factors actually causing the disease or pathologic state).

Predisposing Causes

Predisposing causes are those factors which lower the resistance or increase the susceptibility of the skin to attack. Many eruptions are secondary manifestations of some internal disorder.

Age. Some eruptions develop only at certain periods of life. Ichthyosis, impetigo neonatorum and epidermolysis bullosa appear in infancy. Verruca vulgaris, impetigo contagiosa, ecthyma and tinea capitis are primarily diseases of childhood. The adolescent boy or girl is prone to develop acne vulgaris, seborrhea oleosa and psoriasis. Kraurosis vulvae, carcinoma and senile keratoses are conditions commonly seen in the aged.

Sex. Lupus erythematosus, chloasma, Paget's disease of the nipple and herpes gestationis occur most commonly in women.

Race. The importance of race as a predisposing factor in the cause of disease has diminished in the past three decades. Because of intermarriage, pure racial characteristics have been greatly diluted. It is not true that pemphigus vulgaris is a disease limited to the Jewish race or that psoriasis and epitheliomas do not occur in the black race. It is true, however, that persons of black extraction are prone to develop keloids, acne keloid, dermatosis papulosa nigra and granuloma inguinale.

Heredity. Ichthyosis, trichoepithelioma, psoriasis and keratosis palmaris et plantaris are familial conditions. There is also a hereditary tendency to the development of the "hay fever-asthma-eczema" syndrome.

Season. Miliaria rubra, solar erythema, larva migrans, and insect bites are most commonly seen during the summer months. Cold weather produces or aggravates conditions such as ichthyosis, psoriasis and winter eczema.

Occupation. An occupational dermatosis may be defined as an eruption produced by a substance or substances encountered by the patient during the course of his work. A previously existing eruption aggravated by working conditions is also considered by state industrial accident commissions as a compensable occupational disease.

Geography. Different geographic areas have different endemic diseases. Many animal vectors disseminating infectious disease have a limited geographic range.

Organic Disease. Erythema nodosum, purpura, tuberculosis cutis, atopic eczema, xanthomata, furunculosis, urticaria pigmentosa, erythema multiforme, pseudoxanthoma elasticum and many other lesions are cutaneous manifestations of systemic disease.

Precipitating Causes

Trauma. Trauma inflicted by physical violence, chemical burns, sunlight, heat and physical therapy may produce an eruption. Externally produced injury is frequently a means of introducing pathogenic microorganisms into the skin.

Animal Parasites. These frequently cause skin eruptions which have characteristic morphologic features. *Pediculus capitis, Pediculus pubis* and *Pediculus corporis* are insects which bite and suck blood but do not inject a foreign substance. The body louse (*P corporis*) transmits epidemic typhus, trench fever and other infections by introducing its fecal matter into its bite.

    Cimex lectularius (bed bug) makes its home in crevices of furniture and uses the human body for feeding purposes. A transitory wheal develops following the bite (caused by chemical injected by the insect). The lesions are extensive and heavily crusted. Secondary pyogenic infection frequently develops.

    Pulex irritans (flea) is one of the more common causes of papular urticaria in children. The lesions are

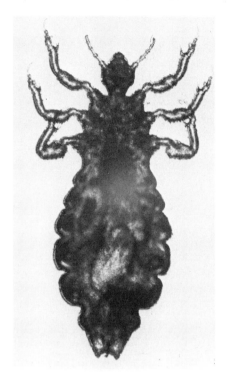

Body louse

Crab louse

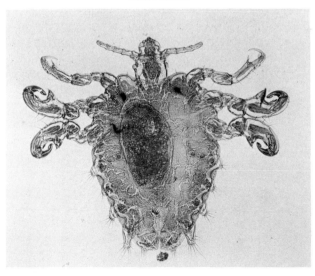

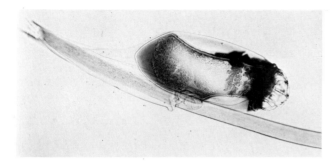

Crab louse ovum (x150)

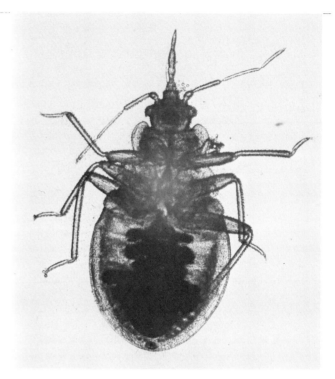

Bedbug (x26)

small papules or vesicopapules. Intense pruritus occurs because of the irritating substance injected by the insect. Fleas transmit endemic typhus, bubonic plague and other infections.

Tunga penetrans (chigoe) is a flea. The female of the species burrows into the skin, producing a large papule with a central puncture blocked by a portion of the body of the parasite. Extensive secondary infection and gangrene may result from chigoe infestation. This condition, which is limited to tropical areas, primarily involves the feet.

Ancylostoma braziliense and *Gasterophilus hemorrhoidalis* cause "creeping eruptions" called larva migrans. The larvae of the insects produce a continuous, red, tortuous, thread-like burrow just beneath the stratum corneum marking their line of migration.

Entamoeba histolytica may produce cutaneous involvement by extension or inoculation. An amebic dermatitis may develop in the skin following a surgical procedure on a visceral abscess. Extension of rectal disease onto the skin about the anus may produce extensive ulcers or furuncles. Amebic ulcers in the skin are irregular purulent lesions with undermined ragged edges. The organism may be recovered from the ulcers.

Trichinella spiralis causes cutaneous lesions resembling erythema multiforme, "rose spots," or scarlatiniform erythema. Edema of the eyelids, petechiae and urticaria are also common findings.

Wuchereria bancrofti causes human filariasis, a tropical disease. The scrotum, breasts and lower extremities may develop elephantiasis. Lymphadenitis and funiculitis also occur.

Latrodectus mactans, the black widow spider, produces a painful edematous lesion which may also be purpuric. Systemic symptoms including tremors, numbness, vomiting and general malaise are frequently violent. Fatalities are rare.

Tick bites may produce cutaneous nodules which do not resolve when the acute inflammatory reaction subsides. In this country, *Dermacentor andersoni* and *Dermacentor variabilis* are vectors of Rocky Mountain spotted fever and tularemia.

Sarcoptes scabiei (itch mite). The female of the species burrows under the skin and deposits eggs and

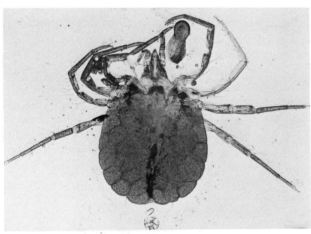

Chigger

Flea

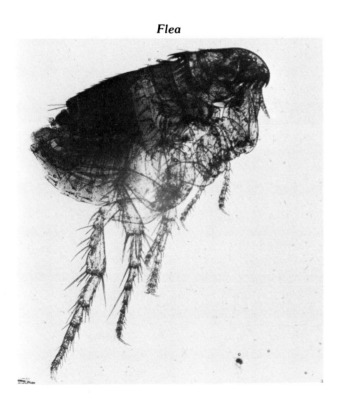

fecal matter. The male usually lives on the skin or under the epidermis outside the burrows.

Pyemotes ventricosus (grain itch mite) attacks people who work with grain. It produces papular or papulovesicular urticaria with intense pruritus and sometimes fever.

Trombicula irritans is the common American chigger. Only the larvae of these mites are parasitic. The adult mite lives on woody decaying substances. During the summer months they are commonly found in the grass, bushes and fields. The lesions produced are hemorrhagic papules. Pruritus is intense.

Euproctis chrysorrhoea (larva of the brown-tail moth) causes caterpillar dermatitis, common in Massachusetts and other parts of New England. The pruritic, erythematous dermatitis and urticaria are caused by the irritation and toxicity of caterpillar hairs.

Culicidae (mosquitoes) have numerous species and produce pruritic, urticarial lesions caused by the injection of venom. Some patients develop severe generalized allergic reactions to mosquito bites.

Hymenoptera include bees, hornets, wasps and some members of the family of ants. These insects may produce prolonged urticaria and serious systemic illness because of the venom injected.

Viruses. Viruses are organized, living bodies which are not visible under the ordinary microscope.

Smallpox, alastrim, milkers' nodules, varicella, rubeola, rubella, herpes simplex, herpes zoster, Kaposi's varicelliform eruption, warts of all types, molluscum contagiosum, lymphogranuloma venereum and cat scratch disease are among the many dermatoses caused by viruses.

Rickettsiae. Unlike viruses, these intracellular parasites are visible with standard microscopic techniques. Epidemic typhus, murine typhus, Rocky Mountain spotted fever, rat-mite dermatitis and rickettsial pox are caused by specific rickettsiae.

Bacterial Infections. Staphylococcic infections include impetigo, furuncles and carbuncles, cellulitis, folliculitis and secondary pyogenic infection of eczematous eruptions.

Streptococcal infections include secondary pyogenic infection of previously existing dermatoses, impetigo contagiosa, ecthyma, erysipelas, scarlet fever, gangrenous balanitis and other dermatoses.

Erysipelothrix rhusiopathiae causes erysipeloid.

Pasteurella tularensis causes tularemia. The organism usually enters the body through a minor abrasion or tick bite. The tularemic chancre frequently develops about the fingers and hands. Many different types of cutaneous lesions may complicate the systemic picture of this disease.

Hemophilus ducreyi is the gram-negative bacillus which causes chancroid. This condition is described in Chapter 9: Sexually Transmitted Diseases.

Treponema pertenue is the spirochete which causes yaws, a tropical disease. *Treponema pallidum* is the spirochete which causes syphilis. This is also discussed in Chapter 9.

Fungi. The mycoses, both superficial and deep, are caused by fungi. The superficial mycoses include tinea capitis, epidermophytosis, tinea versicolor and other cutaneous lesions which do not have systemic manifestations. Among the deep mycoses are histoplasmosis, blastomycosis, coccidioidomycosis and sporotrichosis. See Chapter 6: Mycology.

Metabolic Disorders. The dermatoses attributable to metabolic disorders include the xanthomas, Addison's disease, acanthosis nigricans, gout, amyloidosis, hemochromatosis, calcinosis, porphyria and pellagra.

Allergy. Endogenous allergic reactions are attributable to the existence of a state of specific hypersensitivity to some injected, ingested or inhaled substance. The clinical manifestations vary and include such morphologic lesions as purpura, erythema multiforme, urticaria, exfoliative dermatitis and scarlatiniform eruptions. Exogenous causes of allergic reactions include a large variety of substances which come in contact with the skin and to which a patient may become sensitized.

Congenital Abnormalities. These include ichthyosis, nevi, congenital ectodermal defect, epidermolysis bullosa, polydactyly, mongolian spots and disturbances of growth.

Vascular Lesions. Those which produce skin changes include embolism, thrombosis, arteritis, phlebitis, arteriosclerosis and angiospasm.

Hematopoietic Disorders. Those disorders producing eruptions include lymphosarcoma, Hodgkin's disease, lymphatic or myeloid granulocytic leukemia and monocytic leukemia. The skin lesions include petechiae, pigmentation, stomatitis, herpes zoster, furunculosis, lichenified dermatitis and urticaria.

Emotional Disturbances. These are capable of producing or aggravating dermatoses. Psychogenic stimuli produce neurotic excoriations, factitious dermatitis, trichotillomania, pruritus ani and pruritus vulvae, delusions of parasitosis and other conditions. Chronic dermatoses such as eczema, dermatitis herpetiformis and psoriasis are frequently aggravated by psychogenic stimuli.

Neoplastic Diseases. These include epitheliomas (basal cell, squamous cell and transitional), sarcoma of the skin, multiple hemorrhagic sarcoma of Kaposi, lymphoblastomas, melanomas, metastatic malignancies in the skin, eosinophilic granulomas and other malignant and nonmalignant tumors.

Dermatoses of Undetermined Origin. These include granuloma annulare, scleroderma, lichen sclerosus et atrophicus, psoriasis, pityriasis rubra pilaris, lupus erythematosus, pemphigus vulgaris, pseudoxanthoma elasticum and many other conditions.

Endocrine Dysfunction. Cutaneous changes are frequently observed as a manifestation of endocrine gland malfunction. In some instances the skin lesions are the first clinical evidence of disease.

Autoimmune Disease. Alterations in immunoglobulins are associated with the development of lupus erythematosus, pemphigus vulgaris, scleroderma and bullous pemphigoid.

CHAPTER | 4

Diagnostic Procedures

A combination of history, physical examination and judicious use of laboratory procedures is necessary to make a dermatologic diagnosis. The examiner must be a competent observer, having a thorough knowledge of subjective and objective symptoms. In many instances, the impression gained from physical examination contradicts the history obtained from the patient. A systemic method of examination is essential.

Medical History

The history should be obtained with the same care used in obtaining information from a patient with a systemic disease. Poorly organized interrogation seldom elicits the necessary information. Occupational disease, allergic dermatoses, infectious diseases, psychogenic disorders and constitutional diseases require different types of questions.

Subjective symptoms are disturbances of sensory perception which are not seen or felt by the examiner. These are pruritus, burning, pain, formication, tingling, hyperesthesia, anesthesia and paresthesia. These symptoms vary in degree and intensity with the individual patient. The emotional stability of the patient must be considered in the evaluation of such complaints. A psychotic person who has delusions of parasitosis may have intense pruritus even though no parasites are present, whereas a phlegmatic individual with scabies may complain of only slight discomfort.

Physical Examination

As part of the general examination, the practitioner should consider the gait, manner of speech, presence or absence of tremors, and the general color and tone of the skin. The opportunity to diagnose the focus of a patient with an endocrinopathy is best presented at the initial interview. The examiner should attempt to estimate the patient's physical age by considering the condition of the hair, elasticity and general condition of the skin, and the presence or absence of arcus senilis. A complete physical examination is desirable. Careful scrutiny of the disrobed patient in good light is essential. Daylight is the most satisfactory source of illumination. A daylight electric bulb is satisfactory but light produced by the ordinary incandescent bulb or fluorescent tube distorts color and may alter the appearance of objective symptoms.

The practitioner should record the distribution and arrangement of the lesions, and the gross characteristics of the eruption.

Objective Cutaneous Lesions. Primary and secondary objective symptoms or signs are apparent to the practitioner. A thorough knowledge of these objective

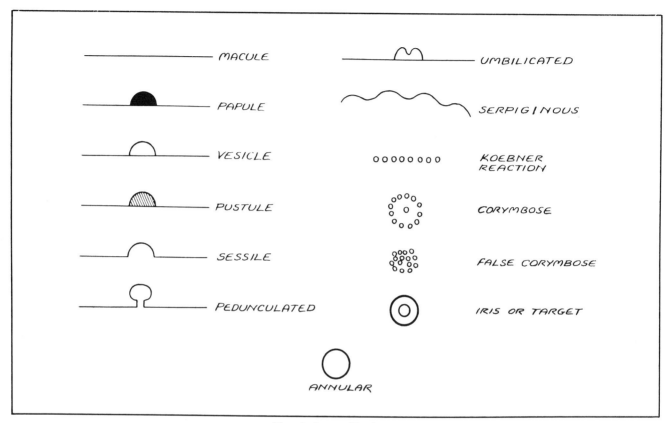

Morphology of lesions

lesions is necessary to arrive at a morphologic diagnosis. Objective symptoms are divided into primary and secondary lesions.

Primary Lesions. A macule is a lesion of the skin which is neither raised nor depressed. A papule is a solid elevation in the skin. A vesicle is an elevation of the skin filled with serum. A pustule is an elevation of the skin filled with pus.

Combinations of primary lesions may exist, *eg,* maculopapule, papulovesicle, vesicopustule.

Secondary Lesions. Scales are fragments of the stratum corneum. They may be profuse and silvery white as in psoriasis, scant and adherent as in lichen planus, or oily and yellowish as in seborrheic dermatitis.

Crusts are coagulation products of blood, serum, pus or combinations of these. The appearance of the crust may be complicated by local medications.

Excoriations are "scratch marks." These are factitious linear disruptions in the continuity of the skin. The presence of excoriations indicates the subjective symptom of pruritus.

Fissures are cracks in the skin secondary to loss of tone. Fissures are commonly observed in eczematous processes such as atopic dermatitis. Rhagades are fissures seen in congenital syphilis and vitamin deficiencies and occur in radial arrangement at muco-cutaneous orifices (*eg,* commissures of lips).

Scars represent healing of a wound or ulcer by fibrous tissue. Atrophic scars, observed in discoid lupus erythematosus and other conditions, develop without preceding ulceration.

Depigmentation or hyperpigmentation may develop following an inflammatory reaction.

Ulcers are localized, circumscribed disruptions in the continuity of the skin extending below the basal layer. Ulcers heal with scar formation.

An erosion is a superficial denudation of the skin. It may arise *de novo* or following the rupture of a vesicle. A nodule is a large elevation of the skin (>5 mm diameter). A bulla or pustule is a large vesicle (>5 mm diameter).

Configurations. Configurations of lesions are frequently of great importance in establishing a morphologic diagnosis.

Annular lesions are ringed lesions in which the periphery and central portion differ in appearance. There are 14 relatively common dermatoses in which annular lesions may appear.

Umbilicated lesions are those which have a central depression. They are commonly seen in molluscum contagiosum, lichen planus and varicella.

Serpiginous lesions have undulating margins. The arciform border is formed of several lesions which have become confluent. This phenomenon is observed in psoriasis, nodular serpiginous syphilid and other conditions.

A discrete lesion is one which is isolated. They may be small, large, single or multiple.

A confluent lesion is composed of several smaller lesions which have coalesced.

An iris lesion, composed of multiple concentric rings, is commonly seen in erythema multiforme. It is also called a "target lesion."

Linear grouping of lesions is characteristic of dermatitis venenata, nevus unius lateris, lichen planus, lichen nitidus and verruca plana juvenilis. This phenomenon may also be observed in psoriasis.

Characteristic groups of vesicles occur in herpes simplex, herpes zoster, dermatitis herpetiformis and dermatitis venenata.

A pedunculated lesion is one in which the base is smaller than the body of the lesion.

A sessile lesion slopes into the normal skin and has a broad base.

A nummular lesion is flat-topped, circinate and elevated (coin-shaped).

Laboratory Aids in Diagnosis

Biopsy. The histopathologic picture of many dermatoses is not specific, and it is important that the clinician recognize the limitation of biopsy as an aid in diagnosis. Great judgment should be exercised in the selection of the lesion to be examined. Biopsy is an essential diagnostic procedure in many patients with dermatoses, and in all lesions in which a malignant change could be possible. The biopsy specimen should be studied by someone who is experienced in interpreting dermal histopathology.

Several methods may be used for the removal of a skin specimen for study:

Simple Excision. Procaine solution (1%) is injected around and under the area to be excised. The specimen is transfixed by the hypodermic needle used in infiltrating the skin with procaine. The section of tissue is removed to the depth of the subcutaneous tissue (at least 2-3 mm) by making an incision on either side of the transfixing needle. The biopsy wound is closed with sufficient sutures to insure a good cosmetic result.

Dermal Biopsy Punches. These vary in size from 2-8 mm in diameter. The area to be biopsied is infiltrated with 1% procaine solution, the biopsy punch is pressed into the lesion by a circular motion to the depth of the subcutaneous tissue, the specimen is grasped by forceps, and freed with scissors. Although this is a rapid method of obtaining tissue, the elliptical excision described in the preceding paragraph is preferred by the authors. A biopsy should be taken gently

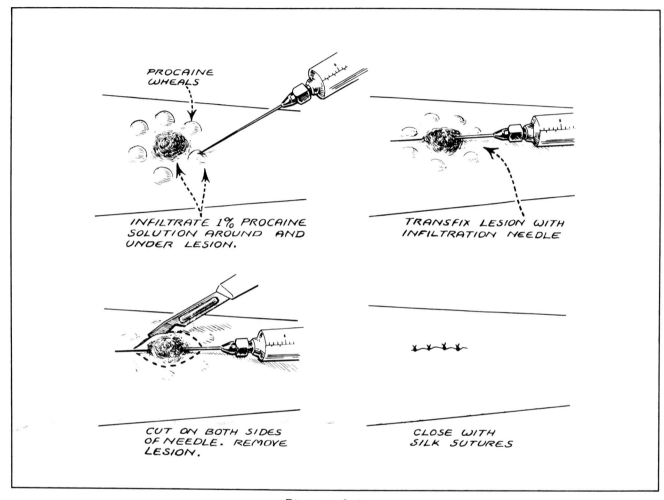

PROCAINE
WHEALS

INFILTRATE 1% PROCAINE
SOLUTION AROUND AND
UNDER LESION.

TRANSFIX LESION WITH
INFILTRATION NEEDLE

CUT ON BOTH SIDES
OF NEEDLE. REMOVE
LESION.

CLOSE WITH
SILK SUTURES

Biopsy technique

to avoid artefacts. It should then be placed in a clean bottle containing 5-10% formalin solution. An adequate clinical description should accompany the biopsy specimen to the laboratory.

Studies for Fungi. Identification of common dermatophytes may be made with a minimum of laboratory equipment. Direct examination of scales, hair, vesicles or nail scrapings may be performed with the use of a 20% solution of potassium hydroxide, a slide and cov-erslip, and a microscope. Sabouraud's or Mycosel® culture media, ready for use, may be obtained commercially.

Direct Examination. Hair, scales, vesicles or nail scrapings are placed in the center of a glass slide and covered with a coverslip. A drop of 20% potassium hydroxide solution is placed at the margin of the coverslip and allowed to contact the specimen by capillary attraction. The moistened specimen is allowed to

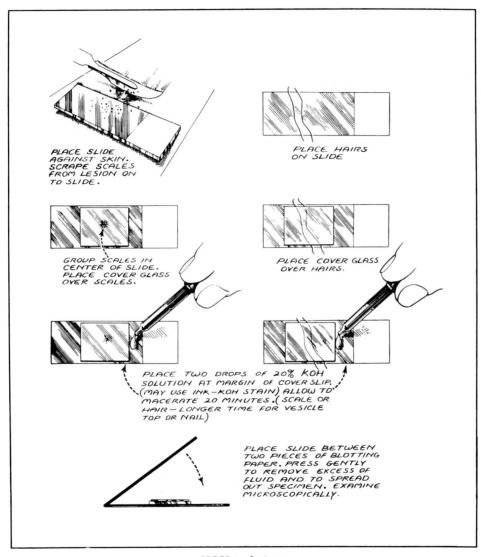

PLACE SLIDE
AGAINST SKIN.
SCRAPE SCALES
FROM LESION ON
TO SLIDE.

PLACE HAIRS
ON SLIDE

GROUP SCALES IN
CENTER OF SLIDE.
PLACE COVER GLASS
OVER SCALES.

PLACE COVER GLASS
OVER HAIRS.

PLACE TWO DROPS OF 20% KOH
SOLUTION AT MARGIN OF COVER SLIP.
(MAY USE INK-KOH STAIN) ALLOW TO
MACERATE 20 MINUTES.(SCALE OR
HAIR—LONGER TIME FOR VESICLE
TOP OR NAIL)

PLACE SLIDE BETWEEN
TWO PIECES OF BLOTTING
PAPER. PRESS GENTLY
TO REMOVE EXCESS OF
FLUID AND TO SPREAD
OUT SPECIMEN. EXAMINE
MICROSCOPICALLY.

KOH technique

macerate for a variable time, depending on the density of the material to be examined. Scales should macerate for 10-15 minutes, vesicle tops for 1-2 hours, hair for 15-20 minutes, and nail scrapings from 12-24 hours. The maceration time may be reduced by gently warming the wet preparation. The slide preparation is placed between two pieces of blotting paper and gently pressed to express the excess potassium hydroxide or stain and spread the specimen. Reduced light is used for the microscopic examination.

Culture Methods. A culture on fungal medium should be made from all cases of suspected mycotic infection regardless of the direct examination results.

The Wood light consists of ultraviolet rays with a peak wave length at 365 nanometers filtered through nickel oxide glass. Purple electric bulbs also transmit ultraviolet rays in the region of 365 nm; this is a photoflood lamp covered with a layer of cobalt. These lamps become hot and occasionally explode; therefore, they must be handled with caution.

The Wood light is one of the most practical methods used for identification of *Microsporum audouini* and *M canis*. It is valuable for screening school children for the presence of tinea. Infected hairs exhibit brilliant green fluorescence.

Not all fungus infections of the scalp show fluorescence. This is particularly true of trichophyton infections of the hair. This modality produces golden yellow to dark brown fluorescence in the lesions of tinea versicolor and coral red fluorescence in erythrasma. Many other organic and inorganic substances also fluoresce when exposed to the Wood light.

The Wood light is also of value in the diagnosis of pediculosis capitis. The ova glow with a grayish fluorescence.

Skin Tests. Patch tests, scratch tests and intradermal tests are frequently employed to determine the etiology of allergic dermatoses.

Patch Tests. The patch test is the method used to determine skin sensitivity to contact allergens such as poison ivy, medicaments, resins and cosmetics.

The suspected allergen is placed on a piece of nonwoven soft bandage and applied to an area of skin with occlusive tape. The upper back is the preferable testing site. The piece of gauze containing the suspected sensitizing substance may be covered with cellophane and sealed with adhesive tape, or with Elastoplast™. Readings are made in 48-72 hours. A positive test may be classified as 1+ (erythema), 2+ (erythema and edema), 3+ (vesiculation and erythema) or 4+ (necrosis).

The examiner must be sure that he is not using a primary irritant in the performance of this test, or that the concentration of the test material is too great. Volatile substances, such as gasoline, soap, acids and alkalis, may be classified as primary irritants. These substances will produce a reaction in the skin of any individual. A positive reaction to a primary irritant is not an index of hypersensitivity.

Scratch Tests. These are used to determine possible allergic reactions to inhalants, or ingested or injected substances. They are of doubtful value. The tests are usually performed on the lower back, forearms or the sides of the thighs. Using a pointed scalpel, a scratch 6-12 mm long is made for each of the substances to be tested. A drop of 0.1 normal sodium or potassium hydroxide solution is placed over each scratch. A drop of the substance to be tested is placed into the drop of the potassium hydroxide solution and gently mixed with a clean applicator stick or toothpick. After 15 minutes the skin in the tested area is rinsed with sterile water and dried. A control scratch in which only the sodium or potassium hydroxide solution is used must be done with each series of tests. Readings are made in 1, 2 and 4 hours. A positive reaction consists of a wheal 1.5-2 cm in diameter.

Intracutaneous Tests. These are performed by injecting 0.1 cc of the test material intradermally into the skin of the forearm or the upper back, using a tuberculin syringe or a small hypodermic syringe. The test substance must be injected superficially so that a wheal is produced. The readings are made at a variable interval depending on the type of material used in the test.

Routine Blood Studies. Blood chemistries, hemograms, sedimentation rate and electrophoretic patterns should be done whenever indicated. In view of the fact that most of these tests are expensive, they should not be performed on every patient who visits the office or the clinic. These tests are usually not necessary in scabies, pediculosis, pityriasis rosea, psoriasis, alopecia areata, verruca vulgaris, epidermophytosis and impetigo contagiosa. In conditions such as cutaneous xanthomata, eosinophilic granuloma, gout, erythema multiforme, erythema nodosum, tuberculosis, lupus erythematosus and blastomycosis, special studies are definitely indicated.

Roentgen Studies. It is necessary to have routine X-ray studies of the chest and skeletal structures in xanthomatosis, sarcoidosis, tuberculosis, blastomycosis, eosinophilic granuloma and other systemic diseases manifested by skin lesions.

Diascopy. A diascope is a thick glass slide which is pressed against the skin for the purpose of observing changes other than an inflammatory reaction. Its primary value lies in the clinical study of lupus vulgaris, where the yellowish brown color of the nodule is made visible by the use of this test.

Bacterial Studies. Bacterial studies should be performed on resistant pyogenic infections. Initial cultures may be made on blood agar. The identification of the causative organism should be made by a competent bacteriologist. Disc diffusion or tube dilution sensitivity tests should be performed to determine the antibiotic of choice for the systemic treatment of resistant pyogenic infections.

Serologic Studies. Serologic investigation can aid in establishing the cause of an infectious process. VDRL, fluorescent antibody treponemal absorption (FTA-ABS) and *Treponema pallidum* immobilization (TPI) tests are used in syphilis and will be discussed in Chapter 9. Antistreptolysin O (ASO), antihyaluronidase and anti-DNase B tests are helpful in infections produced by Group A beta-hemolytic streptococci. Complement fixation, hemagglutination, neutralization and flocculation tests are employed in other diseases. When an infectious process is suspected, it is always best to save paired sera so that retrospective diagnoses are possible.

Cytologic Examination. Epidermal scrapings and cytologic preparations are valuable. Molluscum contagiosum may be diagnosed by squash preparations of the extracted molluscum body. Wright's stain examination of vesicular fluid contents in viral diseases (Tzanck test) may reveal clumped giant cells with diagnostic inclusion bodies. Aspirates of bullae may contain acantholytic cells and epidermal foreign bodies as fiberglass spicules. Cytologic imprints of mycosis fungoides or lymphomatous plaques can be diagnostic.

Electron Microscopy. Rapid ultramicroscopic examination for viral particles by the negative staining technique can be completed within hours. Electronmicroscopic examination of the dermal-epidermal junction can be decisive in classifying a case of epidermolysis bullosa or in detecting amyloid fibers.

Immunofluorescence. In the last 15 years immunofluorescence of some eruptions, particularly bullous and connective tissue diseases, has proved to be an important diagnostic measure. Direct immunofluorescence is performed by using the patient's own skin as substrate for the reaction with fluorescin-conjugated antihuman globulin. Indirect immunofluorescence is a more complex test in which the patient's sera is incubated with a normal section of substrate (human skin or monkey esophagus). After completion of this reaction, the slide is washed and flooded with fluorescin-conjugated antihuman globulin then examined under the fluorescent microscope. These tests may be more specific by employing antibodies to the various immunoglobulins or components of complement rather than unpurified tagged antihuman globulin. The specific results of these procedures will be discussed under the individual disease headings.

Cell Culture. Skin tissues may be grown *in vitro* as cell organ cultures in order to isolate viruses or to study their enzyme content in various metabolic disorders. It is difficult to keep epithelial cells growing for any prolonged period of time without having fibroblasts overgrow the culture.

CHAPTER 5

Dermal Histopathology

The history and clinical findings are important aides in the interpretation of many skin biopsies. The microscopic findings of some dermatoses are pathognomonic; however, many dermatologic entities do not have diagnostic histopathological pictures, and in such situations the biopsy may only confirm or disprove the clinical impression.

The examiner should follow a routine in studying sections of skin so that some diagnostic point may not be overlooked. The section should first be examined using the reverse ocular technique. The general structure of the epidermis, relative thickness of the keratin layer, presence of acanthosis, gross architecture of the epidermis, and the pattern of the dermatosis may be visualized in this manner. The section is then studied to determine whether it is thickened or decreased. The presence of parakeratosis, plugging, Munro abscesses or other changes which may be present should be noted. The examiner should observe the thickness of the stratum lucidum where present, and the presence of an increase or decrease in the thickness of the granular layer. He should carefully study the rete (prickle cell layer) for the presence of edema (intracellular or extracellular), balloon degeneration, acanthosis, infiltration, mitosis, dyskeratotic cells, absence of prickles and other possible alterations. The cells in the basal layer of the epidermis should be examined for mitosis, pigmentation, acantholysis, exocytosis and other pathologic changes. After the study of the epidermis has been completed, the examiner should proceed to note changes in the papillary layer of the dermis such as liquefaction at the junction of the basal layer and the papillary portion of the dermis. Changes in the midportion of the dermis, the deeper layers of the dermis and, finally, those in the subcutaneous tissue or fatty layer should be noted. The type of cellular infiltrate (perifollicular or perivascular) should be recorded. The hematoxylin-eosin stain is usually satisfactory for demonstration of changes in collagen or elastic tissue but occasionally special stains must be used. Sebaceous glands, blood vessels, sweat glands and hair follicles should be studied for pathologic changes.

Glossary of the More Common Dermal Histopathology Terms

Acantholysis is a loss of coherence and polarity of epidermal cells due to degeneration of the intracellular bridges. Acantholysis may be due to a lack of resistance in the prickle cells in a circumscribed area which allows fluid to collect between the cells. The acantholytic cell (dying cell) becomes enlarged and spherical. The peripheral cytoplasm becomes basophilic and forms a halo about the enlarged, deeply stained nucleus.

Acanthosis denotes an increase in the thickness of the prickle cell layer of the epidermis. This may be caused by an increase in the number of the individual rete cells or to an increase in the size of the cells.

Atrophy is an acquired decrease in size of a portion of the body, of an organ, of an individual tissue or of individual cells. It is manifested by repression, or partial to complete disappearance of structural elements. It is caused by gradual loss in volume, actual destruction or transformation into degenerative products. Atrophy is usually evidenced in the epidermis by flattening at the dermal junction and loss of rete pegs.

Basophilic degeneration refers to the blue staining of the connective tissue when hematoxylin-eosin stain is used. It is found in such conditions as lupus erythematosus and actinic dermatitis.

"Cellules claires" are found in and about the basal layer of the epidermis. They are thought to be related to melanocytes, dendritic cells or the tactile cells of Merkel-Ranvier.

Collagen is the normal fibrillar connective tissue found in the corium.

"Corps ronds" and grains are dyskeratotic cells occurring in the prickle cell layer. These are characteristically found in keratosis follicularis.

Dyskeratosis signifies a defect in keratin formation. Dyskeratotic cells are those which undergo abnormal keratin formation.

Epithelial giant cell is an abnormal or large multinucleated epithelial cell.

Epithelioid cells are derived from the reticuloendothelial system and resemble epithelial and endothelial cells.

Exocytosis designates the invasion of inflammatory cells in the epidermis.

Foreign body giant cells are multinucleated macrophages in which the nuclei are grouped in the center of the cell.

Granuloma is a broad term which covers subacute or chronic inflammatory processes that are circumscribed and contain various cell types in circum-

ferential layers. It excludes both the acute exudative process and tumors and is observed in syphilis, tuberculosis, leprosy and the deep mycoses.

Histiocytes are connective tissue cells of the reticuloendothelial system and have phagocytic properties.

Hyperkeratosis is an increase in thickness of the stratum corneum.

Hyalin degeneration means that the connective tissue has become homogenous and is stained more intensely than normal by eosin.

Hyperplasia is an increase in cellular elements.

Hypertrophy indicates an increase in size of individual cells which subsequently produce enlargement of the involved part.

Karyorrhexis describes nuclear dissolution.

Lacunae are small, slit-like, intra-epidermal vesicles, usually lined by a layer of basal cells. They often contain desquamated, acantholytic epidermal cells which have lost their prickles because of degenerative changes or partial keratinization.

Langhans' cells are multinucleated giant cells seen in tuberculosis and other granulomas. The nuclei are arranged in an arciform manner at the periphery of the cells.

Liquefaction degeneration describes the type of dissolution of the basal cell layer observed in lichen planus, lupus erythematosus and some other conditions. The cytoplasmic contents are destroyed leaving intact cell membranes.

Macrophages are histiocytes which have phagocytized particulate matter or microorganisms.

Molluscum bodies are large intracytoplasmic inclusions which contain the virus of molluscum contagiosum.

Munro abscess is a microscopic collection of leukocytes found in the stratum corneum at the granular layer. These occur in psoriasis.

Necrobiosis is a peculiar type of connective tissue degeneration observed in necrobiosis lipoidica diabeticorum and granuloma annulare in which the tissue retains its grossly identifiable form.

Nuclear dust is fragments of basophilic nuclei

scattered intracellularly. These changes are especially visible in regions where leukocytes are concentrated.

Parakeratosis indicates retention of nuclei in the cells of the stratum corneum. This is observed in some scaling dermatoses.

Pautrier's abscess is a microscopic epidermal collection of infiltrate cells seen in mycosis fungoides. The same type of cells which form the infiltrate in the corium are in the abscess.

Pseudoepitheliomatous hyperplasia is a benign increase in epidermal elements observed in chronic inflammatory dermatoses and may resemble prickle cell carcinoma.

Pyknosis means shrinking of the cell nucleus.

Senile or *actinic degeneration* refers to changes in the elastic tissue observed in the skin of the elderly. The affected fibers in the papillary dermis are basophilic.

Spongiosis indicates intercellular edema of the epidermis.

Touton giant cells are xanthoma cells in which multiple nuclei are grouped around small islands of nonfoamy cytoplasm.

Tubercles are characteristic groups of cells found in tuberculosis and sarcoidosis.

Xanthoma cells are histiocytes which have one or more nuclei. These cells contain phagocytized lipoid material.

CHAPTER 6

Mycology

Fungi are plant-like microorganisms which have no roots, leaves or stems. They do not contain chlorophyll and they can utilize either living or dead organic matter for food. Fungi exist in two main morphological types: yeasts and filaments. The yeasts tend to be oval or spherical and form colonies which are soft in their consistency. Asexual reproduction is by a budding process, ie, blastospore formation. The filamentous fungi form branching tubular structures called hyphae. These intertwine to form a mycelium, which is visible to the eye as the thallus, or fungus colony. The hyphae of the so-called bread and water molds (Phycomycetes) are usually nonseptate, ie, they have no cross walls. Therefore, the protoplasm is free-flowing and the hyphae are said to be coenocytic. The hyphae of the other classes (Basidiomycetes, Ascomycetes and Deuteromycetes) are septate.

Very important in the identification of fungal isolates is the recognition of the sporulation process. Two classes of spores are produced: sexual and asexual. Sexual spores are rarely important in the diagnosis of pathogenic fungi, most of which are contained in the class Deuteromycetes (Fungi Imperfecti). It is characteristic of the members of this class that only their asexual sporulation process is known. Common laboratory contaminants as well as pathogenic fungi are found in this class.

Two categories of asexual spores are recognized: thallospores and conidia. Thallospores are reproductive structures formed directly as modifications of the mycelium. There are three types of thallospores. First, the blastospore is formed by a budding process. Blastospores are commonly seen in the yeasts. Second, the chlamydospore is a thick-walled spherical cell which may occur as a terminal enlargement of a hypha, or it may occur laterally or within a hypha, in which case it is said to be intercalary. Some yeasts, such as Candida albicans, also form chlamydospores when cultured on appropriate media. Third, the arthrospore is a thick-walled rectangular cell formed by a segmentation process; little or no expansion of the hyphal diameter occurs. Arthrospores are usually seen in chain formation. Their presence is important in identifying fungi such as Geotrichum candidum and Coccidioides immitis.

Conidia are usually produced on specialized hyphal structures called conidiophores from which they are freed by abstraction at the point of attachment. However, they may form directly on the hypha. Microconidia are relatively small and usually single-celled; they vary in shape from spherical through egg-shaped to club-shaped. Macroconidia are larger and usually multicellular by reason of cross septations; they vary in shape from tubular through spindle-shaped to club-shaped. Shapes and size of the candida help identify the species. Asexual spores of *Phycomycetes,* such as *Mucor* and *Rhizopus,* are contained in a spherical *sporangium* at the top of a *sporangiophore* and are termed *sporangiospores.*

Mycologic Diagnostic Methods

Direct Microscopic Examination. The specimen (scales, vesicle tops, hairs, nail shavings, pus, *etc*) is placed in the center of a glass slide; two drops of 10-20% potassium hydroxide are added, and a coverslip is placed over the specimen. The preparation should be gently warmed to hasten clearing. Positive direct examinations may reveal hyphae and arthrospores, budding yeasts or sulfur granules, depending on the organism present. Improvements over brightfield microscopy for observing such preparations include dark phase microscopy and fluorescence microscopy; in the latter case acridine orange, present in a concentration of 1:10,000, is an excellent fluorochrome for revealing fungal structures.

Nail specimens treated with potassium hydroxide should be kept in a moist chamber overnight to dissolve the keratin. Hair requires 15- 20 minutes to clear, vesicle tops may require 1-2 hours, and scale may be examined immediately. Spinal fluid should be centrifuged and the sediment examined. If *Cryptococcus neoformans* is suspected, an India ink wet mount should be prepared.

Stains. The hematoxylin-eosin technique can be used to visualize hyphal components in tissue sections and is necessary for determining the nature of the inflammatory response. However, special stains are necessary before such sections can be judged negative for mycoses or actinomycoses. The Gram stain is very useful for staining *Nocardia* sp and *Actinomyces israelii;* it is especially valuable for staining the cells of *C albicans* and other yeasts found in sputum, oral lesions, vaginal secretions, cerebral spinal fluid, *etc.* The acid-fast staining technique is sometimes required to differentiate *Nocardia* from *Actinomyces,* the former being acid-fast. Aqueous sulfuric acid (1%) is used as the decolorizing agent. The periodic acid-Schiff (PAS) stain is an excellent procedure for demonstrating fungal elements in any specimen material including nail scrapings, skin scrapings, pus, sputum, *etc.* The Giemsa stain is useful when a specimen is suspected of containing *Histoplasma capsulatum.* The most useful stain of all for demonstrating fungal components in tissue is the Gomori methenamine-silver nitrate procedure. A specific stain is Mayer's mucicarmine procedure for *Cryptococcus.*

Culture Methods. Commonly used media for the cultivation of fungi from various specimen materials include Sabouraud's agar and Emmon's agar. The former is more inhibitory toward bacterial contaminants because of its low pH of about 5.6, but the latter, having a pH near neutrality, is more favorable for the cultivation of *H capsulatum* and *Blastomyces dermatitidis.* Such media have been made more selective for the isolation of pathogenic fungi through the addition of the antimold agent cycloheximide and the antibacterial agent chloramphenicol. These media are commercially available. Incubation is at room temperature. A very valuable medium for the presumptive identification of dermatophyte isolates is dermatophyte test medium (DTM). This contains cycloheximide to restrict fungal contaminants, and gentamicin and chlortetracycline hydrochloride to inhibit bacterial growth. In addition, phenol red is present as a pH indicator; dermatophytes produce an alkaline reaction turning the medium red. Most contaminating fungi and bacteria that are able to grow produce an acid reaction, and the medium remains yellow. Dermatophyte test medium is an excellent medium for the office practice of dermatophyte mycology.

Classically, corn meal agar has been used to stimulate chlamydospore production by *C albicans;* however, *germ tube* production is more dependable for the presumptive identification of this organism. Germ tubes are formed at 37°C in serum and on a variety of solid media such as rice infusion-oxgall-Tween 80 agar. After incubation at 37°C for 3 hours to check for germ tube production, the culture is then incubated at room temperature to allow for chlamydospore production. Corn meal agar with 1% dextrose can be used to differentiate *Trichophyton rubrum* (red-purple pigment) and *Trichophyton mentagrophytes* (no pigment). *Microsporum audouini* does not grow on rice medium; *Microsporum canis* does. Thioglycollate broth can be used to culture *A israelii* from specimens that are normally sterile; broth media should not be used for specimens containing a mixed microbial flora. *Nocardia asteroides* grows on the surface of broth media, forming a pellicle. *Actinomyces* and *Nocardia* will not grow on media containing antibacterial agents. Blood agar media incubated at 37°C are useful for demonstrating the parasitic phase of dimorphic fungi such as *H capsulatum* and *B dermatitidis*. It is advantageous to incubate such cultures under increased CO_2 tension. Cultures of filamentous fungi are identified through an examination of their gross and microscopic characteristics. Yeast and actinomycete isolates may require a determination of their biochemical characteristics, *ie*, fermentation, assimilation and enzymatic reactions, before they can be speciated.

Animal Inoculation. Intravenous, intracerebral and intraperitoneal inoculations of laboratory animals aid in determining the pathogenicity of an isolate as well as establishing the parasitic phase of dimorphic fungi. For intraperitoneal inoculation, suspending the inoculum in 5% hog gastric mucin may increase the chances of establishing an infection.

Filtered Ultraviolet Light (Wood light). Ultraviolet light filtered through cobalt nickle glass (peak wavelength—3,650 Å) is used in a darkened room as a diagnostic aid in presumptively diagnosing such entities as: tinea (pityriasis) versicolor (dull brown fluorescence), erythrasma (reddish fluorescence) and tinea capitis due to *M audouini* and *M canis* (infected hairs fluoresce with a bright green color; hairs infected by other fungi do not fluoresce).

Serologic and Immunologic Tests for the Mycoses. Tests available for the serodiagnosis of histoplasmosis include: the complement fixation test, using both yeast phase and mycelial antigens; the immunodiffusion test; and the latex agglutination test. Indirect immunofluorescence using the patient's serum or specific antiserum is also a valuable diagnostic procedure. For coccidioidomycosis similar procedures are available; in addition, a tube precipitin test is highly specific and very valuable for detecting early active disease. The yeast cell agglutination test (tube or slide) and the latex agglutination test are very sensitive and quite specific for sporotrichosis; indirect immunofluorescence is also beneficial. Complement fixation and immunodiffusion procedures have been standardized for paracoccidioidomycosis (South American blastomycosis). In the case of North American blastomycosis, currently available antigen preparations are of no value; they lack sensitivity and specificity. For cryptococcosis the classic procedures used to test for circulating antibody are seldom successful during active disease; instead, testing for circulating capsular antigen is much more likely to be successful, and this is commonly done with a latex agglutination test. Immunofluorescent procedures are also helpful.

Skin test agents with a high degree of sensitivity and specificity are available for histoplasmosis (histoplasmin) and paracoccidioidomycosis (paracoccidioidin). In cases of North American blastomycosis, the skin test agent, blastomycin, is not dependable. Caution is required when using histoplasmin, since it has been shown that the skin testing histoplasmin-positive individuals may stimulate increased complement fixation titers. This phenomenon has not been recorded for the other skin test agents mentioned.

Dermatophytoses

Dermatophytoses are fungus infections of keratinous tissues (hair, skin and nails) caused by the dermatophytes, which are members of three genera: *Trichophyton, Microsporum* and *Epidermophyton*.

Tinea Pedis (epidermophytosis, athlete's foot, ringworm of the foot). Interdigital spaces and soles of the feet are affected. The condition may be acute, subacute or chronic. Most cases are caused by *T rubrum, T mentagrophytes,* and *Epidermophyton floccosum*. The acute condition is vesicular and edematous. Secondary pyogenic infection may cause systemic symptoms. The subacute stage is primarily vesicular. The chronic stage produces fissures and macerations between the toes. Dry, hyperkeratotic, scaling areas may be present on the sides and soles of the feet. The third and fourth interdigital spaces are commonly involved. Tinea pedis occurs universally, but is more common in tropical and temperate climates. It is said to be the most common mycosis of man.

Differential diagnosis. The presence of branny, furfuraceous, flaky patches or patches of vesicles over the soles, plus fissures and macerated soggy epidermis in interdigital areas is suggestive of tinea pedis. Hyperkeratotic plaques on the heels and balls of the feet may occur. The condition must be differentiated from: atopic dermatitis, contact dermatitis, pustular psoriasis, dyshidrosis, hyperhidrosis, pyoderma, candidiasis, drug reactions, *etc.* Demonstration of hyphal components in skin preparations and culture of the fungus proves the diagnosis of tinea pedis.

Onychomycosis (ringworm of the nail, tinea unguium). The etiology of dermatophytic onychomycosis is multiple, but *T rubrum, T mentagrophytes* and *C albicans* are most commonly involved. Infectious agents associated with mycosis elsewhere on the host are often those associated with nail invasion. Affected nails become thickened, brittle, distorted and discolored; there is a heavy accumulation of detritus beneath the nail plate when dermatophytes are involved. This usually does not occur with *C albicans*.

Differential Diagnosis. This condition must be differentiated from psoriasis, onycholysis, pachyonychia congenita, exfoliative dermatitis, eczema, dystrophy following trauma, bacterial infections and contact irritants. Nail infections are the most difficult to treat and show no tendency to spontaneous cure. Scrapings and cultures are essential for accurate diagnosis.

Tinea Cruris (jock itch, ringworm of the groin, eczema marginatum). Tinea cruris is a fungus infection of the crural, genital and perianal areas caused by *E floccosum,* various *Trichophyton* species and *C albicans.*

The lesions are usually well-defined, with elevated borders surrounding the reddish, scaling areas of dermatitis; the eruption spreads peripherally and vesicles or vesicopustules may be seen in the margins. The eruption is usually bilateral, but not necessarily symmetrical. The axillae may become involved and present a picture similar to that of the groin.

Differential Diagnosis. The sharp margination and active periphery are characteristic of tinea cruris; however, when the marginated appearance is absent other conditions such as neurodermatitis, contact dermatitis, psoriasis, seborrheic dermatitis, erythrasma and candidiasis must be considered. Scrapings and cultures are needed to help establish the etiology.

Tinea Corporis (ringworm of the body, tinea circinata, tinea glabrosa). Tinea corporis involves the glabrous skin and the resulting lesions may vary from those of simple scaling through scaling with erythema to deep granulomata. The disease is of worldwide distribution and the etiology is associated with species of the *Trichophyton* and *Microsporum* genera. The classic lesion is an annular macule with an elevated, erythematous margin and central scaling. The periphery may show the presence of vesicles and pustules. Lesions may be single or multiple. Animals are frequently vectors of this common infection in children.

Differential Diagnosis. Tinea corporis is to be differentiated from psoriasis, pityriasis rosea, granuloma annulare, neurodermatitis, secondary syphilis, annular lichen planus, seborrheic dermatitis, contact dermatitis, drug eruptions and erythema annulare centrifugum. Demonstration of the fungus by wet mount and/or by culture establishes the diagnosis.

Tinea Imbricata (tokelau; scaly ringworm; tinea circinata tropical; Burmese, Chinese, India ringworm). This is a disease of the tropics. The lesions are characteristic concentric scaling rings. There is little if any inflammatory response, yet pruritus may be intense. The nails and hair are usually spared. The etiologic agent is *Trichophyton concentricum.* Mixed infections may occur involving *T rubrum, E floccosum* or other dermatophytes. The infection resists treatment.

Differential Diagnosis. The clinical appearance of tinea imbricata is so characteristic that it can seldom be confused with other diseases.

Tinea Barbae (tinea sycosis, barber's itch, ringworm of the beard). This is a chronic infection of the bearded area of the face and neck which may be superficial, resembling tinea corporis, or deep, involving the hair follicles. The deep infection is a pustular folliculitis with abscess formation and kerion-like lesions. Draining sinuses may develop and involve the surrounding tissue. Various species of *Trichophyton* and *Microsporum* are involved, more commonly *T rubrum, T mentagrophytes, Trichophyton verrucosum* and *M canis.* The Wood light would be beneficial in diagnosing the latter.

Differential Diagnosis. Tinea barbae must be differentiated from contact dermatitis, alopecia areata, seborrheic dermatitis, sycosis vulgaris, pustular syphilis, anthrax, actinomycosis, halogen dermatitis and cystic acne.

Tinea Capitis (ringworm of the scalp, tinea tonsurans). This is a fungus infection of the scalp and hair caused by species of *Trichophyton* and *Microsporum*. In children the disease is caused more often by species of *Microsporum*. The hairs become brittle, break off or fall out producing circumscribed areas of partial alopecia covered with adherent dry scales. Infections with *M canis* and *Microsporum gypseum* may produce edematous inflammatory lesions called *kerion. M audouini* usually causes dry scaly lesions. Hair infected with *M canis* and *M audouini* will fluoresce brilliant green when illuminated with filtered ultraviolet from the Wood light in a darkened room. Hairs infected with *gypseum* do not fluoresce. *M canis* and *M gypseum* are transmitted to man from animals. *M audouini* is transmitted through human contact.

Tinea capitis caused by *Trichophyton tonsurans* and *Trichophyton violaceum* results in "black dot" ringworm in both adults and children. Infected hairs break off at the level of the scalp and the spores within the hair stump (*endothrix* infection) give the appearance of a "black dot," and do not fluoresce.

Tinea Favosa (favus, honeycomb ringworm). Tinea favosa is a chronic type of tinea capitis in which characteristic cup-shaped crusts (*scutula*) are formed. These are yellowish and are composed of masses of mycelia and epithelial debris. Hairs are trapped in the scutulum and fungi are found deep in the hair follicle. The inflammatory infiltrate is more intense than that seen in tinea capitis. The lesions have a musty odor. Considerable scarring and permanent alopecia frequently result. The infection may occasionally involve the glabrous skin and the nails. The usual etiologic agent is *Trichophyton schoenleini;* however, *T violaceum* and *M gypseum* are rarely isolated. The disease is most commonly seen in Poland, Russia, Europe, the Balkans, the Mediterranean basin and in the Bantu region in South Africa. It occurs rarely among native-born North Americans, but endemic foci have been recognized in Virginia, Kentucky and on the Gaspé penninsula of Quebec.

Differential Diagnosis. The diagnosis of tinea favosa is apparent when the following triad exists: typical yellowish scutula, a musty odor and a dull green fluorescence of hairs under Wood light. Discoid lupus erythematosus, pseudopelade, psoriasis, impetigo, folliculitis decalvans, trichotillomania and secondary syphilis must be included in the differential diagnosis. Isolation of the etiologic agent proves the diagnosis.

Epidermophytoses

Epidermophytoses are superficial infections limited to the stratum corneum. The etiologic agents involved have a predilection for this substrate and are not associated with hair and nail infections.

Tinea Versicolor (pityriasis versicolor, chromophytosis, liver spots, tinea flava, dermatomycosis furfuracea). This is a superficial, chronic fungus infection which appears as fawn colored, scaly macules on the trunk. Occasionally lesions develop in the groin, axillae, arms, thighs, neck, face and scalp. The lesions produce a dull greenish-brown fluorescence under Wood light. Exposure to sunlight may result in an apparent hypopigmentation of the lesion areas because of resistance to the normal tanning process and the bleaching potential of this agent. A slight pruritus may develop. The etiologic agent has been designated as *Pityrosporon orbiculare*. This organism is lipophilic and can be cultured on Sabouraud's agar containing olive oil. However, cultural proof of etiology is not required, inasmuch as the appearance of the organism in skin scrapings is pathognomonic—a combination of yeast-like cells and tortuous bacillary cells which may show branching. The forms are easily seen in KOH wet mounts, and the PAS stained specimens.

Differential Diagnosis. Tinea versicolor must be differentiated from chloasma, tinea corporis, erythrasma, secondary syphilis, pityriasis rosea, vitiligo, seborrheic dermatitis and other pigmentary disorders. Appropriate microscopy confirms the diagnosis.

Erythrasma. This is a chronic infection of the stratum corneum caused by a bacterium, *Corynebacterium minutissimum*. The lesions usually appear in the axillae, toewebs and genitocrural areas, but may be seen in other intertriginous areas. They appear as serpiginous, erythematous maculopapules with a scant amount of greasy scale. A characteristic coral-red fluorescence occurs under the Wood light. Culture of the etiologic agent is ordinarily not done. Direct microscopic examination of lesion scrapings reveals branching filaments plus bacillary and diphtheroidal forms about 1μ in diameter. These are readily distinguished from *P orbiculare* and the hyphae and arthrospores of the dermatophytes.

Differential Diagnosis. Erythrasma can be differentiated from tinea versicolor through appropriate microscopy. Erythrasma is limited to intertriginous areas. Tinea cruris shows a more acute inflammatory reaction. Wood light fluorescence is characteristic for erythrasma.

Tinea Nigra Palmaris (tinea nigra, pityriasis nigra, keratomycosis nigricans palmaris, cladosporiosis epidermica). This is an asymptomatic infection of the stratum corneum usually limited to the palmar aspects of the hands. The etiologic agent is *Cladosporium wernecki*. The lesions are sharply delineated, brown to black macules without raised borders, scaliness or vesiculation. Erythema and inflammation are absent. Microscopy of skin scrapings reveals masses of darkly pigmented, multi-branched hyphae. The infection responds readily to treatment with Whitfield's ointment; 2% salicylic acid, tincture of iodine and 3% sulfur also are effective.

Differential Diagnosis. The infection must be differentiated from contact dermatitis, melanoderma of Addison's disease, pigmented nevus, hyperchromia, syphilis, tinea versicolor and malignant melanoma. Microscopy and culture prove the diagnosis.

Trichomycoses

Trichomycoses are infections of hair caused by microorganisms which have a predilection for this substrate and are not associated with skin and nail infections.

Black Piedra (tinea nodosa, trichomycosis, trichomycosis nodosa). A fungus infection in which hard black nodules are formed along the hair shaft. The infection is limited to the scalp, beard and mustache. It starts under the cuticle and then spreads as an ectothrix growth, eventually encircling the hair shaft. The concretions are firmly adherent and vary in size from microscopic to large visible nodules. The etiologic agent is *Piedraia hortae*. Crushed granules reveal closely packed, highly septate, dark brown hyphae. Fusiform, slightly curved ascospores are found; the in vitro growth is greenish-black to black, and a reddish soluble pigment is produced. Culture is rarely necessary to prove diagnosis.

Differential Diagnosis. Black piedra must be differentiated from trichorrhexis nodosa and the nits of pediculosis capitis. Microscopic examination leads to the diagnosis.

White Piedra (tinea nodosa, trichosporosis, Beigel's disease, chignon disease). The granule formed in white piedra is softer than that in black piedra. It occurs on the beard and moustache. The concretion may form in the same manner as in black piedra, or the etiologic agent, *Trichosporon cutaneum*, may penetrate the hair shaft and form endothrix nodules along the axis, weakening the hair at these points, which leads to breakage. The nodules are light brown in color, and are composed of septate, branching hyphae, arthrospores and blastospores. Ascospores are not formed. Colonies of *T cutaneum* are yeast-like when young, becoming wrinkled, leathery and integument-like with age. Hyphae, arthrospores and blastospores are formed.

Differential Diagnosis. Differential diagnosis involves trichomycosis axillaris, trichorrhexis nodosa and the nits of pediculosis capitis. Microscopic examination leads to the diagnosis.

Trichomycosis Axillaris (lepothrix, trichomycosis nodosa, trichonocardiosis axillaris). This is an infection of the axillary and pubic hair. The concretions may be yellow, red or black. The red and black varieties are due to associated pigment-producing micrococci. The etiologic agent is *Corynebacterium tenuis*. The shaft of the hair is involved, but not the hair base or root. The concretions are soft, but adherent. The hair appears lusterless and breaks easily. The nodules on the hair are composed of delicate short, bacillary cells embedded in a mucilaginous material. Culture is not required for diagnosis.

Differential Diagnosis. Trichomycosis axillaris must be differentiated from white piedra, black piedra, trichorrhexis nodosa, monilethrix and the nits of pediculosis capitis. Microscopic examination leads to the diagnosis.

Candidiasis

Candidiasis is caused by species of the genus *Candida*. Usually the etiologic agent is *C albicans*; however, *Candida stellatoidea, Candida tropicalis, Candida krusei, Candida parapsilosis, Candida guilliermondi,* and *Candida pseudotropicalis* are sometimes encountered. Infections may involve the skin, mouth, genitalia, nails or gastrointestinal tract. Systemic disease can also occur, as well as allergic reactions. These organisms are primarily opportunists, seldom causing primary infections. They occur normally in small numbers in the alimentary tract and on mucocutaneous membranes. *C albicans* is rarely isolated from normal human skin; however, trauma and environmental change can lead to rapid colonization. The source of infections by *Candida* sp in most instances is probably endogenous.

Mucocutaneous Candidiasis. Oral candidiasis (thrush) results in the formation of creamy white patches scattered over the mucous membranes. Involved are the tongue (glossitis), mouth (stomatitis), lips (cheilitis) and commissures of the lips (perleche). Vulvovaginal candidiasis is characterized by a creamy discharge accompanied by inflammation and pruritus. The perineum and the inguinal area may be involved. The condition is commonly seen in diabetes, in which it is related to the high sugar content in blood and urine, and in pregnancy, where it is correlated with the increased glycogen present in the vaginal epithelium. Balanitis and balanoposthitis may result when the conjugal partner has candidiasis. Perianal candidiasis results in pruritus ani and may be a complication of systemic antibiotic therapy. The surface of the lesion is macerated and covered with a moist, whitish film.

Cutaneous Candidiasis. Intertriginous candidiasis involves vesicopustular, erythematous, moist areas and is most commonly seen in the axillae, inframammary areas, umbilicus, gluteal folds, the groin and interdigital spaces. Paronychia is a painful swelling of the periungual tissue. Onychia is characterized by thickening, discoloration, distortion and crumbling of the nail plates. Candidal lesions involving toes resemble tinea pedis caused by the the trichophytons. Moist, erosive lesions of the interdigital spaces of the fingers are called erosio interdigitalis blastomycetica.

Generalized Candidiasis. Extensive lesions may develop in the gastrointestinal tract, lungs, liver, spleen, endocardium and the meninges. Arthritis has been reported and pneumonic consolidation may occur.

Differential Diagnosis. The diagnosis of cutaneous and mucocutaneous candidiasis is relatively simple to establish by microscopy and culture. Direct examination will differentiate candidiasis from dermatophytosis, seborrheic dermatitis, geographic tongue, lichen planus, leukoplakia, tertiary syphilis and pyo-derma. The production of germ tubes and chlamydo-spores on rice infusion-oxgall-Tween 80 medium by the yeast isolate presumptively identifies *C albicans*.

Mycology of the Dermatophytes

Species of *Trichophyton* attack hair, skin and nail tissue. When invading hair, some species are of the endothrix type; others are ectothrix. Branching hyphal components are seen in infected skin and nails; chains of arthrospores may be formed. Colonies may be cottony, granular, powdery or glabrous. Pigmentation may be present. Microconidia are single-celled and are produced in grape-like clusters, or singly from a lateral position. Macroconidia are multicellular, smooth-walled, and are clavate to fusiform to cigar-shaped. Nodular bodies, chlamydospores, racquet hyphae and coiled hyphae may also be seen.

Species of *Microsporum* attack hair and skin. They are ectothrix in the invasion of hair. Some species cause infected hair to fluoresce under Wood light. Branching, segmented hyphal components are seen in skin. Colonies may be cottony, wooly, matted or powdery. Pigmentation varies from white to buff to brown. Microconidia are single-celled and are born laterally on hyphae either sessiley or on short conidiophores. Macroconidia are multicellular, rough-walled (when mature) and spindle-shaped. Their form and size are important in speciation. Racquet hyphae, pectinate hyphae, nodular bodies and chlamydospores may be formed.

There is but one species of *Epidermophyton, E floccosum*. It attacks only skin and nails. Its appearance in infected materials cannot be differentiated from that of *Trichophyton* and *Microsporum*. Colonies may be velvety to powdery with radiating folds. Pigmentation varies from white to yellow to brown. Microconidia are not formed. Macroconidia are multicellular, thin-walled, smooth-walled, and clavate. Chlamydospores, coiled hyphae, racquet hyphae and nodular bodies may be seen.

Trichophyton mentagrophytes (finea pedis, tinea corporis, tinea capitis, tinea barbae) is an ectothrix infection. The colonies vary from cottony to granular to powdery, produce white to yellowish to tan to red-dish-brown pigmentations, and are urease-positive. The fungus perforates human hair *in vitro*. On culture mount numerous microconidia are present in grape-like clusters with moderate numbers of macroconidia.

Trichophyton verrucosum (tinea corporis, tinea capitis, tinea barbae), an ectothrix infection, is ac-quired from cattle. The colonies are slow-growing, heaped, glabrous and contain minimal aerial hyphae. The pigmentation varies from white to yellow ochre and colony growth is enchanced at 37°C. Neither micro-conidia nor macroconidia are produced on Sabouraud's agar. Chains of chlamydospores develop at 37°C.

Trichophyton megnini (tinea barbae, tinea cor-poris, onychomycosis) is an ectothrix infection. The colony is cottony to velvety and develops radial grooves. This organism produces pink to violet color on obverse side of the culture tube. A nondiffusible red pigment appears on the reverse side. Microconidia and macroconidia are produced. An absolute requirement for histidine helps to separate the colonies of this species from those of *T rubrum*. This organism is a rare species found in Europe and Africa.

Trichophyton tonsurans (tinea capitis [black dot], tinea corporis, tinea barbae, onychomycosis) is an endothrix infection. Cultures of the organism produce variable growth showing heaped or sunken colony growth with folds. The colonies are velvety to pow-dery, varying in color from white to cream, yellow, red or brown. The reverse side of the tube may show red-dish pigmentations. Growth may be thiamine-depend-ent. On culture mount microconidia are usually abun-dant and variable in size and shape; balloon forms may be seen. Macroconidia are rare. Chlamydospores are common.

Trichophyton violaceum (tinea capitis [black dot], tinea corporis, onychomycosis) is an endothrix infection. Colony growth is slow with a heaped, folded or glabrous morphology. Deep violet pigmentation appears on both obverse and reverse sides of the tubes. Strains rapidly become pleomorphic. Microconidia and macroconidia are rarely produced on culture mounts. There is a partial growth requirement for thiamine.

Trichophyton schoenleini (tinea favosa, favus) is an endothrix infection. The colonies may be heaped, glabrous, waxy or cerebriform in appearance. They are slow growing but may grow better at 37°C. Colony color varies from yellowish-white to brownish in color. On culture mounts microconidia are rare and macroconidia are not produced. Hyphal branches may have characteristic swollen (nail head) tips.

Trichophyton rubrum (tinea corporis, onychomycosis, tinea pedis, tinea barbae) rarely invades the hair. Colony is slow growing, cottony and white. The reverse side of the culture tube develops a reddish to purple nondiffusing pigmentation. Numerous microconidia are produced in primary cultures; macroconidia are rare. Chlamydospores, racquet hyphae and nodular bodies are seen. *T rubrum* is urease-negative and does not perforate human hair *in vitro*. (See *T mentagrophytes*.)

Trichophyton concentricum (tinea imbricata) does not invade the hair. Colony is raised, folded and convoluted. The colonies are glabrous and white at first, becoming brownish to coral red with time. The hyphae are distorted; microconidia and macroconidia are not present. This organism may be in reality a variety of *T schoenleini*. Growth is stimulated by thiamine.

Microsporum audouini produces tinea capitis of the ectothrix type. Infected hairs fluoresce under Wood light. There is a slowly growing, white to gray or tan colony containing velvety, aerial mycelium. Radiating furrows may form on the surface of the culture. Microconidia and macroconidia are rarely seen on culture mount. When macroconidia are produced they are bizarre in shape. Thick-walled terminal or intercalary chlamydospores are helpful in making an identification.

Microsporum canis produces tinea capitis of the ectothrix type and tinea corporis. The infection is ac-
quired from household pets. Infected hairs fluoresce under Wood light. The fungus grows rapidly, producing a white to yellowish-brown colony with cottony to wooly aerial mycelia. The obverse of the culture tube is colored deep yellow to reddish-brown. Large, multiseptate, thick-walled, rough-surfaced, spindle-shaped macroconidia are produced in abundance on primary isolation. There are 6-15 cells per macroconidium. Slender, clavate microconidia are produced.

Microsporum gypseum produces tinea capitis of the ectothrix type. Infected hairs do not fluoresce. The colonies grow rapidly, producing a powdery surface due to prodigious sporulation. The colony color is buff to cinnamon to brown. Microconidia and macroconidia are produced. The latter are not as sharply spindle-shaped as those of *M canis*. Four to 6 compartments exist per macroconidium. They are thin-walled and have a roughened surface. The source of this fungus is soil.

Epidermophyton floccosum does not invade hair. Tinea cruris, tinea pedis, tinea corporis and onychomycosis result from the invasion of this microorganism. Early colony growth is white in color and granular, becoming velvety and powdery in texture. Pleomorphism of the culture occurs. This phenomenon is marked by conversion to sterile, white cottony overgrowth. Microconidia are not produced. The macroconidia observed on culture mount are smooth-walled, multiseptate and clavate. Chlamydospores are frequently abundant.

The Deep Fungus Infections

Actinomycosis (lumpy jaw, streptotricosis, leptotricosis). This infection in man is a chronic suppurative and granulomatous disease. It is customarily classified as: cervicofacial, thoracic and abdominal and is characterized by the formation of abscesses which spread by extension to involve contiguous tissues. Multiple, draining sinus tracts develop which break the skin and exude serosanguineous fluids containing "sulfur granules" containing the pathogen and other bacteria. The etiologic agent in most cases is *A israelii,* now considered to be an endogenous filamentous bacterium rather than a fungus. The organism is a normal anaerobic inhabitant of the oral cavity, ordinarily leading a parasitic but nonpathogenic existence. Gram-positive, branching filaments about 1 μ in diameter are found in lesion materials; these are not acid-fast. Laboratory diagnosis involves culturing the organism at 37°C under anaerobic conditions on Sabouraud's medium or in thioglycollate broth in the case of uncontaminated surgical specimens. A israelii is catalase-negative, a finding which helps differentiate it from similarly appearing anaerobic diptheroids, which are catalase-positive. Other anaerobic actinomycetes such as *Actinomyces naeslundii*, *Bifidobacterium eriksonii* and *Arachnida proprionicus* have produced actinomycosis in man.

Nocardiosis. This is an acute or chronic suppurative disease, primarily occurring as a pulmonary infection. Systemic disease and mycetomas may develop. "Sulfur granules" may be discharged in the exudate from the cutaneous lesions as in the case of actinomycosis. *N asteroides*, *Nocardia brasiliensis* and *Nocardia caviae* are the etiologic agents. They are exogenous, aerobic, filamentous bacteria. In stained smears of sputum and other specimen materials they are seen as delicate, branching, gram-positive, weakly acid-fast filaments. The agents may be cultured on Sabouraud's agar, blood agar and in broth media, where they form a pellicle. Isolates may vary considerably in their pigmentation from chalky buff through yellow to deep orange and must be differentiated from mycobacteria.

North American Blastomycosis (Gilchrist's disease). This entity is a chronic, suppurative and granulomatous disease which occurs primarily as a pulmonary infection, a chronic cutaneous disease or a systemic disease. Cutaneous lesions may be the first evidence of systemic infection. Pulmonary blastomycosis may mimic tuberculosis or neoplasm. The etiologic agent is the dimorphic fungus *B dermatitidis*. This agent replicates *in vivo* and *in vitro* at 37°C on blood agar as a single, budding thick-walled yeast with the bud attached to the parent cell by a wide septum. At room temperature on Sabouraud's agar, *B dermatitidis* proliferates as a slowly growing colony which is variable in appearance, ranging from glabrous to white and cottony. Culture mount examinations reveal oval to round or piriform microconidia measuring 3-5 μ diameter. These structures are sessile or attached to the hyphae by conidiophores of varying lengths. Chlamydospores are seen in older cultures.

South American Blastomycosis (paracoccidioidomycosis, paracoccidioidal granuloma, Lutz-Splendore-Almeida disease). This is a chronic granulomatous disease of the skin, mucous membranes and lymph nodes, which may also become a systemic disease. The etiologic agent is *Paracoccidioides brasiliensis*, a dimorphic fungus which produces a multiple, budding yeast phase in infected tissues and in vitro on appropriate media at 37°C. This fungus produces a filamentous colony with microconidia similar to those produced by *B dermatitidis* at room temperature. The organism has been isolated from soil in South America and thus the disease is endogenous to South and Central America. Histological sections of infected tissue show giant cells containing organisms which, in the absence of multiple budding yeast cells, resemble those of North American blastomycosis. Skin tests (paracoccidioidin) and serologic examinations such as the complement fixation and precipitin tests are useful diagnostic aids.

Coccidioidomycosis (coccidioidal granuloma, valley fever, San Joaquin fever, Posada-Wernicke disease). This mycosis usually occurs as an upper respiratory infection of variable severity. It rarely progresses to a chronic pulmonary or systemic disease. The etiologic agent, *C immitis*, is probably the most infectious mycotic agent. Most people living in endemic areas eventually acquire the infection. Coccidioidomycosis is endemic in the southwestern United States, northern Mexico and selected areas of Central and South America. *C immitis* is a soil organism where it produces highly infectious arthrospores capable of becoming airborne when the soil is disturbed. These spores are also produced in abundance on artificial media, so great care must be exercised with this organism in the laboratory. The pathologic sections of *C immitis* infections show large (20-60 μ in diameter), thick-walled spherules which contain numerous endospores when mature.

Histoplasmosis (Darling's disease). Like coccidioidomycosis, histoplasmosis is a highly infectious disease occurring primarily as a pulmonary infection. In rare cases it transforms into a progressive, chronic, malignant disease with anemia, fever, leukopenia, splenomegaly and hepatomegaly. In pulmonary histoplasmosis the characteristic method of healing is by calcification. The etiologic agent is the dimorphic fungus *H capsulatum,* a soil organism. *In vivo* it parasitizes the cells of the reticulo-endothelial system as a yeast-like organism resembling *Leishmania* with no parabasal bodies. Wright's or Giemsa stains should be used to demonstrate the yeast phase within large mononuclear cells and occasionally within polymorphonuclear cells. The organism is easily grown on artificial media. At room temperature microconidia are produced as well as large, thick-walled, single-celled tuberculate macroconidia. The latter are presumptive evidence for speciation. Some strains readily convert to the yeast phase at 37°C on appropriate media; animal inoculation is required for identification of recalcitrant strains.

Sporotrichosis. This mycosis usually occurs in the lymphocutaneous form following trauma. An indolent ulcer is formed at the site of trauma, usually the hands. Ultimately multiple subcutaneous nodules, which ulcerate and produce a discharge, appear along the course of draining lymphatics. The etiologic agent is *Sporothrix schenckii* which is ubiquitous in nature. Sporotrichosis is considered an occupational hazard of greenhouse workers, rose fanciers, nurserymen and farmers. In addition to the lymphocutaneous form, localized cutaneous, mucocutaneous, pulmonary and disseminated infections are recognized. *S schenckii* may be difficult to recognize by Gram stain in direct smears; however, PAS, methenamine-silver nitrate and immunofluorescence techniques are very effective. The organism is readily cultivated, producing a glabrous, wax-like colony at room temperature within several days. In vitro characteristic rosettes of microconidia are produced. At 37°C the parasitic yeast phase is produced. Specific diagnostic tests are the sporotrichin skin test, the yeast cell agglutination test and the latex agglutination test.

Cryptococcosis (European blastomycosis, torulosis, Busse-Buschke disease). Cryptococcosis is caused by the encapsulated yeast, *Cryptococcus neoformans.* The primary infection is pulmonary; however, in debilitated or leukemic patients, systemic manifestations develop. The organism has a strong predilection for the central nervous system, thus accounting for the most commonly recognized form of the disease, meningitis. Symptoms include headaches, vertigo, nuchal rigidity, vomiting and subsequent mental disturbances. Cutaneous and mucocutaneous lesions may appear as manifestations of systemic disease. *C neoformans* is found in nature wherever pigeon droppings are found. The organism is readily grown as a mucoid colony on Sabouraud's agar at both room temperature and 37°C. The India ink wet mount is used to demonstrate the encapsulated organism in cerebral spinal fluid. A latex agglutination test is used to detect capsular antigen in body fluids. Direct and indirect immunofluorescent techniques are available for detecting both antigens and antibodies. Amphotericin B is the drug of choice for treatment; untreated cases are invariably fatal.

Mycetoma (madura foot, maduromycosis). This is a chronic infection involving lesions that develop into tumefactions with draining sinus tracts and ''grain'' production. Usually the feet are involved, but occasionally the hands and buttocks are attacked. The etiology is varied involving actinomycotic agents such as: *Actinomyces, Nocardia, Actinomadura* and *Streptomyces;* and *ecemycotic* agents such as: *Allescheria, Madurella, Acremonium, Phialophora, Currularis, Leptospira* and *Cephalosporium.* Noting grain color is of some help in making a diagnosis. The condition is of worldwide distribution but more common in the tropical and subtropical zones where shoes are not worn. *Monosporium apiospermum,* the imperfect stage of

A boydii is the etiologic agent most frequently found in the United States. It is readily cultivated, producing a white aerial mycelium which turns dirty gray on aging. Characteristic ovoid to pyriform microconidia are produced terminally on short to long conidiophores.

Chromomycosis (chromoblastomycosis, verrucous dermatitis). This disease is characterized by the development of warty, verrucoid, cutaneous nodules, usually confined to the feet and legs. The etiology is varied and involves a variety of dematiacious (darkly pigmented) fungi, which gain entrance to tissue by way of trauma. Early lesions may appear as "ringworm;" however, over a period of weeks and months hyperplasia causes an elevation of these areas above the surrounding skin. These nodules have a cauliflower-like appearance. Advanced lesions may become pedunculated, rising several millimeters above the skin. Lymphatics may become blocked leading to elephantiasis of the extremity. The principal fungi causing chromomycosis are: *Fonsecaea pedrosi*, *Fonsecaea compactum*, *Phialophora verrucosa* and *Cladosporium carrioni*. Other *Phialophora* and *Cladosporium* species are rarely encountered. *Fonsecaea pedrosi* is the most common etiologic agent. In early lesions the organism appears as distorted hyphal elements. In advanced lesions the round, thick-walled, dark brown bodies, which divide by septation, are seen. These organisms are readily cultivated on Sabouraud's agar at room temperature giving rise to brown to black brittle colonies. Speciation depends greatly on the types of sporulation present: *Cladosporium*, *Acrotheca* and *Phialophora*.

Protothecosis. Protothecosis is caused by species of *Prototheca*. These are achlorophyllous algae which are thought to be closely related to the green alga, chlorella. They are ubiquitous in nature and have assumed importance as opportunists in debilitated patients. Because of their spherical structure, they have been confused with yeasts and the yeast phase of dimorphic fungi. However, they do not bud, but reproduce by forming endospores, the mother cell becoming a spherule. Verrucous cutaneous and disseminated infections have been recorded in man. In tissues the organism stains well by PAS and methenamine-silver nitrate procedures. The morula, or mulberry, form is pathognomonic. Prototheca are readily cultivated on laboratory media, but may be overlooked because of their relatively slow growth. *Prototheca zopfii* and *Prototheca wickerhamii* are identified with human infection.

CHAPTER 7

Allergy

Allergy is an acquired reaction, a specific alteration in living tissue upon exposure to organic or inorganic substances.

Hypersensitivity is a greater than normal capacity to react. The term may be used synonymously with allergy.

Immunity is a state of resistance to a specific pathogenic agent.

An allergic reaction postulates that (1) the allergen was encountered, in some form, by the patient at a previous time; (2) the patient's response to the subsequent exposure was different from the response to the first exposure; and (3) the alteration in the reactive capacity of the patient was the result of a previous exposure. In allergic states, the incubation period is the time lapse that exists between exposure to a given agent and the first appearance of a characteristic reaction by the sensitized tissue. The reaction time is the period which exists from the moment of exposure of the sensitive tissue to the specific excitant, to the appearance of the first gross tissue change.

Some allergens give rise to specific reactions when used as test materials; poison ivy produces a vesicular reaction in 24-48 hours; aspirin, an urticarial type reaction in 15-30 minutes; and the tubercle bacillus, a papular reaction in 24-48 hours. An accelerated response may be obtained when an incubation period is abbreviated because of increased host reactivity.

Allergy, hypersensitivity and immune reactions have many dermatologic manifestations. Type I, anaphylactic reactions, may be responsible for urticarial eruptions. Antibody (usually IgE) is cell bound as on the surface of mast cells. Bridging of antibody sites by antigen molecules causes release of histamine and other vasoactive substances. These, in turn, cause vasodilation and transudation from blood vessels in the skin producing the urticarial wheal.

Type II, cytotoxic reactions, are best exemplified by autoimmune thrombocytopenia and resulting petechial eruptions. Here, antigen attaches to the cell membrane of the platelet and antibody reacts with it there. With complement acting as mediator, the platelet is destroyed. In the autoimmune bullous diseases, *eg*, pemphigus vulgaris and bullous pemphigoid, various tissues, *ie*, intercellular substances (pemphigus) and basement membrane substance (pemphigoid), serve as antigens causing their destruction and the formation of separation in the skin, either within the epidermis (pemphigus) or at the basement membrane level (pemphigoid).

In type III, hypersensitivity or immune complex diseases, the skin, as well as other organs, is involved because antigen-antibody complexes are trapped within capillaries. Complement is then fixed by these complexes and neutrophil chemotaxis occurs. The target organ, or site of damage, is not only the antigen locus. Type III reactions are clinically demonstrated by the Arthus' reaction, serum sickness and a number of human vasculitis disorders. In lupus erythematosus, immune complexes are deposited within the skin at the basement membrane as well as in the kidney glomerulus, causing cutaneous and glomerular lesions.

Type IV, cell-mediated immune reactions, are the basis of allergic contact dermatitis and tuberculin reactions. Sensitized lymphocytes attack antigens fixed to the skin. The lymphocytes release "lymphokines" which cause such reactions as accumulation and immobilization of macrophages, cytotoxicity and blast transformation in other lymphocytes.

Cutaneous Allergic Reactions

Urticaria. The skin is the shock tissue. There is edema caused by extravasation of fluid and cells through the capillary walls. Clinically there is wheal formation. Reaction time varies from a few minutes to a few hours and is usually accompanied by pruritus. There may be a familial tendency.

Urticarial lesions are induced by foods, drugs, insect allergens, inhalants, foci of infection and other endogenous agents. Contact urticaria is rare but may occur because of transepidermal penetration. Wool, silk, animal danders, animal saliva and such drugs as bacitracin may be responsible for this condition. Physical agents such as heat, cold, light and pressure may cause urticaria. In urticaria pigmentosa, manipulation of cutaneous lesions composed of accumulations of mast cells produces urticarial lesions. In dermatographia, pressure seems to release histamines from cutaneous mast cells. In some cases, this tendency can be passively transferred suggesting IgE mediation. In many cases this is not possible, suggesting some nonimmunologic mechanism of histamine release.

Scratch and intracutaneous tests are used as diagnostic measures. Care must be exercised in intracutaneous testing in order to prevent severe anaphylactic reactions. Scratch testing is safer and less expensive, but is not as sensitive as intracutaneous testing. The initial local red reaction (erythema) at the site of trauma starts in 3 seconds and reaches its maximum in 45 seconds; it is independent of the nerve supply, as it is caused by vasodilation. The second phase, flare, is manifested by intensification and spread of the erythema through an axone reflex and is caused by the dilatation of the arterioles. The third phase is local increased permeability of blood vessels which produces edema and is also due to the action of histamine primarily on venules. This triple response (of Lewis) may be elicited by three types of substances: (1) primary urticariogenic substances such as histamine, morphine, atrophine or scopolamine; (2) stroking of the skin (dermatographia); and (3) true allergic urticarial sensitivity.

Atopic Dermatitis. The term atopy literally means "without place." Patients with atopic dermatitis usually have a family history of other atopic disorders such as allergic rhinitis, asthma, migraine, urticaria or gastrointestinal disturbances. Eosinophilia is a common finding. Serum IgE levels may be elevated although the level of IgE does not always vary with severity of the disease process. Positive intracutaneous tests or scratch tests and passive transfer antibodies (Prausnitz-Küstner test) may be demonstrated. Anaphylactic reactions may develop in patients with atopy, necessitating caution in administering foreign proteins, particularly penicillin antigen with the elaboration of skin sensitizing (IgE) antibodies.

It is not clear how the immunologic abnormalities in patients with atopic dermatitis translate into the chronic disease entity we know as atopic dermatitis. When exposed to antigen, skin sensitizing antibodies produce a wheal and flare (triple response) reaction. The typical eruption in atopic dermatitis is a chronic one with erythema, scaling, hyperpigmentation and lichenification occurring predominantly in the flexural areas of the body. These changes are mediated by rubbing and scratching in response to chronic pruritus. Perhaps the chronic release of small amounts of histamine and attendant rubbing and scratching are responsible for the clinical disease. Many factors unrelated to allergy *per se* modify the disease. Thus, temperature extremes, exercise, sweating, exposure of the skin to irritants and emotional tension tend to exacerbate pruritus and the dermatitis in susceptible patients. In some patients, emollient preparations are helpful. In others, the opposite is true and greasy preparations aggravate the condition.

Multiple pharmacologic abnormalities are present in atopic dermatitis. There is an increased sensitivity to alpha adrenergic agents with rapid and prolonged vasoconstriction occurring in response to these agents or to cooling and vasodilatation occurring slowly in response to heat. Stroking the skin produces so-called "white dermatographia" with prolonged vasoconstriction at the site of the stimulus instead of the usual vasodilatation. Acetylcholine, when injected into normal skin produces vasodilatation. In atopic patients, vasoconstriction occurs. Histamine and kinins also produce less than the expected vasodilation on injection.

Immunologic abnormalities also occur. Cell-mediated immunity appears to be deficient in atopic patients. Circulating T and B lymphocytes are reduced in number. Pyoderma and widespread cutaneous viral infections such as herpes simplex and vaccinia occur. Superficial fungus infections and warts occur with great frequency in atopic individuals. Recent evidence suggests that these patients are unresponsive to beta adrenergic agents and consequently unable to control their release of inflammatory mediators from the dermal cells.

Skin testing is not an absolute, definitive diagnostic measure. Atopic individuals have a propensity to react to many injected test allergens but may not react to them on clinical contact. There is a strong psychogenic component which may modify the clinical reaction to the allergen.

Eczema. The term eczema is a morphologic, not a specific diagnostic, term. Eczema may be atopic, seborrheic or contact. In the acute phase, the eruption is macular, papular or vesicular, dry or moist, and has an erythematous, edematous base. It may be uniform or multiform, discrete or confluent, ill-defined or partially defined. Crusting may or may not be present. As the eruption becomes chronic, the skin becomes thickened and lichenified because of accentuation of the normal skin lines. The lesions may be dull red or hyperpigmented. Secondary pyogenic infection may complicate the picture. An area of chronic eczema may become acutely inflamed.

Atopic dermatitis is an eczematous condition. Testing is done by scratch or intradermal methods which cause an immediate urticarial response. Inhalants and ingestants are the substances most frequently used in testing. Extreme caution must be exercised in intracutaneous testing because of the possible production of a severe constitutional reaction. In childhood the approximate ratio of positive reactions to foods vs inhalants is 2.5:1; in adolescence, inhalants predominate. A positive scratch, intradermal or Prausnitz-Küstner test is of no significance if a reaction is not obtained on clinical exposure to the allergen. Approximately 50% of patients with atopic dermatitis have other atopic diseases, and it is seldom possible to recognize the offending allergen in these cases. Multiple allergens may be responsible for the production of clinical symptoms in a single individual.

Contact Dermatitis. Contact dermatitis may be caused by a primary irritant or a sensitizing substance. A primary irritant produces its response by actual physical damage to the skin. Examples of primary irritants are strong acids, alkalis, phenol and mustard gas. Some substances act as primary irritants or allergens, depending upon the concentration which comes in contact with the skin.

Contact dermatitis is a cell-mediated immune reaction. The antigen is a simple chemical (hapten) conjugated with a larger carrier protein, presumably a normal component of the epidermis or dermis. Some degree of carrier specificity can be demonstrated. Sensitization is thought to occur in the regional lymph nodes where the antigen-carrier protein is caused by lymphatic vessels. Sensitized lymphocytes are produced, and then react on subsequent exposure to the antigen. Contact allergic reactions differ from contact irritants in two ways: not all of the population is susceptible, and prior contact with the sensitizer is a prerequisite for the disease.

Detailed history and careful observation are important steps in the investigation of allergic contact dermatitis. The sensitizing material may be contacted at home, at work, at play or in transit. Allergic contact dermatitis is usually eczematous; however, substances such as silk or morphine may cause an urticarial response.

The patch test is the diagnostic method of choice. Patch testing is performed by placing the moistened, suspected agent on the skin of the patient and covering it with a nonmedicated band-aid or an Elastoplast.® Volatile agents such as perfume are left uncovered. In 24-48 hours, the covering is removed and the intensity of the reaction recorded. A delayed positive test may not appear for 72 hours after the application of the test substance. A positive reaction varies from simple erythema to bleb formation and necrosis.

Patch testing must be carefully performed. A test material must be in proper dilution, since it may act as a primary irritant in 5% concentration or as a true sensitizer in 3% concentration. The positive test must be interpreted in the light of previous exposures.

The most common contact sensitizers include metal (particularly nickel, chromates and mercurials), topical medications including neomycin and benzocaine, lanolin, preservatives such as parabens, ethylenediamine, formalin, paraphenylenediamine, turpentine and rubber ingredients (mercaptobenzothiazide) and thirams.

Drug Eruptions. Drug eruptions may be allergic or toxic. Toxic manifestations will occur if the dose is large enough or the medication has a cumulative effect or both. Evidence on which a diagnosis of an allergic drug eruption is based includes: (1) previous tolerance to the drug; (2) small doses elicit a response; (3) a cutaneous response different from that produced by its usual toxic or pharmacologic action; (4) different drugs may elicit the same response; (5) regardless of the dose, an allergic response cannot be caused in all persons; (6) the absence of cumulative effects; (7) the ability of a drug to cause a specific reaction not produced by its isomer; and (8) the fulfillment of the criteria of the incubation period and spontaneous flare.

Simple chemicals and drugs may mimic the manifestations of diseases caused by microorganisms or other allergens. There are variations in species susceptibility and immunity to simple chemicals just as there are to microorganisms.

Drugs have different degrees of ability to sensitize. A drug may cause different types of eruptions; *eg,* salicylates may cause toxic erythema, urticaria, erythema multiforme or purpura. There is a tendency for certain drugs to produce a characteristic response: iodides and bromides usually cause follicular lesions; phenolphthalein and antipyrine produce erythema multiforme or fixed eruptions. Drug reactions are not always caused by the substance administered, but may be caused by its metabolites. Moreover, more than one allergen may be present in a "drug," thereby accounting for a polymorphic eruption if the active agents react differently.

Skin tests are of no value except in the eczematous drug eruptions. The diagnosis of a drug eruption is based on the type of reaction caused by a specific drug, the locations in which the eruption appears, the circumstances under which exposures may occur and knowledge of the sensitizing potentials of apparently unrelated drugs.

Fixed Drug Eruptions. The site of the eruption, but not the reaction, is fixed. The lesions are oval or round erythematous patches, occasionally associated with edema, but always leaving hyperpigmentation when the acute lesion subsides. They may be single or multiple. The original eruption may be macular, urticarial or bullous; less commonly herpetiform, necrotic, nodular or follicular.

The involved sites may lose reactivity, partially or completely, temporarily or permanently, but new areas may become sensitized. Polyvalent sensitivity may exist; a site which reacts to antipyrine may also erupt when phenolphthalein or barbiturates are given.

There is no association with heredity or general health. The peripheral blood vessels are the reactive site. Patch tests with the offending agent are negative on uninvolved areas but may be positive at the previous site of the skin lesion. Systemic challenge with the suspected drug is required to establish the diagnosis.

Allergic Dermatoses Caused by Physical Agents. Abnormal reactions to light may be caused by light alone (sunburn, polymorphous light eruptions), by light plus an exogenous agent (phototoxicity, photoallergy), or by light in combination with an abnormal endogenous chemical (porphyrias). In addition, certain diseases such as systemic or discoid lupus erythematosus and reactivation of herpes simplex are aggravated by sun exposure.

Phototoxic eruptions involve the absorption of light by a chemical or drug and the transference of its energy to vulnerable tissue. Tetracycline is a common cause of phototoxicity. The term phototoxicity suggests that given enough of the sensitizing agent and light, anyone will get the reaction, *ie*, allergy is not involved. Generally, the sunburn spectrum of ultraviolet light (290-320 mμ UVB) is implicated in most, but not all, phototoxic reactions which resemble an accentuated sunburn. Phototoxicity can be produced by topical re-action of light with coal tars or psoralens.

Photoallergy is frequently caused by longer wavelengths of ultraviolet light (320-400 mμ UVA). The reactions are more diverse in character and can appear eczematous or papular. Unexposed areas are sometimes involved. Sulfur drugs, phenothiazines and halogenated salicylanalides contained in some deodorant soaps are capable of causing photoallergy.

Photoallergic responses appear only after a suitable incubation period and thereafter may be reproduced within 24 hours. They cannot be produced on all individuals.

Polymorphous light eruptions include: (1) erythema with or without edema; (2) erythema multiforme; (3) acute or chronic eczema; and (4) papular urticaria or prurigo. No detectable exogenous agent is involved. Exposure to sunlight may cause transient erythema (occasionally associated with edema) lasting from several minutes to an hour. Erythema multiforme–like eruptions are more commonly seen and are difficult to distinguish from acute lupus erythematosus. An eczematous response with papules and vesicles is a frequent development. Single, pink, indurated plaques with telangiectasia, lichenification and scaling may occur on the cheeks and neck. The mechanism of this disease or group of diseases is not clear.

In the future, some patients may be found to have photoallergy and others phototoxicity.

CHAPTER | 8

Occupational Dermatoses

An occupational dermatitis is a skin eruption produced by contact with a material or materials which a patient handles during the course of his work. A previously existing dermatosis which has been aggravated by such materials is also classified as an occupational disease, even though the factor that caused the original eruption was not related to the job in any way. The State Industrial Accident Commissions in the United States report that skin eruptions constitute approximately 60% of all medical diseases reported to the compensation boards. The increase in incidence of industrial dermatoses during the past 25 years may be attributed in part to the introduction of many synthetic materials. Practically every substance used in modern industry is either a potential sensitizer or a primary irritant. The industrial dermatologist is a specialist in his own right and must possess the qualities of safety engineer, clinician and chemist, as well as a knowledge of forensic medicine.

There are many facets in the problems of industrial dermatology which require careful scrutiny. If a person who has psoriasis, seborrheic dermatitis or an eczematous eruption is employed in an industry where he is subjected to contact with oil, soap, chemicals or inhalants, the original condition may be aggravated by such contact, and therefore be considered by the State Industrial Accident Commission as an occupational disease. Preemployment examinations are of great value in excluding persons with such conditions. If an individual sustains a minor injury during the course of his work, and is treated by the plant nurse with an antiseptic ointment or solution, or one of the antihistamine ointments to which he is sensitive, a reaction may develop which will be far more extensive than the original minor injury. If the physician, first aid person, or nurse at the plant applies some sensitizing medication to a nonoccupational disease or injury, the dermatitis which develops is considered an occupational illness, and is compensable. Before any medication is prescribed for a suspected occupational disease, the diagnosis should be established and the relationship of the eruption to the industry should be proved.

Unfortunately, some industrial physicians consider a dermatitis as occupational merely because the type of work the patient does is frequently productive of eruptions in fellow workers. It is possible that the dermatitis which developed may have been caused by some nonindustrial exposure to substances such as hair dye, toilet articles, paint, household detergents, plants or materials handled during the pursuit of a hobby. Careful patch testing may exclude these things, although a positive patch test does not necessarily mean that the substance which produced the test reaction was responsible for the development of the dermatitis. The test substance may have been a primary irritant. A negative patch test is not necessarily conclusive evidence that the dermatitis is nonoccupational. The areas tested may not be hypersensitive and the test never accurately reproduces the actual conditions under which the patient worked.

The physician should have first hand knowledge of the type of work the patient does and the industrial hazards involved. In order to gain this information it may be necessary to visit the scene of operations and personally investigate the situation.

Causes of Occupational Dermatoses

1. Plants of various types, including fruit, vegetables, weeds and flowers are capable of producing a state of hypersensitivity. Dermatitis venenata due to rhus plants may develop in graveyard employees, telephone linemen and gardeners.

2. Fiberglass workers are irritated by the small spicules that become lodged in the skin.

3. Epoxy resins are common sensitizers. These substances are employed in many industries as sealants or glues. They are only sensitizers, however, before they have completely dried.

The synthesis of plastic substances involves the use of sensitizing and irritating substances such as phenolformaldehyde resin, melamine, sulfonamides, colors, hardeners and other chemical substances. The dermatitis which develops is rarely the result of contact with the finished product but is caused by handling of the component parts.

4. Nickel dermatitis is common in patients who handle any metallic alloy containing this element.

5. Specific trauma produces lesions such as fissures on the fingertips, observed in those who pack glassware in stripped paper, or calluses on the palms of carpenters.

6. Specific infections are observed, such as erysipeloid in fishermen, sporotrichosis in gardeners and pyoderma on the fingers of butchers.

7. Insect bites are observed in poultry workers, animal handlers and farmers.

8. Chemical substances may produce occupational dermatoses of various types. Strong acids and alkalies are primary irritants and produce burns; other chemicals are sensitizing substances and produce eruptions similar to poison ivy dermatitis. Serious and sometimes fatal sequelae may follow prolonged exposure to inorganic arsenic, chromic acid and other chemicals.

9. Various reactions other than sensitization to the finished product may be encountered in the synthetic rubber industry. One of the component parts of synthetic rubber, agerite alba, may produce depigmentation of the normal skin. Temporary hair loss is another hazard of the rubber industry.

Prevention of Occupational Dermatoses

1. Preemployment history and physical examination.

2. Evaluation of all possible industrial hazards in the plant with establishment and enforcement of safety regulations.

3. An adequate, well-trained medical department to diagnose and treat the dermatitis at the time it develops.

4. Establishment of the occupational origin of the disease and avoidance of treatment of nonoccupational diseases at the person's place of employment.

5. Proper use of diagnostic procedures such as patch tests.

6. Removal of the individual from contact with the suspected causative agent the day the dermatitis develops.

CHAPTER 9

Sexually Transmitted Diseases

The designation "sexually transmitted disease" has replaced the term "venereal disease" in recent years, and now includes a number of other diseases that can be spread by sexual contact. Warts, type 2 herpes simplex infections, nonspecific urethritis and infectious hepatitis, as well as syphilis, gonorrhea, chancroid, granuloma inguinale and lymphogranuloma venereum, are included in this category. Although statistical figures are difficult to verify, it is quite obvious that due to various social, economic and medical factors, the incidence of all sexually transmitted diseases is rising. Since cutaneous lesions are part of the clinical picture in most of these diseases, the practitioner must become familiar with their dermatologic manifestations.

Syphilis

Syphilis is a chronic relapsing disease caused by the spirochete *Treponema pallidum,* and is characterized by long periods of apparent quiescence during which the only evidence of disease is a positive serologic test. The organism is transmitted by direct contact with the infectious lesions of early syphilis and becomes systemic within hours. *T pallidum* is a highly refractile, spiral organism, 6-20 μ in length with 6-20 equidistant, regular spirals. The organism has a characteristic rotation on its long axis and in the live state is visible only by the use of the darkfield microscope.

Following an incubation period which varies from 7-90 days, the primary lesion, or chancre, may appear. The initial lesion may be small, large or evanescent. Chancres in women are rarely seen. For purposes of classification, untreated disease is either early (first two years) or late (after two years). The infectious lesions occur only in the early stages and destructive lesions in the late stage. The disease is not hereditary but may be transmitted to the fetus *in utero* during and after the fifth month of pregnancy.

Histopathology of Syphilis. The fundamental histopathologic findings in all clinical lesions of syphilis consist of a perivascular infiltrate of plasma cells and lymphocytes, thickening of vessel walls and obliterative endarteritis. The early infiltrate of polymorphonuclear leukocytes in primary syphilis is replaced by plasma cells and lymphocytes. In secondary syphilis, the cellular infiltrate extends deep into the cutis. It is difficult to distinguish the chronic granulomatous picture of late syphilis from that of tuberculosis. The characteristic pathologic changes include vascular occlusion, central caseous necrosis surrounded by epithelioid cells and foreign body giant cells, and a peripheral plasma cell infiltrate.

Primary Syphilis. The primary lesion, or chancre, is the first clinical lesion to appear and develops at the site of treponemal inoculation. It is usually a single,

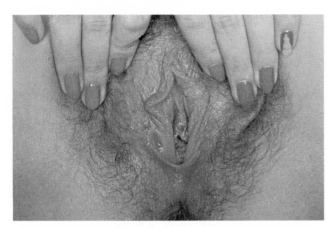

Chancre of the vulva

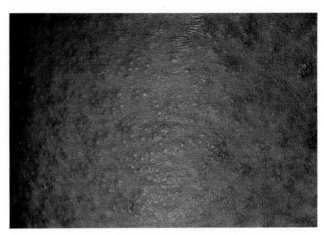

Secondary syphilis

relatively painless, indurated ulcer with a firm, clean base; however, some initial lesions may be superficial and evanescent. Chancres may also be multiple and painful. Most initial lesions occur on the genitalia but may also develop at the anus, mouth, lips, nipples and fingers. In women, the chancre may occur on the cervix and is frequently overlooked unless a speculum examination of the vagina is performed. The chancre will heal spontaneously in 2-10 weeks if left untreated.

The appearance of a positive serologic test depends upon the development of an immunologic response which occurs several weeks after the onset of the chancre. Therefore, a darkfield microscopic examination for *T pallidum* is the only definitive means of establishing the diagnosis of primary and secondary lesions.

Secondary Syphilis. From several weeks to 6 months (average, 3 weeks) after the appearance of the chancre, the patient may develop one or more signs of secondary syphilis. During this period of generalized spirochetemia, every organ of the body is invaded by *T pallidum*.

The cutaneous lesions are usually symmetrical and nonpruritic and may be macular, papular or pustular. Macular lesions are nonscaling, usually pinkish in color, partially defined and may simulate pityriasis rosea. Papular secondary syphilis lesions may form characteristic reddish-brown groups of small papules (false corymbose), annular, papular, perioral lesions or larger lenticular papules. Annular lesions, which usually occur on the face, show central clearing and a raised grooved border forming broken or incomplete circles. Moist hypertrophic eroded papules (condylomata lata) occur in the perianal and other intertrigi-

Secondary syphilis

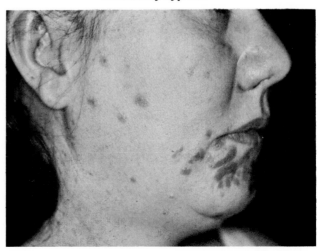

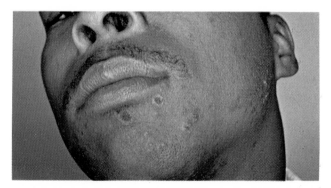

Annular lesions

nous areas. These flat papular lesions are covered by a grayish membrane and are teeming with spirochetes. Pustular syphilis is an uncommon manifestation and is usually seen in blacks. Ecthymatous secondary lesions, which are rare, occur late in the secondary period.

More than one type of lesion may be seen in the same patient. The palms and soles may show infiltrated reddish-brown macules. A patchy, "moth eaten" alopecia may appear concurrently with other lesions or as

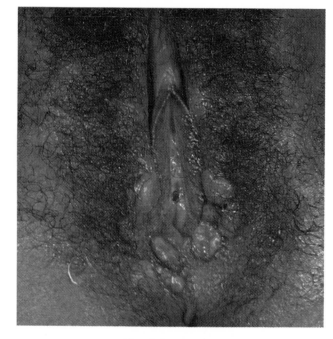

Condylomata lata

Ecthymatous secondary syphilis

Papular secondary syphilis

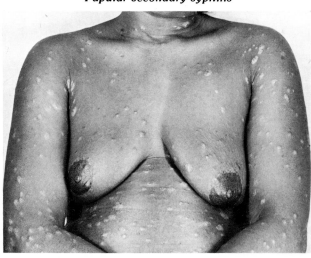

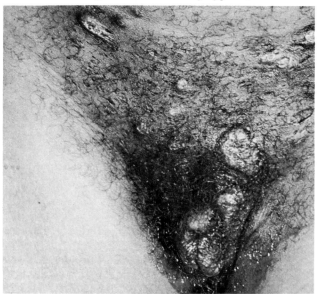

the sole manifestation of secondary syphilis. Iridocyclitis may occur and usually responds well to treatment. Mucous patches are highly infectious erosive lesions of the mouth and vagina. Deafness may occur either due to swelling of the eustachian tube from pharyngitis or swelling of the sheath of the eighth nerve. Mild systemic symptoms of malaise, fever, headache and sore throat are frequent. Generalized lymphadenopathy with multiple firm, rubbery movable nontender nodes is usually present in secondary syphilis. Hepatitis and meningitis are also manifestations of this stage of the disease. An immune complex type of nephritis may also occur. There are reported cases of nephrotic syndrome ranging from mild transient proteinuria to gross hematuria, azotemia and hypertension. All manifestations respond well to antisyphilitic therapy.

The serologic test for syphilis is invariably positive in high titer in secondary syphilis.

Latent Syphilis. If secondary syphilis is not treated, the lesions involute in approximately 4-12 weeks and the patient enters a stage of asymptomatic infection, detectable only by serologic tests. During the first two years of infection, this stage is known as early latent syphilis, and afterward is called late latent syphilis. This arbitrary division was established for prognostic and epidemiologic purposes. The patient more readily transmits the disease during the early period. Also, serologic reversal is more likely to occur in patients who are treated in the early stage. In late latent syphilis, the serologic test may remain positive for life, even though the patient has been adequately treated. Determination of the time interval of latent syphilis depends greatly on a careful history of primary or secondary lesions, and through investigation of previous serologic tests such as would be found on previous hospitalizations, marriage certificates, employment and military induction physicals.

Approximately two-thirds of untreated patients will remain in the stage of late latency. The remainder will exhibit cutaneous or systemic late manifestations of the disease.

Late Cutaneous Syphilis. Cutaneous lesions of late syphilis are known as gummas. These may be solitary or multiple. A solitary gumma begins usually as a subcutaneous nodule which undergoes liquefaction necrosis, forming a punched out, relatively painless ulcer. This may slowly heal followed by another nodule appearing at the periphery tending to gradually enlarge the area of involvement. Nodular serpiginous syphiloderm and nodular ulcerative syphiloderm are other forms of gummatous syphilis.

Cardiovascular Syphilis. The cardiovascular system is commonly affected by late syphilis but may not become clinically manifest for 10-40 years after the primary infection. The T pallidum invades the small arteries causing an obliterative endarteritis. The vasa vasorum of the great vessels are involved resulting in a weakening and scarring of the muscular coat and a tortuous and dilated vessel. The aorta is most often involved but the process can also affect the myocardium and aortic valves.

Uncomplicated Syphilitic Aortitis. Mild aortic involvement may result in minimal loss of elasticity and fibrosis with some dilatation. The condition may be asymptomatic and difficult to diagnose by physical examination. A loud tambour-like second sound in the absence of hypertension or atherosclerosis in a patient with a positive serologic test for syphilis should make the examiner suspicious of syphilitic aortitis.

Aortitis occurs more frequently in blacks than whites. It is found in adults with inadequately treated acquired syphilis and is extremely rare as a late manifestation of congenital syphilis.

Stenosis of the coronary ostea may cause symptoms of angina or vague complaints of substernal pressure. Pain may radiate to the face or epigastrium. There may be no electrocardiographic evidence of the disease. Aortic insufficiency may or may not be present.

Aortic insufficiency is usually due to dilatation of the aortic ring rather than primary valvular involvement. It is frequently asymptomatic until the patient has the first episode of heart failure. Paroxysmal nocturnal dyspnea may be present and the patient may complain of pounding in the head, roaring in the ears or postural dizziness. Differential diagnosis from hypertensive and arteriosclerotic cardiovascular disease is often difficult. The pulse pressure is widened with the diastolic pressure low giving a pistol shot sound over the femoral artery. A blowing, high pitched decrescendo diastolic murmur heard at the base may be accentuated by leaning the patient forward in expiration. Electrocardiographic changes are not specific. X-ray examination shows left ventricular hypertrophy possibly with calcification in the first part of the aorta (unusual in nonsyphilitics).

Specific therapy of cardiovascular syphilis is probably of little value. The patient should be treated with supportive measures: digitalis, low salt diet, limited fluids, nitroglycerine, rest, sedation and diuretics.

Aneurysms of the thoracic aorta are more common than aneurysms of the carotid, subclavian or innominate arteries. Syphilitic aneurysms are saccular and may grow to a large size, occasionally eroding through the chest wall or vertebrae. Signs or symptoms may be absent or pronounced, depending on the location of the aneurysm. The most common site of involvement is the ascending aorta. Diagnosis is made by routine X-ray procedures and physical examination.

Neurosyphilis. Abnormal spinal fluid findings occur in 10-30% of all patients with early syphilis but of these, only a few develop clinical neurosyphilis. Laboratory abnormalities, in most patients, represent invasion rather than involvement, and demonstrate the body's reaction to the generalized spirochetosis. Adequate therapy of early syphilis protects the patient against neurosyphilis but inadequate therapy may predispose to neurorecurrence or late forms of symptomatic neurosyphilis. Neurosyphilis seems to be more common in whites.

Nonparenchymatous neurosyphilis implies involvement of the blood vessels in the meninges.

Meningitis may occur spontaneously in the first two years of infection or may even follow adequate treatment. It is characterized by cranial nerve palsies, papilledema or convulsions. Spinal fluid findings include pleocytosis and positive complement fixation tests although the total protein may be within normal limits. It responds well to treatment.

Vascular neurosyphilis results from obliterative endarteritis of the small branches of the middle cerebral or other arteries. Symptoms are those of a focal vascular accident, the clinical syndrome depending on the area involved. Since these are vascular lesions, the cerebrospinal fluid may be negative. The diagnosis should be suspected in a young normotensive patient whose serologic test for syphilis is positive. Response to treatment is usually good, without sequelae.

Meningovascular neurosyphilis is the most frequently encountered form of symptomatic neurosyphilis, combining the symptoms of meningitis with the effects of vascular damage: epilepsy, cranial nerve palsies, anisocoria, fixed pupils or vascular accidents. Prognosis is usually good following adequate therapy. The spinal fluid findings vary.

Asymptomatic neurosyphilis is diagnosed by laboratory findings on spinal fluid. Patients with untreated or adequately treated syphilis showing no clinical manifestations of disease must have a spinal fluid examination done to rule out asymptomatic involvement of the central nervous system. The fluid is checked for elevation of cell count, protein, complement fixation and fluorescent antibodies.

Gumma of the Brain may be single or multiple. Symptoms are similar to those of other tumors of the central nervous system and vary with the location. The blood serologic titer is usually high and the complement fixation reactive.

Parenchymatous neurosyphilis may be inflammatory or degenerative.

General paresis, also known as general paralysis of the insane, encephalomalacia or syphilitic encephalomyelitis, is a destructive inflammatory process which, if untreated, will eventually kill the patient. Early symptoms include irritability, fatigability, forgetfulness, personality changes, headaches, weight loss, disturbed sleep and loss of competence. Later, the memory becomes grossly impaired, judgment becomes defective, and the patient suffers from emotional instability, lack of insight, confusion, disorientation, delusions and convulsions. Objective signs of paresis are: pupillary abnormalities; perioral tremor; hyperreflexia; dysarthria; tremors of the tongue, hand and face muscles; and positive Babinski's reflexes.

The blood serologic test is invariably positive in high titer and the spinal fluid is strongly positive. Paresis usually develops 5-25 years after onset of the disease.

The most common type of paresis is simple deterioration in which there is a gradual loss of the finer qualities of personality which distinguish the individual. Expansive mania, paranoia and agitated depression also occur in paresis. Lissauer's paralysis begins as focal epilepsy and is then associated with hemiparesis and aphasia. Untreated patients with paresis die from intercurrent infection or in status epilepticus.

Juvenile paresis occurs in late congenital syphilis, between the ages of 6 and 15 years.

Paresis responds to treatment with penicillin.

Tabes dorsalis or locomotor ataxia is a degenerative disease of the posterolateral columns which usually begins 20 or more years after infection. Cerebral involvement is limited to papillary abnormalities, extra-ocular motor palsies and primary optic atrophy.

Argyll-Robertson pupils are fixed to light but react slowly to accommodation. They are persistently micotic and react poorly to mydriatics. The visual pathways are intact.

Early symptoms of tabes dorsalis are lightning pains, paresthesias, urinary disturbances such as dribbling and hesitancy, diminished libido, cystometric evidence of lost bladder tone, diminished or lost deep tendon reflexes, and diminished vibratory and position sense. Later, incontinence and nocturnal bed-wetting may occur, as well as visceral crises (gastric, rectal, bladder or laryngeal), difficulty in walking, cord bladder, trophic joint changes (Charcot's joint) and ataxia.

Since tabes dorsalis is a degenerative disease, the spinal fluid findings may be normal. *T pallidum* is not found and the disease responds poorly to treatment.

Primary optic atrophy may occur independently or be associated with tabes dorsalis. The optic nerve head degenerates producing complete blindness. Treatment is ineffective.

Erb's spastic paraplegia is a degenerative involvement of the anterior horn cells and anterolateral tracts. The motor paralysis of extremities and bladder does not respond to treatment.

Adie's syndrome simulates tabes dorsalis but has no relation to syphilis. The symptom complex includes hyporeflexia of the lower extremities and pupils

Charcot joint of late syphilis

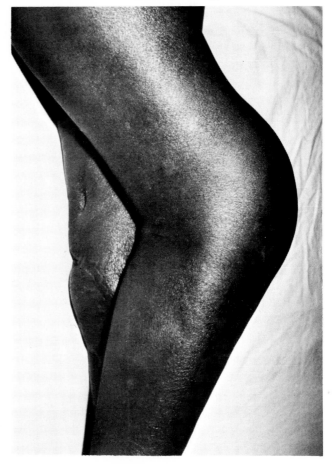

which react to neither light nor accommodation.

Interpretation of Serologic Tests for Syphilis. The diagnosis of syphilis depends on careful evaluation of the patient's physical status, history and laboratory findings. In no instance should the diagnosis of syphilis be made on the sole basis of a single unconfirmed serologic test. The only *definitive* diagnosis is observing the *T pallidum* under the darkfield microscope.

Serologic tests for syphilis fall into two categories: nonspecific or reagin tests and *Treponema*-specific tests.

The nonspecific serologic tests basically measure a reaction between a lipoidal antigen and a nonspecific mixture of antibodies called reagin. This reaction binds complement and effects an indicator system. The indicators vary with the test and may result in flocculation (VDRL), complement fixation (Kolmer), or agglutination (rapid plasma reagent). These tests may be quantitated by diluting the serum and reporting the highest dilution at which a positive test is obtained as its titer. Quantitative tests, when properly interpreted, are of value in determining the activity of infection or results of therapy.

The *Treponema*-specific serologic tests utilize the treponema as the antigen. The original test was the *Treponema pallidum* immobilization (TPI) test which used live spirochetes and measured their immobilization by serum containing specific antibodies. This cumbersome test is no longer available and has been replaced by the fluorescent treponemal antibody absorption (FTA-ABS) test which utilizes a lyophilized Reiter strain of *T pallidum* as the antigen. The serum is absorbed first with Nichols strain *T pallidum* to absorb out common treponemal group antigen and is then applied to the slide. Fluorescein labeled antihuman globulin is applied and fluorescence will occur at the site of specific antigen-antibody reaction. *Treponema*-specific antibodies appear slightly earlier in the course of disease and may remain positive for the rest of the patient's life. This test (FTA-ABS) is of little use in determining the activity of disease. A more recently developed test, the treponemal hemagglutination (TPHA) test measures specific antibodies and can be performed with automated laboratory equipment.

Biologic false-positive tests for syphilis do occur. Temporary false-positive reactions may occur during pregnancy, following immunization, and during acute febrile infectious diseases such as mononucleosis, leprosy, malaria, hepatitis, measles, chickenpox and upper respiratory infections. Chronic biologic false-positive (BFP) serologic reactions may occur in systemic lupus erythematosus and other connective tissue diseases. Long-term follow-up of patients with chronic BFP reactions reveals a very high incidence of collagen vascular disease.

Congenital Syphilis. Although syphilis is not hereditary, the fetus may be infected in the uterus of an untreated mother after the sixteenth week of pregnancy. Adequate treatment of the infected mother early in the course of the pregnancy will prevent the development of the disease in the infant.

A newborn, infected infant may have a bullous eruption of the extremities and diaper area. This is the only phase of the disease in which vesicular lesions appear. Cutaneous lesions similar to those of secondary syphilis may be present. Other early signs include hepatosplenomegaly, bloody rhinitis and periostitis. A serologic test on cord blood may only reflect crossover of the mother's positive serologic test for syphilis (STS), so a darkfield microscopic examination of skin lesions or tests on the infant's venous blood should be done. The FTA-ABS test measures treponemal specific macroglobulin that is presumably produced by the fetus. The presence of this serum macroglobulin is thought to indicate the presence of active infection in the newborn.

Late manifestations of congenital syphilis do not appear until later in childhood or after puberty. These include interstitial keratitis, eighth nerve deafness, hydrarthrosis (Clutton's joint), Hutchinson's teeth and mulberry molars. Interstitial keratitis may occur at any period of the patient's life and probably represents a hypersensitivity response. Hutchinson's teeth are wide-spaced peg-shaped, notched upper central incisors. Mulberry molars contain multiple small cusps and defective formation.

The cardiovascular system is not involved in late congenital syphilis. Congenital neurosyphilis does occur and varies in its manifestations.

Syphilis and Pregnancy. The fetus does not become infected until after the fourth month; therefore, treatment of maternal syphilis before the fifth month prevents transmission of infection to the child. Treatment of the mother also treats the fetus and may be instituted as late as the eighth month. Treatment with penicillin during any pregnancy will prevent fetal syphilis in subsequent pregnancies, unless the mother is reinfected.

Treatment. Early infectious syphilis may be treated with procaine penicillin G, 600,000 units daily for 10 days. The patient may also be treated with two weekly doses of 2.4 million units of long-acting benzathine penicillin G. Penicillin-sensitive patients should be treated with 500 mg tetracycline four times a day for 15 days. The treatment for the late stages of syphilis is approximately 10 million units of benzathine penicillin G in divided doses. Patients with neurosyphilis will probably require even larger doses.

The practitioner should remember that reversal of the serologic test may be delayed, or the test may remain permanently positive. A persistently positive serologic test for syphilis following adequate therapy is not an indication for retreatment as long as the titer is low and fixed.

Reactions to treatment include allergic reactions to penicillin and specific reactions associated with the treatment of syphilis. *The Jarisch-Herxheimer reaction* is an intensification of syphilitic lesions or a febrile response, possibly due to endotoxins, in the first 24-48 hours following therapy. *The therapeutic paradox* is irreversible damage produced by contractile scarring in the healing process.

Gonorrhea

Gonorrhea is a disease of the genitourinary tract, caused by *Neisseria gonorrhoeae*. It is the most common infectious disease in the United States.

Gonorrhea in men begins as anterior urethritis 2-4 days following exposure. It is manifested by a thick, yellowish purulent discharge. If the infection is untreated, chronic posterior urethritis develops manifested by a scant mucoid discharge. Complications may include epididymitis, arthritis, prostatitis, conjunctivitis and septicemia. Up to 40% of infected men are believed to be asymptomatic.

In women, gonococcal urethritis may occur but the infection usually begins as cervicitis. Symptoms may be minimal or absent in this stage of the disease. Retrograde infections involve the Fallopian tubes, causing pyosalpinx. Systemic complications may occur. A significant number of patients of both sexes also have involvement of rectum and posterior pharynx.

Diagnosis of gonorrhea in men is made by microscopic examination of a Gram-stained smear of the urethral discharge. The organism is a gram-negative intracellular diplococcus. Culture of the cervical discharge is necessary to diagnose gonorrhea in women. Careful evaluation and culture of the pharynx and rectum of patients with suspected gonorrhea or contacts of these patients is done when the physician suspects orogenital sex or homosexuality.

Treatment. Penicillin is the drug of choice in the treatment of gonorrhea. The dose of 4.8 million units of procaine penicillin is given intramuscularly after a dose of 1 gm of probenicid by mouth. Ampicillin and spectinomycin may also be used successfully. It is imperative to treat all sexual contacts. Cure of the disease does not confer immunity against reinfection. Serologic test for syphilis must be performed, when the patient is treated, and monthly for three months thereafter.

Chancroid

Chancroid is a disease of the genitalia caused by *Hemophilus ducreyi*. The initial lesion is a small papule or vesicopustule which breaks down into a ragged ulcer with undermined edges and a necrotic base. The ulcers are usually multiple, soft and painful. Painful regional lymphadenopathy with the formation of fluctuant buboes is a common occurrence. Balanitis and phimosis are frequent complications.

H ducreyi is a short, nonacid fast, gram-negative bacillus which tends to form chains. About 15% of cases may have concurrent early syphilis; therefore, a darkfield microscopic examination and serologic follow-up are mandatory. The laboratory confirmation of a clinical diagnosis of chancroid depends on the demonstration of the *H ducreyi* on stained smear from the ulcer and culture on eosin-methylene blue agar.

Treatment. Sulfisoxazole, 1 gm every 6 hours combined with 500 mg tetracycline every 6 hours for 14 days, is the therapeutic method of choice. If the patient is sensitive to sulfa drugs, tetracycline is used alone.

Granuloma Inguinale

Granuloma inguinale is a disease limited to the genitocrural area, but its mode of transmission is unknown. It is caused by *Donovania granulomatis* (Donovan body). The condition rarely occurs in white patients.

The initial lesion of granuloma inguinale is a subcutaneous nodule which ulcerates to form a spreading, shallow, indurated, granulomatous ulcer with rolled, undermined edges. It spreads by direct extension without involving lymphatics. The ulcers tend to heal spontaneously, with dense, deforming scars which occasionally obstruct lymphatics, forming elephantiasis or a brawny edema known as esthiomene. The extending granulomatous lesion may cause spontaneous amputation of the genitalia.

The diagnosis is made by the demonstration of Donovan bodies in stained smears (Wright's or Giemsa) from the margin of the ulcer. They appear as small intracytoplasmic encapsulated organisms in large macrophages.

Treatment. Granuloma inguinale responds to treatment with orally administered tetracycline, the drug of choice. Chlortetracycline, oxytetracycline, chloramphenicol and erythromycin are also effective but cause a high incidence of side reactions. Penicillin is of no value in the treatment of granuloma inguinale.

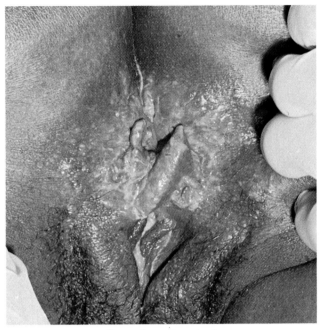

Granuloma inguinale

Herpes Progenitalis

Herpes simplex is the most common genital lesion; it can cause serious sequelae in women.

The onset of the lesion which consists of grouped vesicles on an erythematous base may be heralded by mild paresthesia. The vesicle fluid becomes pustular, then the lesions dry and become crusted. The lesions heal without scar formation. Relapses occur in about 75% of cases and the lesions usually recur on or about the same site. The virus is isolated only in the acute vesicular stage. There is evidence that the herpes virus remains latent in the regional sensory ganglia. Type 1 herpes simplex is most often responsible for lesions of the head and neck; type 2 herpes simplex lesions are most commonly associated with sexual transmission. However, about 15% of patients have lesions in the genital area from which type 1 herpes simplex virus can be recovered.

In women, genital herpes is frequently subclinical or inapparent since the cervix is the chief site of involvement. There is evidence that the herpes simplex virus type 2 may be related to the subsequent development of carcinoma of the cervix.

Diagnosis is made most readily by the morphology of the grouped vesicles. Cytologic examination by PAP smear or Tzanck preparation will show multinucleated giant cells and intranuclear inclusions. Viral culture for identification is necessary for definite diagnosis.

There is no satisfactory curative treatment or prophylaxis.

Lymphogranuloma Venereum

Lymphogranuloma venereum is a viral systemic disease caused by a *Chlamydia (Bedsonia)* organism. The initial lesion is a transient, tiny papulovesicle which is usually neglected. The disease is disseminated through the lymphatic system. In men, large fluctuant inguinal bubos, often grooved by the inguinal ligament, are a common occurrence. In women, the lymphatic drainage is posterior to the deep perirectal and pudendal nodes. This results in an insidious, painless destruction of the labia, rectovaginal fistulas and rectal stricture. The diagnosis is usually made clinically and is confirmed by serologic tests.
Treatment. Sulfonamide, 1 gm four times daily for 2-3 weeks or tetracycline, 500 mg four times daily for a week is the treatment of choice.

Condyloma Acuminatum

Condylomata acuminata (warts) are caused by the papovavirus. In the genital area, warts may grow rapidly into moist, cauliflower-like papillomatous growths. The type of lesion which develops is attributed to heat, moisture and friction. These lesions occur most frequently in intertriginous areas such as under the prepuce, perirectal and vulvovaginal areas. Condylomata may also be present inside the urethra or rectum.
Treatment. Podophyllin is usually effective, but clearing is difficult if reinfection by the sexual partner continues.

Molluscum Contagiosum

Molluscum contagiosum is caused by a poxvirus and is not uncommon in childhood. It consists of multiple, discrete, flesh-colored, dome-shaped, umbilicated papules. Solitary lesions may be quite large and even resemble a basal cell carcinoma. The lesions are contagious and are spread by direct contact. For this reason, when they occur in the genital region of adults, molluscum may be considered a sexually transmitted disease.
Treatment. Removal of the lesions by simple curettage is the treatment of choice.

CHAPTER 10

Psychosomatic Medicine Applied to Dermatology

The relationship of the integument to internal organs and systems is emphasized throughout this text. Infiltrated plaque-like lesions on the legs may indicate thyroid-pituitary disease, and yellow nodules about the elbows or knees are associated with disturbances of lipid metabolism. Erythema marginatum may be the first manifestation of rheumatic fever. These are examples of cutaneous manifestations of organic diseases. Skin conditions which are caused by or influenced by the psyche, and which by their disfiguring appearance cause mental aberrations are of equal importance. The exact role of the psyche in the production or aggravation of these dermatoses is unknown.

Dermatoses Directly Associated with Psychic Disturbances

The objective symptoms of the dermatoses described below are caused by the emotionally disturbed or psychotic patient.

Acarophobia or parasitophobia is a condition in which the patient has delusions of parasite infestation. Pieces of detritus or epithelial debris are forcibly removed by the patient from the skin, often deeply enough to cause ulcers. These particles of material are brought to the doctor with the insistent statement that they were "alive" when removed. Psychotherapy is necessary for these people.

Factitious dermatitis, feigned eruption or malingerer's disease, is deliberately caused by the patient with a desire to gain sympathy, collect compensation or evade undesirable duty. These lesions may be excoriations or may be caused by application of caustic materials, hot metal, *etc,* and frequently have bizarre appearances resembling no previously reported disease.

Neurotic excoriations are the result of unconscious or uncontrollable scratching of accessible areas of the body. The lesions may be widespread or localized to a small area such as the occipital region (localized neurodermatitis).

Trichotillomania is a compulsive pulling or twisting of the hair, sometimes resulting in large bald areas.

Chronic sucking or biting of localized areas by mentally defective patients causes hypertrophied, hyperpigmented lesions with excessive hair growth.

Dermatoses Influenced by Emotional Tension

The role played by the psyche in influencing the course of dermatoses such as dyshidrosis, atopic dermatitis, seborrheic dermatitis, lichen planus and psoriasis is obscure. The objective symptoms are usually intensified during periods of emotional tension, and patients frequently volunteer the information that pruritus increases when they are "upset." Many patients state that the dermatosis causes no discomfort during working hours but begins to itch when they relax physically.

Pruritus ani and pruritus vulvae are prevalent in emotionally tense patients, frequently necessitating the administration of sedatives or tranquilizers as adjunctive therapy.

Although verrucae are virus infections, some authorities believe that the psyche has a peculiar influence on the course of the disease. Not infrequently, especially in growing children, warts may be "hexed off," or cured by the oral administration of placebo or colored medications.

Alopecia areata, functional alopecia in women, seborrheic alopecia, vitiligo and exfoliative cheilitis are caused or aggravated by emotional tension.

Hyperhidrosis, or excessive sweating, is often a manifestation of anxiety or tension.

All allergic dermatoses, including urticaria, exhibit increased symptoms during periods of emotional tension.

Dermatoses In Which the Cosmetic Defect Causes Emotional Disturbances

These include acne (especially where scarring is a prominent feature), multiple neurofibromatosis, rosacea, large nevi, psoriasis, alopecia, bromhidrosis and congenital defects.

CHAPTER 11

Principles of Therapy

Effective treatment of cutaneous lesions is entirely dependent on accurate diagnosis, determination of the causative factor and thorough knowledge of the potential of the modalites employed. As new, more efficient drugs and procedures are developed, many agents become obsolete. In general, the dermatologist employs the same systemic medications used by the internist, the pediatrician and the family practitioner.

Physical Therapy

Radiotherapy. The indications for radiotherapy in dermatology have diminished considerably since the advent of antibiotics and corticosteroids, but the application of ionizing radiation remains an important part of dermatotherapy, and is still the treatment of choice in some benign and malignant dermatoses.

Roentgen rays are generated in vacuum tubes when fast moving electrons are stopped suddenly by impingement against a target. The speed of the electrons is regulated by the voltage which controls the penetrating power or quality of the X rays produced. The materials through which the rays must pass before reaching the surface of the body (filtration) also influence quality by absorbing a relatively high proportion of the softer, less penetrating rays. Radiations generated at 100 peak kilovolts (kvp) or less are adequate for almost all dermatologic purposes.

Intelligent selection of the quality of radiation appropriate for treatment of a given dermatosis depends on understanding of the nature and depth of the pathologic process. It is desirable, perhaps essential, to use as soft a quality as is compatible with adequate treatment of the disease, in order to protect underlying organs and structures from unnecessary radiation. It must be remembered that the effect of ionizing radiation is always damaging, and that successful radiotherapy depends on production of adequate damage to a disease process without causing permanent or irreparable damage to normal tissues. This is especially important over such radiosensitive structures as the eye, gonads and bone marrow. Superficial X rays generated at 50-100 kvp are needed for relatively deep processes.

Beta and gamma rays, from radium and other sources, are used occasionally. Beta rays are electrons which are absorbed superficially at depths depending on the initial energy of the particles and therefore on their source. Within their range of penetration, they evoke intense ionization. Gamma rays are highly penetrating; this power varies with the source. They are usually used in dermatology at very short source-tissue distances, since their intensity falls off rapidly in accordance with the inverse square law.

There is evidence that ultraviolet rays may also be ionizing, although they are absorbed almost entirely

Dermatologic Therapy Classification

I Physical Therapy

A. Ionizing Radiation
  1. X rays
  2. Grenz rays
  3. Radium
  4. Cathode rays
  5. Electron beam

B. Ultraviolet Rays
  1. UVA
  2. UVB

C. Cryotherapy
  1. Liquid nitrogen
  2. Solid carbon dioxide

D. Baths
  1. Oil
  2. Starch

E. Electrosurgery
  1. Monopolar current (desiccation)
  2. Bipolar current (cutting and epilation)
  3. Galvanic current (electrolysis)

II Topical Therapy

A. Antipruritic Agents
  1. Menthol
  2. Phenol

B. Anti-inflammatory Agents
  1. Fluorinated corticosteroid creams, ointments and lotions
  2. Nonfluorinated creams, ointments and lotions

C. Antifungal Agents

D. Antiacne Agents

E. Cytotoxic Agents

F. Sunscreen Agents

G. Keratolytics

H. Bleaching Agents

I. Parasiticides

J. Depilatories

K. Antiperspirants

L. Destructive Agents

M. Excipients
  1. Oily ointment bases
  2. Vanishing cream bases
  3. Lotion bases
  4. Aerosols

III Systemic Therapy

A. Antibacterial Drugs
  1. Antibiotics
  2. Sulfonamides
  3. Sulfones

B. Antifungal Drugs
  1. Griseofulvin
  2. Nystatin

C. Antimetabolites

D. Sedatives and Tranquilizers

E. Analgesics

F. Antihistamines

G. Corticosteroids

H. Photosensitizing Agents

---

in the upper epidermis. The cumulative effects of sunlight on the skin, such as sailor's skin and keratoses, result from repeated exposures to ultraviolet rays.

The safe use of radiotherapy of any quality or kind demands accurate control of dosage. Every X-ray or grenz-ray machine must be calibrated individually by a radiation physicist, preferably with the power source with which it is to be operated. Calibration should ordinarily be repeated at yearly intervals. X-ray dosage is given in terms of roentgen units and quality. Dosage of beta and gamma radiation may be expressed in roentgen equivalents or in milligram or millicurie-hours, whereas that of thorium X is expressed in microcuries per cubic centimeter and controlled by watching the effect on the disease process.

All ionizing radiations accelerate the aging process in the skin, the degree depending on the quality and amount of the radiation. The ultraviolet rays in sunlight are known to produce premature wrinkling, telangiectasia and keratoses which can eventuate in squamous cell carcinoma. High dosage of grenz rays can cause superficial atrophy and telangiectasia, but has not been reported to produce any of the more severe radiation sequelae. Conventional X rays, beta rays and gamma rays in high doses are capable of causing all of the effects mentioned, plus sclerosis, keratosis, ulcer and carcinoma. These radiations cause pigmentation. The development of any of these undesirable reactions can be diminished considerably by fractionation, using multiple small doses instead of a single massive dose.

Ultraviolet. Phototherapy as a primary or adjunctive measure is of value in the treatment of psoriasis, vitiligo and other dermatoses. While natural sunlight is the most efficient source of ultraviolet rays, its intensity varies with the season and therefore, particularly in the temperate zone, it is better to use an artificial source to deliver measured dosage.

The band of ultraviolet radiation is divided into three sections: UVC (200-280 nm); UVB (280-315 nm); and UVA (315-400 nm). In dermatologic therapy only UVB and UVA are of value. The Goeckerman therapy for psoriasis employs topically applied tar and exposure to a light source which emits both UVA and UVB. The PUVA (psoralen and UVA) therapy, used in the treatment of psoriasis and other dermatoses, uses a light source which emits only UVA. Systemically administered psoralens are used in conjunction with the light therapy in the PUVA technique.

Cryotherapy. This is an effective method of treatment for seborrheic keratoses, actinic keratoses and warts. Liquid nitrogen is the cryogen of choice but solid carbon dioxide may also be used.

Electrosurgery. Some other physical agents also play important roles in dermatologic therapy. Damped high frequency oscillating current is used for the fulguration (external spark) or desiccation (interstitial spark) of warts, moles, keratoses, skin tags and carcinomas.

Bipolar high frequency cutting current may be used for the removal of skin tumors. Its use is not recommended if a specimen is to be submitted for microscopic study because the cut surface is seared and the cells are distorted by coagulation.

Electrolysis, the passage of a small direct current through the tissues so that sodium chloride is hydrolyzed and sodium hydroxide is formed at the negative electrode, may be employed to destroy small moles and superfluous hair.

Baths. Soothing baths using a bland oil or starch are a useful adjunctive measure to relieve subjective symptoms in the treatment of many dermatoses.

Topical Therapy

Ointments are the most frequently prescribed form of external medication and consist of a base and active ingredients. Ointment bases may be divided into those which are water-repellent, water-absorbent, water-miscible (any of the commercially available vanishing creams or emulsion bases) and water-soluble. Vanishing creams are better suited for acute or subacute dermatoses and oily ointments are better for chronic, scaly or dry dermatoses.

Lotions are solutions or suspensions of drugs in aqueous or hydroalcoholic vehicles, to be applied to the skin without rubbing (*eg,* calamine lotion).

Liniments are suspensions or solutions of drugs in oily or soapy vehicles to be applied to the skin by inunction (*eg,* calamine liniment, camphorated oil).

Pastes are emollient, ointment-like preparations, which have the ability to absorb moisture (*eg,* Lassar's plain zinc paste).

Wet dressings or compresses are solutions or suspensions applied by saturated dressings to inflamed, edematous or denuded areas to soothe, reduce edema or combat infections (*eg,* Burow's solution).

Dusting powders consist of active medication mixed with inert substances such as talc (*eg,* deodorant powders, prickly heat powders, foot powders).

In general, fatty preparations lubricate skin by sealing in sweat and insensible water whereas aqueous or alcohol preparations dry the integument on repeated application.

Antipruritics. Phenol (0.5-1%) and menthol (0.5-1%) in ointment, cream or lotion bases are effective antipruritic agents.

Cytotoxic Agents. Topically applied 5-fluorouracil in cream or solution (1-5%) is effective in the treatment of actinic keratoses and other superficial premalignant lesions. Its use in cancer is experimental.

Antifungal Agents. Tolnaftate, miconazole, haloprogin and clotrimazole are effective in the treatment of many superficial dermatophyte infections. Nystatin and clotrimazole are effective on topical applications in the treatment of monilial infections. Nystatin and clotrimazole are provided in ointment, cream and lotion bases.

Antibiotic Ointments. These agents are effective, but there is divided opinion about their superiority. However, these preparations are employed as an adjunctive measure in the treatment of pyogenic infections when systemic antibiotics are prescribed.

Corticosteroids. Fluorinated and nonfluorinated corticosteroid creams and ointments are of value in the treatment of many inflammatory dermatoses. The nonfluorinated corticosteroids should have preferential use in children and in the treatment of eruptions in the intertriginous areas. Fluorinated corticosteroids applied under occlusion or in the intertriginous areas frequently cause striae formation.

Parasiticides. Gamma benzene hexachloride in lotion base and as a shampoo is the drug of choice in the treatment of pediculosis and scabies. Crotamiton cream and 12% benzyl benzoate lotion are excellent alternative preparations.

Keratolytics. Salicylic acid is an inexpensive weak acid which denatures protein and acts as a keratolytic. It may be incorporated in oily ointment bases, water-soluble bases, alcohol or in a plaster. The concentration used is determined by the thickness of the keratin layer. Usually 3-10% preparations are used to treat lesions on the trunk and extremities. Plantar corns or plantar warts are treated with a 40% concentration in a plaster.

Sunscreen Agents. Para-amino benzoic acid (5%) in 50-70% alcoholic solution will block light (wavelengths 280-320 nm). The addition of 5-10% titanium dioxide to the preparation will give wider wavelength protection.

Bleaching Agents. Hydroquinone in a concentration of 2-5% in an ointment or cream base is an effective bleach. It may be used in conjunction with a keratolytic agent to increase penetrability.

Depilatories. Sodium thioglycollate in water or glycerin applied topically is the drug of choice.

Antiperspirants. Aluminum salts are the only effective agents which are relatively nonirritating.

Antiacne Drugs. Retinoic acid (0.025-0.1%) in cream, gel or solution and benzoyl peroxide (5-10%) in similar bases are useful in comedo removal. Colloidal sulfur lotions have a mild antibacterial action and have a drying effect on the skin. Topical antibiotics such as clindamycin are currently being used experimentally in this disease.

Destructive Agents. Cantharidin (0.8%) in an acetone-collodion base is a vesicating agent useful in the treatment of warts. Podophyllin (20-25%) in compound tincture of benzoin is a valuable cytotoxic agent for the treatment of condylomata acuminata. This drug has limited value in the treatment of dry lesions.

Systemic Medications

Many dermatoses depend upon systemic therapy for cure or symptomatic control. In general, the same principles apply to the treatment of skin disease with systemic medications as apply to the treatment of other organs.

Corticosteroids. These drugs, administered judiciously in proper dosage, are used in the treatment of lupus erythematosus, pemphigus vulgaris, bullous pemphigoid, allergic dermatoses and other diseases where they will be of value.

	Equivalent Dosage (mg)
Cortisone	25
Hydrocortisone	20
Prednisone	5
Prednisolone	5
Methyl prednisone	4
Triamcinolone	4
Beta methasone	0.6
Dexamethasone	0.75

Type	Example	Available Dose	
Ethanolamines	Diphenhydramine	50	mg
Ethylenediamine	Tripelennamine	50	mg
Alkylamine	Chlorpheniramine	4	mg
Phenothiazines	Trimeprazine	2.5	mg
Miscellaneous	Cyproheptadine	25	mg
	Hydroxyzine		

Antibiotics. The drug selection is determined by in vitro sensitivity tests. The exception to this rule is the use of tetracycline in treatment of acne vulgaris and rosacea.

Sulfonamides. Sulfapyridine, while not the drug of choice, is useful in the treatment of dermatitis herpetiformis.

Sulfones. These drugs are used in the treatment of leprosy and dermatitis herpetiformis.

Antifungal Drugs. *Griseofulvin.* This antifungal drug is derived from *Penicillium griseofulvum* and has been an effective agent against the superficial mycoses for twenty years. It is best used for the treatment of tinea capitis, tinea of the nails and extensive dermatomycoses. Three preparations of this drug are now commercially available: griseofulvin with regular size granules, micronized griseofulvin and ultramicronized griseofulvin. The daily milligram dosage of these preparations differs but there is little evidence that the therapeutic effectiveness of these drugs differs when the recommended daily dose is administered. The side effects of griseofulvin are rare except for nausea, headaches and occasional diarrhea.

Nystatin. This drug has limited value on systemic administration because of its poor absorption from the gastrointestinal tract.

Amphotericin B. This drug is used in treatment of the deep mycoses. Its intravenous use must be carefully monitored.

Photosensitizing Agents. The psoralens (8-methoxypsoralen and trioxsalen) are known photosensitizing drugs which are utilized to augment the effect of natural or artificial light sources. Other than sunburning, there are few side effects. Nausea may be avoided by dividing the dose over a 2-hour period or by administration of antacids.

Antihistamines. The systemic antihistamines may be used to relieve the itching of allergic diseases but their value in the treatment of nonhistamine-related pruritus is questionable.

Sedatives and Tranquilizers. Control of emotional tension by systemic medication has proved to be valuable adjunctive therapy in the treatment of such dermatoses as seborrheic dermatitis, neurodermatitis, lichen planus, psoriasis, pruritus vulvae and pruritus ani.

Barbiturates are effective sedatives when used for a brief period but may become habit-forming with prolonged usage. Tranquillizing drugs such as hydroxyzine, meprobamate, buclizine, diazepams, chlordiazepoxide and phenothiazines are recommended for relief of emotional tension because of their effectiveness and relative safety in administration.

Keratolytics. Oral cis-retinoic acid is an experimental drug in certain ichthyotic and papulosquamous diseases.

Analgesics. Acetylsalicylic acid, meperidene and morphine are used in dermatology as in other specialties. Cutaneous disorders requiring analgesics include sunburn, pemphigus, cellulitis and malignancy.

Anti-metabolites. *Methotrexate* is an effective agent in psoriasis with varying dosage programs. One successful schedule employs 2.5 mg orally every 8 hours for three doses on a weekly rotation. This schedule was designed to block the active replication phase of the epidermal cells. Hematopoietic and hepatic side effects are common.

Azathioprine. 50-150 mg daily is an effective dosage schedule for pemphigus and related blistering diseases. Monitoring of the blood count and liver function tests is essential.

Hydroxyurea. This has been used for psoriasis but it is not a popular agent since several weeks of therapy are required before maximum effect is apparent.

PART TWO
Morphologic Dermatology

CHAPTER 12

Regional Involvement

Anus and Perianal Areas. Atopic dermatitis, neurodermatitis, folliculitis, condylomata lata, condylomata acuminata, tinea cruris, contact dermatitis, furunculosis, pediculosis pubis, moniliasis, intertrigo.

Breasts. Contact dermatitis, tinea versicolor, Paget's disease, folliculitis, scabies, seborrheic dermatitis, eczema.

Chest and Back. Seborrheic dermatitis, acne vulgaris and acne conglobata, pustular folliculitis, tinea versicolor, seborrheic keratoses, active keratoses, psoriasis, pityriasis rosea, miliaria rubra, neurofibromatosis, herpes zoster, dermatitis herpetiformis, keratosis follicularis, pediculosis vestimentorum, urticaria.

Ears. Seborrheic dermatitis, neurodermatitis, infectious eczematoid dermatitis, chondrodermatitis nodularis chronica helicis, contact dermatitis, epitheliomas, pernio, sarcoid, gout.

Eyelids. Contact dermatitis, xanthelasma, hordeolum, seborrheic dermatitis, epitheliomas, molluscum contagiosum, milia, chalazion, atopic dermatitis (and other "eczematous" eruptions).

Face. Acne vulgaris, rosacea, milia, lupus erythematosus, epitheliomas, seborrheic dermatitis, seborrheic keratoses, erythema multiforme, lupus vulgaris, sarcoid, nevi, angiomas, herpes simplex, herpes zoster, secondary syphilis, molluscum contagiosum, chloasma, vitiligo, freckles.

Extremities. Dermatitis venenata, ecthyma, urticaria, psoriasis, lichen planus, erythema multiforme, erythema nodosum, ichthyosis, keratosis pilaris, purpura, stasis dermatitis, atopic dermatitis, scabies, verruca vulgaris.

Genitalia. Syphilis (chancre, condylomata lata, mucous patches), chancroid, lymphogranuloma venereum, granuloma inguinale, condylomata acuminata, balinitis, lichen planus, carcinomas, dermatitis venenata, kraurosis vulvae, moniliasis, neurodermatitis, scabies, herpes progenitalis, tinea cruris, molluscum contagiosum.

Hands and Feet. Contact dermatitis, epidermophytosis, vitiligo, scabies, hyperhidrosis, dyshidrosis, erythema multiforme, eczema, syphilis, dermatitis repens, verruca, paronychia, post infectious desquamation.

Lips and Mouth. Herpes simplex, aphthous stomatitis, leukoplakia, carcinoma, lingua nigra, chancre, mucous patches, Fordyce's disease, urticaria, retention cyst, lupus erythematosus, transitory benign plaques, avitaminosis, lichen planus, contact dermatitis, moniliasis, erythema multiforme, angular cheilitis.

Neck. Lichen simplex chronicus, neurodermatitis, seborrheic dermatitis, dermatitis venenata, papilloma colli, acne keloid.

Nails. Moniliasis, leukonychia, onychia, onychomycosis, paronychia, syphilis, argyria, congenital absence of nails, spoon nails.

Scalp. Alopecia (areata, senile, traumatic, idiopathic, premature), seborrheic dermatitis, keratoses, scleroderma, dermatitis venenata, psoriasis, tinea capitis, lupus erythematosus, pediculosis capitis, verrucae, nevi, sebaceous cysts, folliculitis.

Trunk. Dermatitis venenata, pityriasis rosea, seborrheic dermatitis, atopic dermatitis, lichen planus, urticaria, herpes zoster, syphilis, pediculosis, exanthemata, fungus infections, drug eruptions.

Regional Involvement by Some Diseases

Area	Disease	Other Clinical Features	Complicating Features Produced by Location	Diagnosis
Groin	Psoriasis	Nail pitting, lesions on extensors, scalp and trunk	May become macerated and complicated by candidiasis	Biopsy
	Seborrheic Dermatitis	Lesions on scalp, presternal area and face	May become macerated and complicated by candidiasis	Biopsy
	Candidiasis	May have nail fold involvement, lesions in axillae and perianal area. Satellite involvement near crease. Involves scrotum	May indicate presence of diabetes. Usually aggravated by heat	Culture
	Tinea Cruris	May be unilateral or bilateral. Nails, trunk and interdigital lesions may occur. Starts on thigh, advances into fold	Usually aggravated by heat	KOH preparation and culture
	Intertrigo	Lesions confined to groin crease	Increase in local sweating	Culture
Penis	Syphilis	Single ulcer with satellite nodes. Secondary lesions may or may not be present	None	Darkfield microscopic examination, STS
	Chancroid	Multiple superficial shallow ulcers with fluctuant buboes in the groin	None except in uncircumcised patients who develop phimosis	Gram stain, culture
	Lymphogranuloma Venereum	Transient superficial ulcer accompanied by or followed by inguinal adenopathy and fluctuant buboes	May cause esthiomene (localized elephantiasis) due to lymphatic obstruction	Serologic test
	Granuloma Inguinale	Peripherally spreading ulcer which destroys tissue as it progresses. Not accompanied by lymph-adenopathy	May cause lymphedema from local inflammatory reaction. May destroy the genitalia	Gram stain
	Aphthous Ulcers	Superficial shallow painful ulcers not accompanied by adenopathy	May be initial sign of developing Behçet syndrome	No specific test, diagnostic by exclusion
	Pyoderma	Painful crusted ulcers. Lymphadenopathy may or may not be present	Bacteremia or septicemia	Culture
	Carcinoma	Usually occurs in an uncircumcised patient. May be minor or extensive	Metastases	Biopsy
	Psoriasis	May occur as a single lesion with no evidence of psoriasis elsewhere or patient may have other signs of the disease	Difficulty in diagnosis if this is the only lesion	Biopsy
	Lichen Planus	Usually accompanied by lesions on the buccal mucosa and the extremities	Difficulty in diagnosis if this is the only lesion	Biopsy

Region	Disease	Clinical Features	Complications	Diagnosis
	Scabies	Lesions present between fingers, on wrists and buttocks	Penile lesions characteristically develop in men with scabies	Microscopic examination of scraping
	Balanitis Xerotica Obliterans	Lesions involve the urethral meatus and narrow the orifice	Obliteration of the meatus and urinary retention	Biopsy
	Erythroplasia of Queyrat	Usually a single lesion on the glans	Development of carcinoma	Biopsy
	Herpes Progenitalis	One or more groups of vesicles on corona and glans. Condition is recurrent	Usually none	Tzank smear, viral culture, serology
Nails	Psoriasis	Plates are thickened, pitted, and may be distorted	Difficult at times to differentiate from onychomycosis	Culture to rule out fungus infection
	Lichen Planus	Thickened distorted plates usually have lesions elsewhere	Usually none	Biopsy
	Onychomycosis	Nails broken off in mid-portion. Usually there is evidence of mycotic infection elsewhere	Usually none	Culture
	Candidiasis	Brown discoloration on sides of nail plate. Paronychia also present	Usually none	Culture
	Onycholysis	Separation of nail plates from the bed. One or more nails are involved	Invasion by opportunistic fungi and bacteria	Clinical
Ears	Seborrheic Dermatitis and Neurodermatitis	Lesions on the scalp, trunk and eyebrows	Occasional secondary pyogenic infection growth of opportunistic fungi	Clinical, culture for bacteria and fungi
	Psoriasis	Pitting of nails, lesions on elbows and knees, lesions on trunk	Usually none	Clinical, biopsy
	Chondrodermatitis Nodularis Chronica Helicis	None	Pain or pressure	Clinical
	Epitheliomas	May have actinic keratoses on other exposed areas	None	Biopsy
	Sarcoid	Lesions of sarcoid on the nose, neck and elsewhere	None	Biopsy
	Gout	Evidence of gout on fingers and toes	None	Blood for uric acid, biopsy of tophi
Breasts	Paget's Disease	Usually a single lesion which involves the areola and the normal skin	Although it resembles an eczematous lesion, this is a carcinoma and unless removed will metastasize	Excision of entire lesion for microscopic examination
	Allergic Contact Dermatitis	Usually none	Usually none	Clinical appearance and patch tests to rubber and synthetic materials
	Tinea Versicolor	Usually lesions are present elsewhere on the trunk	Usually none	Microscopic examination of skin scrapings

CHAPTER 13

Differential Diagnosis Charts

History

A good medical history and a thorough physical examination are essential in the treatment of dermatologic disorders. It is also desirable to have confirmation of the clinical diagnosis with properly selected laboratory studies. Rather than allowing randomly selected studies lead to a diagnosis, the physician lets the clinical findings indicate the procedures to be followed.

Important questions relative to the dermatosis are:

1. How long has the eruption been present?
2. Where did the first lesion appear and how did it progress?
3. How long did you have this before you consulted a physician?
4. What did you use for self-treatment before you saw a physician?
5. What medications did the physician prescribe?
6. How faithfully did you follow his instructions?
7. Did the prescribed medication relieve your symptoms?
8. Do you have discomfort (itching, burning or pain)?
9. When is your discomfort most intense? Is it constant? Is it affected by seasonal or environmental changes?

It is important to remember that the history is often misleading and that careful scrutiny will not necessarily support the information obtained from the patient. After the physical examination it is frequently necessary to repeat portions of the history to get the facts. The patient's complaints of itching, burning, pain, formication, hyperesthesia and anesthesia are subjective symptoms and are therefore variable. The history must be evaluated for each individual; a lesion of the same intensity produces different degrees of distress in different patients.

Reaction Patterns

Some dermatoses which have been described as specific diseases are probably morphologic entities representing reaction patterns. The type of cutaneous response elicited by a stimulus cannot be predicted and for some unknown reason, varies in different persons.

Examination

Observe and record the patient's general appearance, gait, manner of speech and general hygiene. Note hair distribution in both men and women. Is the patient a

Annular Lesions

Disease	Sites	Secondary Lesions	Special Characteristics	Etiology	Diagnostic Aids
Macules					
Pityriasis Rosea	Trunk, extremities; rarely on face	Collarette of scale which peels toward the margin	Lesions fall in lines of cleavage; herald patch frequently present; may form papules	Unknown	None
Tinea Circinata	Trunk, face, extremities	Dry scale; elevated crusted margin; vesicles may be present in the margin	May form concentric rings	Fungi	Examination of scrapings, culture
Erythema Multiforme	Palms, soles; may be generalized	None	Iris or target lesions	Drug sensitivity, foci of infection; may be seasonal	Biopsy, immunofluorescence
Seborrheic Dermatitis	Scalp, face, interscapular area, presternal region, genitocrural area	Oily yellowish scale	May form festooned lesions on forehead	Unknown	Biopsy
Purpura Annularis Telangiectodes	Lower extremities	None	Purpuric lesions; persistent brown pigmentation follows involution of lesions	Unknown	Biopsy
Erythema Annulare Centrifugum	Trunk, extremities	Scant peripheral scale	Forms annular lesions which frequently have incomplete margins	Allergy, sarcoid, tuberculosis, fungus infection	Biopsy
Papules					
Secondary Syphilis	Face; particularly about the nose and mouth	Slight scale at margin	Color is brownish-red; each margin is composed of small segments	*Treponema pallidum*	Darkfield microscopic examination, STS
Erythema Multiforme	Palms, soles; generalized	None	Target lesions; macules and vesicles may also be present	Drug sensitivity, foci of infection and seasonal variation	Biopsy, immunofluorescence
Lichen Planus	Flexor surfaces of forearms, genitalia, mouth	Adherent, scant scale	Forms linear groups of lesions; umbilicated lesions and reticulated leukoplakia	Unknown; associated with emotional tension	Biopsy
Urticaria	Generalized	None	Lesions may form pseudopodia and are transitory	Sensitivity reaction or psychogenic physical stimuli	History, clinical appearance
Granuloma Annulare	Usually over bony prominences	None	Lesions may involute after segment is removed for biopsy	Unknown	Biopsy

(continued)

Annular Lesions (continued)

Disease	Sites	Secondary Lesions	Special Characteristics	Etiology	Diagnostic Aids
Sarcoid	About the nose or mouth, hands and elsewhere	Lesions may ulcerate	Frequently associated lesions in bones of fingers and in lungs	Unknown	Biopsy, Kveim test
Psoriasis	Scalp, elbows, knees, trunk; rarely on face	Profuse silvery scale	Linear groups may occur; bleeding points follow removal of scale	Unknown	Biopsy
Pityriasis Rosea	Trunk, extremities; rarely on face	Collarette of scale which peels toward the margin	Lesions fall in lines of cleavage; herald patch frequently present	Unknown	Clinical appearance
Vesicles					
Erythema Multiforme	Mouth, genitalia, trunk	None	Macules and papules may also be present; relapses frequent	May be caused by drug sensitivity, foci of infection, or may be seasonal	Biopsy, immunofluorescence
Pemphigus Vulgaris	Mouth, trunk, genitalia	Crusts, erosions	Nikolsky's sign; patient seriously ill	Autoimmune disease	Biopsy, immunofluorescence
Dermatitis Herpetiformis	Trunk, extremities	Excoriations, blood crusts, hyperpigmentation	May form groups of vesicles; small papules may be present	Unknown; may be related to gluten intake and anti-reticulin antibodies	Biopsy, immunofluorescence, small bowel biopsy
Impetigo Contagiosa	Face and other areas	Blood and pus crusts	No scar or hyperpigmentation on involution	Staphylococcus or streptococcus	Culture, Gram stain, serology
Bullous Pemphigoid	Trunk, extremities	Blood crusts, excoriations	Closely resembles pemphigus	Unknown	Biopsy, immunofluorescence

nail biter? Are there abnormalities in pigmentation? At the same time the physician should evaluate the psyche of the patient.

Good light is essential for the cutaneous examination. The patient should be studied in daylight or with a lamp containing a daylight bulb. A careful inspection is necessary because "minutiae" are often of great importance.

General examination:
1. Skin is normal, soft, thickened, moist, dry, hot or cold.
2. Hair is white, brown, black, gray, red, sparse, or scalp is bald.
3. Nails are pitted, striated, normal, white, with transverse lines, thickened or separated from nail bed.

Specific examination:

1. Search for a primary lesion (macule, papule, vesicle or pustule).
2. Look for special characteristics or configurations (annular, umbilicated, special groups, *etc*).
3. Observe scale formation. (If present, is it profuse or scant, central or peripheral, oily or dry?)
4. Look for scars, areas of hyperpigmentation or depigmentation.
5. Is there erythema (acute or chronic) or tenderness?

6. Is there edema or lichenification?
7. Are lesions well-defined, ill-defined, sessile or pedunculated?

Paint a word picture of the patient's problem and record your findings. Look under the appropriate heading in the following sections, study the lists and consult the differential diagnosis charts to make a clinical impression. Confirm your diagnosis with the indicated diagnostic aids.

Grouped Vesicles

Disease	Sites	Type of Grouping	Subjective Signs	Etiology	Diagnostic Aids
Zoster	Unilateral, following nerve distribution	Round or oval groups of deep, tense vesicles on inflamed edematous base	Not recurrent; pruritus or pain; may have severe postherpetic pain	Same virus which causes varicella	Tissue culture, Tzanck test, biopsy, serology
Herpes Simplex	One or more groups, most commonly occur on lips or genitalia	Round or irregular groups of flaccid superficial vesicles; frequently covered by a serous crust	Frequently recurrent in same site; pruritus	Virus	Tissue culture, serology, Tzanck test, biopsy
Dermatitis Venenata	On surfaces exposed to sensitizer	Linear groups of vesicles on edematous base	Moderate to severe pruritus	Contact sensitivity	Patch tests
Dermatitis Herpetiformis	Trunk, extremities	Annular lesions and ringed groups; postinflammatory melanin deposits	Intense pruritus	Unknown; may be related to antireticulin antibodies	Biopsy, potasium iodide test, patch test, immunofluorescence, small bowel biopsy
Pemphigus Vulgaris	Mucous membranes, face, trunk, extremities	Annular lesions; flaccid vesicles which rupture easily; Nikolsky's sign	Malaise; difficulty in swallowing if mucous membranes are involved	Unknown	Biopsy, immunofluorescence
Lymphangioma Circumscriptum	Any part of body	Round or irregular groups of lymph vesicles covered with hyperkeratosis	None	Congenital	Biopsy
Bullous Pemphigoid	Trunk, extremities	Annular lesions; flaccid vesicles which rupture easily	Intense pruritus	Unknown	Biopsy, immunofluorescence

Linear Groups

Disease	Primary Lesion	Sites	Secondary Lesions	Subjective Signs	Etiology	Diagnostic Aids
Psoriasis	Papule; when scales are removed it is a macule	Elbows, knees, trunk, scalp, nails, palms, intertriginous areas; rarely on face	Profuse, silvery white scale; when removed, bleeding points are present; forms annular lesions	None or moderate pruritus	Unknown	Biopsy
Lichen Planus	Papule; may form annular and umbilicated lesions	Flexor surfaces of forearms, genitalia, mouth, trunk	Scant adherent dry scale	Mild to intense pruritus	Unknown; emotional tension is associated	Biopsy
Verruca Plana Juvenilis	Flesh-colored or light brown papule	Most commonly on the face; may occur on extremities	None	None	Virus	Biopsy
Lichen Nitidus	Papule	Genitalia, face, extremities	None	None	Unknown	Biopsy
Dermatitis Venenata	Vesicle	Exposed surfaces	Blood crusts, serous crusts; secondary pyogenic infection with pus crusts	Intense pruritus	Contact sensitivity	Patch tests
Lichen Striatus	Papule	Usually on the extremities as a continuous unbroken line	Blood crusts	Mild pruritus	Unknown	Biopsy
Toxic Reactions	Macule or papule; usually erythematous	Usually trunk but may be anywhere	Urticaria	Pruritus	Caterpillars, jellyfish	Clinical appearance

Umbilicated Lesions

Disease	Sites	Primary Lesion	Special Characteristics	Etiology	Diagnostic Aids
Molluscum Contagiosum	Any part of the body	A pearly, globular papule	The molluscum body may be expressed from the lesion	Virus	Biopsy, smear of expressed lesion
Lichen Planus	Flexor surfaces of forearms, genitalia, buccal mucosa	A violaceous, flat-topped papule	Linear groups and annular lesions formed	Unknown; emotional tension is associated	Biopsy
Varicella	Generalized	Vesicle, then pustule	Not true umbilication because it is not formed until the vesicle breaks	Varicella-zoster virus	Tzanck test, tissue culture, serology, biopsy
Variola	Generalized	Macule, then papule, then vesicle and finally a shotty pustule	Patient violently ill	Virus	Tissue culture, serology, Tzanck test, biopsy
Parapsoriasis (Mucha-Habermann disease)	Generalized	Papules, macules and vesicles all occurring at same time	Chronic condition; self-limited	Unknown	Biopsy
Herpes simplex (Kaposi's varicelliform eruption)	Localized or generalized	Vesicles and vesicopustules	Occurs in atopic individuals and in exfoliative dermatitis patients	Herpes simplex virus	Tzanck test, tissue culture, serology, biopsy
Zoster	Any part of the body	Vesicles in groups on an inflammatory base; umbilication is not a constant occurrence	Unilateral distribution of lesions	Varicella-zoster virus	Tissue culture, serology, Tzanck test, biopsy
Vaccinia	Localized or generalized	Multiloculated vesicopustule	Follows exposure to vaccination; generalized in atopic patients	Virus	Tissue culture, serology, Tzanck test, biopsy

Excoriated Lesions

Condition	Sites	Primary Lesion	Secondary Lesions	Special Morphologic Features	Diagnostic Aids
Dermatitis Herpetiformis	Trunk	Vesicles and papules	Excoriations, blood crusts, hyperpigmentation	Grouped vesicles, annular lesions, arciform lesions	Biopsy, potassium iodide test, patch test, immunofluorescence
Dermatitis Venenata	Exposed parts of body	Vesicles	Excoriations, blood and serous crusts, secondary pyogenic infection	Linear groups of vesicles on inflamed edematous base	Patch test
Hodgkin's Disease	Generalized	Lichenified macular eruption	Blood-crusted excoriations	Generalized lymphadenopathy. Herpetic eruptions may develop	Biopsy of skin lymph nodes or involved tissues
Leukemia Cutis	Localized or generalized	Lichenified plaques, nodules or tumors	Blood-crusted excoriations	May resemble neurodermatitis	Biopsy of skin, sternal marrow studies, blood count
Neurotic Excoriations	Any area within easy reach of the hands	None	Deep, blood-crusted excoriations	Pink or white scars may be present in addition to new lesions	Psychiatric examination
Pediculosis Capitis (head lice)	Scalp, forehead and back of neck	None	Excoriations covered with serous blood and pus crusts	Ova attached to scalp hair by chitin; live parasites may be found	Microscopic examination of ova attached to hair
Pediculosis Pubis (pubic lice, crab lice)	Pubic area lower abdomen, buttocks, eyelashes, axillae	None	Blood-crusted excoriations and pus-crusted lesions	Parasites are attached to skin and resemble freckles in the pubic area; brownish ova attached to hairs	Microscopic examination of ova attached to hair
Pediculosis Corporis (body lice, cooties)	Trunk	None	Blood-crusted excoriations, furuncles, pus-crusted lesions	Parasites present in seams of clothing	Microscopic examination of parasites

Excoriated Lesions (continued)

Condition	Sites	Primary Lesion	Secondary Lesions	Special Morphologic Features	Diagnostic Aids
Scabies	Between fingers, on palms, wrists, buttocks, male genitalia; not on face	Vesicle	Blood, serous and pus crusts	Dotted line in vesicle (burrow)	Microscopic study of vesicle contents for *Acarus scabiei*
Papular Urticaria	Face, trunk, extremities	Papules and papulovesicles	Blood crusts, scars, secondary pyoderma	Some lesions may have central punctures	Clinical appearance
Atopic Eczema	Face, trunk, flexures	Macule, papule or vesicle	Scales, crusts, fissures, lichenification, secondary pyogenic infection	History of atopy	None
Jaundice	Generalized	Icteric tint to skin and sclera	Linear blood-crusted excoriations	Systemic illness	Liver functions studies, serum bilirubin

Ulcers

Condition	Sites	Morphologic Features	Diagnostic Aids
Blastomycosis	Face, hands, feet, *etc*	Granulomatous ulcer, which slowly spreads peripherally; humerous small pustules in margin of ulcer	Biopsy, culture, direct microscopic examination of exudate
Bromoderma	Legs	Granulomatous ulcer resembling blastomycosis	Biopsy, blood bromide; rule out blastomycosis by direct examination and culture
Chancroid	Genitalia	Papule or vesicopustule which becomes a superficial, irregular, soft ulcer with granular base, covered with pus; inguinal lymph nodes are enlarged (buboes)	Culture, Gram stain of ulcer
Thermal Burn (third degree)	Any part of body	Well-defined ulcer covered with adherent crust, which eventually separates, leaving a red, granulomatous base	History
Frostbite	Ears, nose, fingers, toes	Erythema, edema, blebs, gangrene; resulting ulcers are superficial or deep	History of exposure

(continued)

Ulcers (continued)

Condition	Sites	Morphologic Features	Diagnostic Aids
Roentgen Dermatitis (advanced)	Irradiated area	Ulcer is superficial and is surrounded by a zone of atrophy and telangiectases	Biopsy
Ecthyma	Legs, buttocks, vulva, *etc*	One or more well-defined ulcers, covered with pus crusts and surrounded by zones of erythema; heal by scar formation	Culture, Gram stain, serology
Epithelioma (basal cell)	Face, ears	Begins as small papule or nodule; grows slowly, spreads peripherally; ulcer is usually shallow and dry and is surrounded by a pearly rolled margin	Biopsy
Epithelioma (squamous cell)	Face, lips, hands, *etc*	Resembles basal cell type but grows more rapidly; superficial or deep ulcer with a granulomatous, irregular, fungoid, central portion which bleeds freely on slight trauma	Biopsy
Factitious Ulcers (self-inflicted)	Areas accessible to hands	Single or multiple, sharply defined, regular or irregular, asymmetric, superficial or deep ulcers. Old lesions heal and new ones constantly appear	History, psychiatric examination
Granuloma Inguinale	Genitocrural area, perineum	Papule which ulcerates and spreads peripherally. The ulcer has a granulomatous base and a raised, rolled margin. Marked destruction of skin and subcutaneous tissue	Microscopic examination of Wright's or Giemsa stained smear of marginal tissue for Donovan bodies
Perforating Ulcer of Foot (malum perforans pedis)	Plantar surfaces over first or fifth metatarsophalangeal joints	Lesion begins as callus-like thickening resembling a plantar wart; eventually the callus covers a deep ulcer which may extend to the bone	STS, spinal fluid examination, neurologic examination, blood sugar

Ulcers (continued)

Condition	Sites	Morphologic Features	Diagnostic Aids
Sickle Cell Anemia Ulcer	Lateral aspect of lower third of legs	Round or oval, punched out ulcer with indurated, slightly raised edges and a profuse purulent discharge	Hemoglobin electrophoreses
Stasis Ulcer	Lower third of legs near the ankles	One or more irregular, superficial or deep ulcers with profuse seropurulent discharge. Usually surrounded by a zone of stasis eczema	Clinical appearance
Syphilis (chancre)	Genitalia, lips, nipples, *etc*	A single, hard, indurated ulcer with scant discharge; satellite lymph nodes are enlarged, hard and painless	Darkfield microscopic examination, STS
Syphilis (ecthymatous)	Trunk, scalp, extremities	Large, round, flat pustules with reddish-brown areola; a thick crust forms over the resulting ulcer	Darkfield microscopic examination, STS
Syphilis (gumma)	Legs, forehead, scalp, *etc*	Begins as rounded subcutaneous nodule or tumor which develops central necrosis, sloughs and forms a deep ulcer with precipitous sides (punched out)	STS
Tuberculosis Cutis Luposa (lupus vulgaris)	Face, neck	A round or oval, well-defined, shallow or deep ulcer, which bleeds easily; nodules are present in the margin	Biopsy, culture
Erythema Induratum	Legs, principally on the calves	Begins as deep-seated, slowly growing nodules which ulcerate; ulcers are superficial or deep with little discharge	Biopsy
Unusual Cutaneous Infections (amebic, diptheria, chromobacteria, salmonella, Listeria, anaerobic organisms)	Anywhere	May appear as "bottleneck" abscesses which ulcerate or well-defined lesions	Biopsy, culture on various media

Alopecias

Condition	Sites	Characteristic Lesion	Other Lesions or Conditions Present	Diagnostic Aids
Alopecia Areata	Scalp, beard; may be generalized	Well-defined, non-inflamed areas	None associated with this condition	Biopsy
Male Pattern Alopecia	Scalp of men	Diminution in quantity or absence of hair in parietal area and on crown	None associated with this condition	Physical appearance
Symptomatic or Functional Alopecia	Scalp of women	Diffuse diminution in quantity of hair	Tension, hormonal imbalance	None; mostly telogen hair loss
Secondary Syphilis	Scalp	Patchy, incomplete areas of alopecia; "moth-eaten" appearance	Other lesions of secondary syphilis	Dark-field microscopic examination of a moist lesion, STS
Folliculitis Decalvans and Pseudopelade	Scalp	Atrophic scarred areas of alopecia throughout the scalp	Follicular pustules and papules in the scalp	Biopsy
Lupus Erythematosus	Scalp, face, ears	Atrophic scarred areas of baldness; follicular plugging and marginal erythema present	Lesions of lupus erythematosus on face, ears, nose and elsewhere	Biopsy, lupus erythematosus cell study, antinuclear antibody (ANA) test, immunofluorescence
Seborrheic Dermatitis and Psoriasis	Scalp, face, presternal area, between the scapulae	Areas of partial alopecia covered with oily adherent scale; festooning of lesions on forehead and behind the ears; annular lesions present	Lesions of seborrheic dermatitis on chest, back and in pubic area	Biopsy
Tinea Capitis	Scalp	Most common in young children	None usually, although other lesions may be present	Wood light examination, direct microscopic examination, culture on Sabouraud's medium
Trichotillomania	Scalp	Areas of incomplete alopecia with remaining hairs of varying lengths	Other evidence of emotional strain; onychophagia (nail biting)	None

(continued)

Alopecias (continued)

Condition	Sites	Characteristic Lesion	Other Lesions or Conditions Present	Diagnostic Aids
Favus	Scalp, nails and other areas	Yellowish cup-shaped crusts (scutula); areas of scarred alopecia; has a musty odor	Nails are thick, friable and lusterless; scutula may be present on extremities and trunk	Direct microscopic examination of scale of hair, culture on Sabouraud's medium
Radiation Alopecia (therapeutic)	Scalp	Hair fall in three weeks; regrowth in three months	Underlying disease for which treatment is given	None required, anagen hair loss
Radiation Alopecia (chronic)	Scalp or other irritated area	Atrophy and telangiectasia; skin surface is poikilodermatous	Underlying disease for which radiation was given; basal cell carcinomas may develop	Biopsy
Postfebrile Alopecia	Scalp and generalized	Diffuse hair loss with gradual regrowth when fever subsides; hair loss may not occur until 2-3 months after febrile episode	Underlying disease which caused the fever	Telogen hair loss, biopsy
Perifolliculitis Capitis Abscedens et Suffodiens	Scalp	Dissecting folliculitis of scalp with irregular areas of alopecia and scar formation	Chronic draining sinuses in scalp	Culture
Drug-Induced Alopecia	Scalp and other hairy areas	Diffuse hair loss; gradual regrowth when causative drug is eliminated	None	Biopsy, anagen hair loss
Endocrine Associated Alopecia	Thyrotoxicosis-diffuse through scalp; myxedema-frontoparietal; Addison's disease-diffuse scalp; hypopituitary-diffuse scalp and other hairy areas	Skin may be altered also by endocrinopathy	Other endocrine signs	Endocrine tests
Scleroderma	Scalp or other hairy areas	Telangiectatic scarred skin	May be morphea or generalized scleroderma	Biopsy, ANA
Metastatic Carcinoma	Scalp	Scarred skin; hard subcutaneous nodules	Primary lesions elsewhere	Biopsy
Epithelioma	Scalp	Ulcerative lesion or broad scar	None	Biopsy

Conditions in Which Scale Formation is a Prominent Feature

Macular

Exfoliative dermatitis	Pityriasis rosea	Rubeola (postinflamma-	Seborrhea
Eczema	Pityriasis rubra pilaris	tory)	Superficial fungus
Ichthyosis	Postinflammatory exfoli-	Scarlatina (postinflam-	infections
Pellagra	ation	matory)	
Pityriasis alba			

Papular

Keratosis pilaris	Lichen planus	Secondary syphiloderma	Superficial epitheli-omatosis

Macular or Papular

Atopic dermatitis	Parapsoriasis	Pityriasis rosea	Psoriasis

Hyperpigmentation or Deposits of Foreign Pigment in the Skin

Addison's disease	Café au lait spots of	Freckles	Postinflammatory de-
Argyria	neurofibromatosis	Hemosiderosis	posit of melanin,
Quinacrine dermatitis	Carotenemia	Jaundice	diffuse or localized
Bismuth pigmentation	Chloasma	Riehl's melanosis	Tattooing, acciden-
	Chrysoderma	Mongolian blue spots	tal and intentional

Atrophic Changes

Anetoderma (macular	Kraurosis vulvae	Necrobiosis lipoidica	Scleroderma
atrophy)	Lichen sclerosus et	diabeticorum	Senile cutaneous
Atrophic lichen planus	atrophicus	Poikiloderma vasculare	atrophy
Balanitis xerotica	Morphea (localized sclero-	atrophicans	Subcutaneous fat
obliterans	derma)		necrosis
Congenital hemiatrophy			

Atrophic Scars (Scars Formed without Preceding Ulceration)

Atrophia striae	Lupus erythematosus	Parapsoriasis varioli-	Radiodermatitis (with
Favus	Lupus vulgaris	formis	telangiectasia)
Folliculitis decalvans		Pseudopelade	

Common Nonscaling Conditions

Adenoma sebaceum	Freckles	Lupus vulgaris	Scleroderma
Angiomas	Granuloma annulare	Macular syphilid	Toxic erythema
Chloasma	Gummas	Pseudoxanthoma	Tuberculid
Epithelioma	Keloid	elasticum	Urticaria
Erythema multiforme	Leprosy	Purpura	Xanthomata
Erythema nodosum		Sarcoid	

Eruptions Which Rarely Involve the Face

Dermatitis herpetiformis	Parapsoriasis	Psoriasis	Tinea versicolor
Lichen planus	Pityriasis rosea	Scabies	

Some Systemic Diseases in Which Cutaneous Eruptions Are a Prominent Feature

Addison's disease	Endocrine dysfunctions	Lymphomas	Syphilis
Anthrax	Eosinophilic granuloma	Lymphogranuloma vene-	Thromboangiitis
Avitaminosis	Epiloia	reum	obliterans
Blood dyscrasias	Erysipelas	Meningococcemia	Tuberculosis
Brucellosis	Gout	Porphyrias	Tularemia
Candidiasis	Hemochromatosis	Rheumatic fever	Typhus
Chancroid	Infectious exanthemata	Rickettsial diseases	Ulcerative colitis
Chemical poisoning	Infectious mononucleosis	Rocky Mountain spotted	Variola
Deep mycoses	Leprosy	fever	Visceral malignancies
Dermatomyositis	Leptospirosis	Sarcoid	Xanthomatosis
Diptheria	Lupus erythematosus	Scleroderma	Yaws

Cutaneous Pigmentary Changes

Pigment	Color	Sites	Extent	Subjective Symptoms	Associated Systemic Disease
Iron (hemosiderosis)	Dark red or red-brown	Legs, thighs, buttocks	Varies from small discrete areas to extensive lesions	Usually none	Schamberg's disease, Majocchi's disease, drug reactions and stasis
Silver (argyria)	Gray or blue-gray	Generalized, including sclera and nail beds	Always generalized	Usually none except the emotional distress caused by the cosmetic defect	The condition for which the silver salt was administrered
Gold (chrysiasis)	Bluish-gray or purplish color	Exposed skin only	Localized to exposed areas	As above	The condition for which the gold salt was administered
Bismuth and Mercury	Blue-gray	Gums, trunk, extremities	May be localized to the gums or the extremities and trunk or both	Painful mouth, difficulty in chewing; skin lesions cause moderate to intense pruritus	The condition for which the bismuth salt was given
Melanin	Light brown to dark brown to black or blue	On any part of the body; usually the photoexposed areas are accentuated initially	May be the small lesions of melasma or extensive lesion on all parts of the body	Usually none except embarrassment due to the cosmetic defect	Some hereditary syndromes, Addison's disease, systemic malignancy, porphyria, malignant melanoma, chronic infections

Dermatoses Associated With Internal Malignancy

Condition	Site of Lesions	Onset	Primary Lesion	Site of Tumor	Type
Peutz-Jeghers Syndrome	Buccal mucosa, hands, feet	Slow	Macular pigment spot	Small intestine	Polyposis, adenocarcinoma
Gardner's Syndrome	Trunk, extremities	Slowly progressive	Papular lesions and cysts	Colon	Polyposis, adenocarcinoma
Palmar and Plantar Keratoderma	Palms, soles	Slowly progressive	Diffuse hyperkeratosis	Esophagus	Carcinoma
Arsenical Keratoses	Palms, soles	Slowly progressive	Multiple verrucous papules	Viscera	Carcinoma
Bowen's Disease	Any part of the body	Slow	Brownish maculopapules	Viscera	Carcinoma
Dermatomyositis (adult)	Generalized cutaneous lesions	Rapid	Varies: urticaria, macules and papules	Viscera	Carcinoma
Erythema Figuratum	Trunk, extremities	Slow	Tortuous gyrate macules	Viscera	Carcinoma
Erythroderma	Generalized	May be slow or rapid	Diffuse infiltrated macules	Generalized	Lymphoma
Acanthosis	Axillae, groin, popliteal spaces, antecubital fossae	Insidious	Verrucous hyperpigmented papules	Viscera	Carcinoma
Multiple seborrheic keratoses (Leser-Trélat)	Trunk	Sudden	Dark brown to black papules	Viscera	Carcinoma
Acquired Ichthyosis	Trunk, extremities	Insidious	Dry scaling macules	Generalized	Hodgkin's disease

Immunofluorescence

Disease	Direct	Indirect
Lupus Erythematosus	In involved skin, IgM, IgC and complement are in a fibrillar pattern at the dermal-epidermal junction. Occasionally some fluorescence is found around cutaneous blood vessels. Similar changes are found also in uninvolved skin of approximately 40% of patients with SLE.	Same
Pemphigus (all types)	Antibody is demonstrable against the epithelial and mucosal intercellular cement in almost all direct specimens. The titer of this antibody should be greater than 1-10.	Same in 95% of cases.
Bullous Pemphigoid	Linear binding of IgG and complement to basement membrane is present on involved and uninvolved skin. Occasionally IgM may be present. Titers of antibody do not correlate with the severity of the disease.	70% of patients have antibody against basement membrane.
Dermatitis Herpetiformis	Normal skin or skin adjacent to the lesion has immune complexes of IgA and complement in a granular band dermal papillae beneath basement membrane. Other immune globulins may also be present. These changes may occasionally be present in involved skin.	Rarely positive
Benign Mucous Membrane Pemphigus	Same as bullous pemphigoid.	Usually negative
Lichen Planus	Large hematogenous deposits of IgG, and sometimes IgM and IgA are present in the upper dermis corresponding to the Civatte bodies which are antibody coated epidermal cells.	Negative
Herpes Gestationis	Properdin, C3 and C5 can be found at the lamina lucida of the basement membrane and along the anchoring fibrils of the dermis.	HG factor: a heat labile factor capable of depositing C3 on the normal skin basement membrane.
Vasculitis	Immunoglobulin and complement may be deposited in the blood vessels of involved skin of patients with early lesions of necrotizing vasculitis.	None

CHAPTER 14

Macular Eruptions

Acrodynia

Synonym. Pink disease.

Sites of predilection. Hands and feet of infants and children.

Objective signs. The hands and feet are markedly edematous and there is diffuse erythema. Cyanosis of the distal portions of the extremities, together with generalized hyperhidrosis and vesiculation, are late sequelae. Secondary pyogenic infection frequently develops. Profuse miliaria rubra may occur on the trunk.

Subjective symptoms. Severe pain, pruritus and fever. The child is irritable and his general health deteriorates.

Etiology. The condition may be the result of mercury ingestion.

Histopathology. Not diagnostic.

Diagnostic aids. History and physical examination.

Relation to systemic disease. The condition may indicate an underlying disorder of the hypothalamus or sympathetic nervous system.

Differential diagnosis. Raynaud's disease, dermatitis venenata, pellagra.

Therapy. Good supportive care and sedation is valuable. Topical antibiotic ointments and systemic antibiotic therapy when indicated. Ganglionic blocking agents may be needed for the automatic dysfunction. A course of BAL may be needed.

Addison's Disease

Synonym. None.

Sites of predilection. The cutaneous lesions are usually generalized.

Objective signs. The earliest lesions may be marked depigmentation or hyperpigmentation. Eventually the skin develops a bronze color caused by the deposit of melanin in the basal layer of the epidermis. The pigmentary changes are most marked over the face, groin, axillae, aerolae, creases of the palms or soles, genitalia and mucosae. Patients with Addison's disease are prone to develop vitiligo.

Subjective symptoms. The cutaneous lesions are asymptomatic. The systemic symptoms are lassitude anorexia, weight loss, postural hypotension and general malaise.

Histopathology. There is a marked nonspecific increase in the deposit of melanin in the basal layer.

Diagnostic aids. History and physical examination, hemogram, blood electrolytes, urinary steroid excretion studies, ACTH stimulation test, flat film of the abdomen looking for calcification of the glands.

Etiology. Primary suprarenal insufficiency.

Relation to systemic disease. Addison's disease is systemic. Some cases may be caused by other diseases such as tuberculosis or histoplasmosis.

Differential diagnosis. Melasma.

Therapy. Dioxycorticosterone acetate pellet implantation, systemic fludrocortisone, supportive measures.

Albinism

Synonym. None.

Sites of predilection. Generalized.

Objective signs. The skin of the entire body is depigmented and hypersensitive to light. The hair is white, yellowish or has a reddish tint. The absence of melanin in the choroid causes the eyes to look pale blue and produces photophobia. Albino skin in the young adult is frequently the site of keratoses, epitheliomas, melanomas and other degenerative changes. Nystagmus may be present. Partial albinism may develop in more than one member of the family.

Subjective symptoms. Photophobia.

Etiology. Congenital. There is a block in the formation of melanin from its precursors due to a relative lack of the enzyme tyrosinase. Several forms of this disease, each with different enzyme deficiencies, exist.

Histopathology. An absence of melanin in the basal layer.

Diagnostic aids. History and physical examination. Examination of the skin and hair bulb for dopa.

Relation to systemic disease. Mental retardation, deafness or other congenital defects.

Differential diagnosis. Clinical appearance is characteristic in this condition.

Therapy. Avoidance of exposure to sunlight. Judicious use of sunscreen agents. Genetic counseling is advised.

Angioma, Benign Acquired

Synonym. Senile angioma, DeMorgan's spots.

Sites of predilection. Trunk.

Objective signs. These are small, bright red or purplish papules, which vary from 1-3 mm in diameter. The papule may be composed of dilated blood vessels or it may be filled with fluid blood. The lesions occur most commonly on the trunks of middle-aged or elderly persons.

Subjective symptoms. None.

Etiology. Unknown.

Histopathology. The epidermis over these lesions is atrophic. Elastic tissue is greatly diminished. There are densely packed groups of dilated capillaries.

Diagnostic aids. Clinical appearance, biopsy.

Relation to systemic disease. None.

Differential diagnosis. Nevus araneus, vascular nevus.

Therapy. Electrodesiccation.

Argyria

Synonym. Silver poisoning.

Sites of predilection. Generalized.

Objective signs. The entire integument exhibits localized, slate blue, permanent hyperpigmentation. This same type of pigmentation may be observed in the lunulae of the nails, sclerae and mucous membranes.

Subjective symptoms. None.

Etiology. Ingested silver salts or continued application of silver colloidal suspensions to the nasal mucosa or pharynx.

Histopathology. Numerous, very fine, refractile granules are found in the membrana propria of the sweat glands, elastic tissue fibers and nerve bundles. These fine granules are seen best with the darkfield microscope.

Diagnostic aids. Biopsy, history and clinical appearance. Chemical determination of silver in the skin can be performed.

Relation to systemic disease. The underlying pathologic state which was treated with silver compounds.

Differential diagnosis. Melasma, postinflammatory pigmentation.

Therapy. None effective.

Atrophy, Cutaneous, of the Aged

Synonym. Senile atrophy.

Sites of predilection. Generalized. The most characteristic changes are seen on the exposed portions such as the face, neck and hands.

Objective signs. The skin is dry and irregularly depigmented, with brownish macules, fine bran-like scale, telangiectasia and loss of elasticity. Actinic keratoses are commonly present on the face and hands.

Subjective symptoms. Pruritus, poor tolerance to soap, bruising.

Etiology. The aging process and chronic sun exposure.

Histopathology. Atrophy of the skin appendages and the subcutaneous tissue. Senile elastosis develops in the corium and the elastic tissue takes the bluish color of the hematoxylin-eosin stain.

Diagnostic aids. Biopsy, clinical appearance.

Relation to systemic disease. Other manifestations of advancing age.

Differential diagnosis. Eczematous eruptions.

Therapy. Avoidance of wind and sun. Use of lubricant creams and sunscreens on the skin. Avoidance of soap when dryness is a problem.

Candidiasis

Synonym. Moniliasis, thrush.

Sites of predilection. Oral mucosa, genitalia, infra-mammary region, groin and axillae, perianal area, interdigital spaces, nail folds.

Objective signs. The infection may be present in fissures at the commissures of the lips (perlèche). These radial grooves become erythematous and are occasionally covered with a whitish film. On the oral mucous membranes, the tongue, the vagina and under the prepuce, white curd-like deposits are present which form a confluent film. Forcible removal of this membrane may cause bleeding. In infancy thrush may precede chronic crusting granulomas on the face, scalp or flexural areas. In the inframammary regions, the groin or where perianal areas are involved, the skin is bright pink and is covered with a whitish film. The area presents a macerated appearance. Painful fissures may develop in the flexural creases and small satellite lesions appear at the periphery of the eruption. When the nail folds are involved, there is swelling and the nail fold is separated from the proximal portion of the nail. On gentle pressure, caseous material may be expressed. The nail plates become discolored and the margins present a greenish-brown color. This yeast infection is a common complication of seborrheic dermatitis in infants and may involve the folds of neck, scalp, trunk and especially the diaper area. When this complication occurs, the skin is moist, erythematous and covered with a faint whitish film.

Subjective symptoms. Pruritus and pain.

Etiology. *Candida albicans.* Occasionally some of the other species of *Candida* may cause this condition. Heat, humidity and friction may be predisposing factors.

Histopathology. The histopathologic changes are governed by the extent of the infection and the tissues involved. A mild to severe inflammatory infiltrate is present. There may be focal areas of suppuration with microabscesses, hyperkeratosis, acanthosis and edema.

Diagnostic aids. Culture and biopsy.

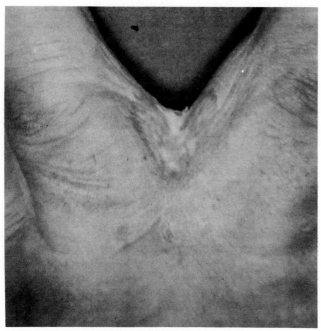

Interdigital candidal infection

Relation to systemic disease. Candidiasis frequently occurs in debilitated or immunosuppressed individuals. It may develop as a complication of broad spectrum antibiotic therapy. Candidiasis occurs as a complicating feature of diabetes mellitus. Cutaneous candidiasis may become a systemic disease in which there is visceral involvement.

Differential diagnosis. Leukoplakia, mucous patches of secondary syphilis, mycotic infection of all types, seborrheic dermatitis, psoriasis, acrodermatitis enteropathica.

Therapy. Local lesions will respond to treatment with topical applications of Mycostatin® or clotrimazole. Mycostatin® is ineffective on systemic administration and clotrimazole should not be used systemically because of the severe adverse reactions it produces. Amphotericin B is the drug of choice for treatment of systemic candidiasis.

Carotenemia

Synonym. None.

Sites of predilection. Generalized.

Objective signs. This condition most commonly occurs in infants and young children. The skin has a diffuse yellow color which is most prominent on the palms and soles. The sclerae are not involved.

Subjective symptoms. No cutaneous subjective symptoms.

Etiology. Excessive intake of foods containing large amounts of carotene, *eg,* orange juice, carrots.

Histopathology. Nonspecific.

Diagnostic aids. History relative to systemic disease, clinical appearance, serum carotene.

Relation to systemic disease. Carotene is normally converted into vitamin A. In myxedema and diabetes this conversion is impaired and carotene accumulates in the skin.

Differential diagnosis. Jaundice. Lycopenemia (ingestion of chemicals found in tomatoes), quinacrine pigmentation.

Therapy. Reduce the intake of carotene (normally found in carrots, oranges, squash, pumpkin, sweet potato and eggs).

Comedones

Synonym. Blackheads.

Sites of predilection. Face, ears, back, chest.

Objective signs. Small black or gray plugs in follicular orifices. These plugs may be readily expressed and are whitish and caseous with black ends. The plug consists of condensed sebum and epidermal debris. The black portion of the plug is not caused by dirt but is a deposition of melanin. Many comedones become acne papules and pustules. Large comedones resembling cysts or neoplasms develop in the elderly.

Subjective symptoms. The psychogenic effect produced by the presence of lesions.

Etiology. Specific causative factors are unknown.

Histopathology. Keratin plug in the pilosebaceous

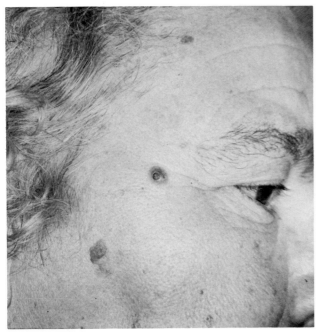

Giant comedo

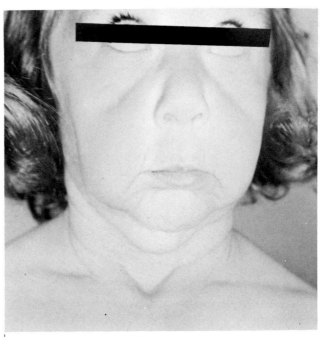

Cutis laxa

orifice with dilatation of the gland by sebaceous material.

Diagnostic aids. Demonstration of the sebaceous plugs by expression, biopsy.

Relation to systemic disease. The condition is common at puberty and is related to hormone activity. It is a common occurrence on the faces of patients who have severe elastic tissue changes from chronic actinic damage.

Differential diagnosis. Clinical appearance is characteristic.

Therapy. Expression of comedones. Lotions or gels containing benzoyl peroxide or retinoic acid.

Cutis Laxa

Synonym. Dermatochalasis, chalazodermia, dermatomegaly.

Objective signs. The condition is present at birth, and presents sagging folds of skin on the face and trunk. The affected child has the appearance of advanced old age. General physical development is normal but affected men have infantile genitalia and are impotent. Children are mentally alert and life expectancy is normal.

Subjective symptoms. The cutaneous lesions do not produce discomfort. The child may be embarrassed by the abnormal appearance.

Etiology. A genodermatosis—an autosomal recessive gene.

Histopathology. The elastic fibers in the dermis are shortened and show granular degeneration. The mucopolysaccharide content of the skin is greatly increased.

Diagnostic aids. Biopsy.

Relation to systemic disease. None.

Differential diagnosis. Ehlers-Danlos syndrome, neurofibromatosis.

Therapy. None is effective.

Dandruff

Synonym. Seborrhea sicca.

Sites of predilection. Scalp, eyebrows.

Objective signs. Scant or profuse, dry or oily, whitish or yellowish-white, flaky scales are scattered throughout the hair. The scales vary from 1-3 mm in diameter. In severe cases an adherent collection of scale may form about the orifice of the hair follicle. The condition varies in severity from a moderate amount of scale to the profuse scaling noted in seborrheic dermatitis.

Subjective symptoms. None to moderate pruritus.

Etiology. Unknown. Scaling is a normal physiologic phenomenon; however, in diseased states the production of scale becomes accelerated.

Histopathology. Hyperkeratosis and exfoliation.

Diagnostic aids. Rule out the presence of fungus infections by the use of scrapings and culture.

Relation to systemic disease. None usually.

Differential diagnosis. Psoriasis, fungus infections.

Therapy. An antiseborrheic shampoo two to three times weekly. A corticosteroid lotion or spray is applied to the scalp daily. If scaling in the scalp is profuse it may be desirable to use a scalp lotion containing 2-3% salicylic acid in 50% alcohol. Anthralin containing pomades are useful in severe cases.

Dermatitis, Factitious

Synonym. Feigned eruption, malingerer's disease, dug-out disease, delusions of parasitosis.

Sites of predilection. Any area of the body which can be reached by the hands.

Objective signs. Objective symptoms vary with the type of irritant which has been used. If a substance such as phenol, mineral acid or a caustic has been applied to the skin, the lesion may be edematous and reddish, surrounded by a zone of darker erythema and scale or serous crusting. Various stages in the evolution of lesions, varying from acute to chronic, may be present. All the lesions are well-defined and too geometrically

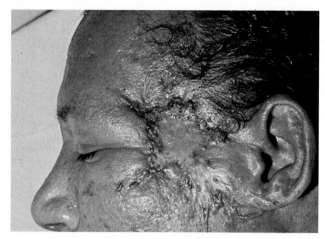

Factitious dermatitis

perfect to be natural in origin. Areas of erythema, vesiculation, necrosis and ulceration occur.

In many patients there are well-healed scars, healing lesions covered with adherent crusts and fresh lesions covered with blood crusts. These represent areas in which the patient has picked out pieces of skin with the fingernails or some sharp instrument.

Subjective symptoms. Those produced by the mental aberration of the patient. Some patients will complain of a crawling sensation under the skin (formication). Another common complaint is that of a parasite on or burrowing under the skin. Patients state that the itching is so intense that they must dig out the parasite.

Etiology. Mental illness. Malingerers may intentionally injure the skin in order to obtain compensation or gain sympathy.

Histopathology. The microscopic picture is not diagnostic.

Diagnostic aids. If the traumatized area or areas are covered with occlusive dressings containing some bland, therapeutically inactive substance, such as sterile petrolatum, the lesions will heal. When the dressings are removed the patient will reproduce the lesions in the same site.

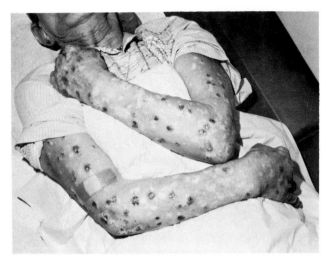

Factitious dermatitis

Relation to systemic disease. The condition is an indication of mental illness.

Differential diagnosis. Syphilis, tuberculosis, occupational diseases, allergic eruptions, drug eruptions.

Therapy. Psychotherapy. Antibiotics may be necessary for secondary infection.

Dermatomyositis

Synonym. None.

Sites of predilection. Any part of the body.

Objective signs. The eruption is polymorphic, often beginning with recurrent edema of the face and extremities. The first lesions may appear on the eyelids and then extend over the cheeks, face, neck and shoulders. A bluish-pink halo (heliotrope) may develop about the eyes. Small, scaly, bluish-red macules develop over the bony prominences and the skin becomes pigmented and atrophic. Telangiectasia or petechiae can be seen around the nails. In some patients the lesions resemble those of systemic lupus erythematosus, poikiloderma or scleroderma. Later, cutaneous manifestations resemble urticaria, erythema multiforme, erythema nodosum or erysipelas.

A low-grade intermittent fever and sweating is a common symptom. The characteristic feature of this condition is the development of nonsuppurative myositis which leads to progressive weakness. In advanced cases walking is impossible and the head droops when the patient is lifted. Mild forms of the condition may become chronic or show complete remission. There is definite tenderness of muscles early in the disease; then muscular atrophy develops.

Subjective symptoms. Cutaneous symptoms vary from mild pruritus to severe pain over the involved areas. There is marked pain and tenderness in the muscles. In advanced cases the patient has difficulty in raising himself to a sitting position. He has weakness of all muscle groups, especially those about the eyes and the limb girdles.

Etiology. This condition has been associated with the collagen-vascular group of diseases. There is an increased association with an internal malignancy in adults who acquire this disease.

Histopathology. The histopathologic picture of skin lesions is nonspecific. A muscle biopsy shows perivascular infiltration with lymphocytes, plasma cells and polymorphonuclear leukocytes. The muscle fibers become edematous, undergo degenerative changes, finally become homogeneous and are replaced by fibrosis.

Diagnostic aids. Muscle biopsy, ANA, electromyogram, urinary myoglobin, antimyoglobin antibodies, serum CPK, LDH, SGOT.

Relation to systemic disease. Splenomegaly. The heart may be involved and death from heart failure may ensue. Involvement of the diaphragm and intercostal muscles may lead to bronchopneumonia or suffocation.

Differential diagnosis. Scleroderma, lupus erythematosus, erythema multiforme, erythema nodosum, poikiloderma.

Therapy. Nonspecific. Corticosteroids may give symptomatic relief. Cures have been observed if an underlying malignancy is extirpated.

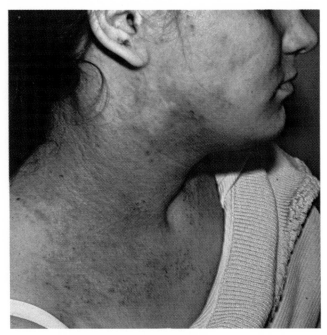

Atopic dermatitis

ECZEMA

The word eczema is a morphologic, not a specific diagnostic, term. An eczematous eruption may be observed with atopic, seborrheic or contact dermatitis. The condition may be acute, subacute or chronic (neurodermatitis). The development of an eczematous eruption can be associated with many factors: an allergic state, focal infection, psychogenic factors or chronic local irritation. Regardless of the causative factor, the basic clinical picture is that of an ill-defined, confluent, acutely or chronically inflamed eruption which exhibits serous exudation, scaling, excoriations and fissure formation. The clinical appearance varies with the age of the individual, site of involvement, causative factors and duration of the eruption.

Eczema, Atopic Dermatitis (in Children)

Synonym. Tetter, seven-year itch.

Sites of predilection. Face, scalp, antecubital fossae, popliteal spaces, trunk, neck, dorsal surfaces of hands and the genitocrural area.

Objective signs. An ill-defined, pink to red, confluent, macular eruption whose surface may be covered with a variable amount of dry scale is characteristic. The lesions become slightly thickened. Excoriations and blood crusts are frequently present and the involved area may be moist or covered with a serous crust. Secondary pyogenic infections or *Candida albicans* infections may occur. Later, a marked accentuation of the normal skin markings (lichenification) caused by thickening of the epidermis and the cellular infiltrate occurs. Fissures may develop, especially on the dorsal surfaces of the hands and fingers. The course of this disorder is punctuated with remissions and exacerbations. The eruption usually begins between the ages of 6 months and 2 years. Exacerbations may occur at any time.

Subjective symptoms. Severe pruritus, pain and loss of sleep.

Etiology. A familial trait. Family history is usually positive for one of the atopic diseases (asthma, hay fever or dermatitis). Hypersensitivity to ingested, injected or inhaled substances has been hypothesized. A relative T-cell hypofunction has been identified in this disorder. Patients with atopic dermatitis frequently develop superimposed contact dermatitis caused by overzealous local therapy. Lesions can be aggravated by emotional stimuli, changes in temperature or humidity, streptococcal infection or drug allergies.

Histopathology. The microscopic picture varies with the stage of the eruption. There is edema of the epidermis and the upper cutis, without frank vesiculation. Vascular dilatation and round-cell infiltration are also present. Moderate acanthosis may be present.

Diagnostic aids. History and physical examination; patch, scratch and intradermal tests are of doubtful value. Immunoglobulin E levels in the serum seem to reflect the severity of the disease in the individual patient. Eosinophilia is common.

Relation to systemic disease. These patients frequently have or develop urticaria, hay fever or asthma. Serious superinfection with vaccinia and herpes simplex viruses occurs.

Differential diagnosis. Fungus infections, contact dermatitis, pityriasis rosea, psoriasis. It is frequently difficult to distinguish between atopic and seborrheic dermatitis in children.

Therapy. The therapy of atopic dermatitis should be kept individualized and simple. The important features are:

1. *Good Nursing Care.* It includes removal of offending stimulants and the institution of health measures such as a balanced diet, good ventilation and removal of emotional disturbances whenever possible. Irritating clothing should be discarded. Bathing with soaps should be restricted to areas that are dirty; simple bathing or soaking with water or oil may be substituted. All extraneous topical agents should be eliminated.

2. *Sedation.* This is best accomplished with antihistamines which also have an antipruritic effect. Tranquilizers or other sedatives may have to be used in selected cases.

3. *Topical Therapy.* The ointments or creams of choice are topical corticosteroids, which are applied without plastic occlusion. Potent or fluorinated corticosteroids may be used sparingly in severe cases, but as soon as feasible, a switch to topical hydrocortisone should be made. Topical antipruritic agents containing 0.5% menthol in emollient cream or an oil can be effective in mild cases.

4. *Systemic Therapy.* Systemic corticosteroids should be restricted to extreme cases of extensive involvement and used only for short periods because of possible complications which include growth retardation in children.

Secondary infection with pyogenic bacteria should be treated with the appropriate systemic antibiotic as determined by in vitro sensitivity tests. Secondary candidiasis may be counteracted with topical clotrimazole or nystatin in cream or lotion bases.

Patients with eczema should not be vaccinated with vaccinia virus for smallpox prophylaxis. Indeed, they should not be in close contact with a normal person who has been vaccinated. Direct contact with active herpes simplex lesions on other persons should also be avoided.

In chronic lesions, 1-3% crude coal tar or solution of coal tar in petrolatum or Lassar's paste is frequently an effective preparation. The commercially available coal tar distillate ointments are efficient and stainless; commercially available corticosteroid ointments and creams reduce erythema and lichenification. One percent phenol crystals in olive or cotton seed oil, and menthol (0.1-0.5%) in alcohol, vanishing cream or lotion base are *effective antipruritic preparations.*

Atopic dermatitis in a child

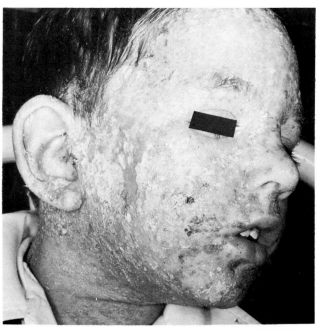

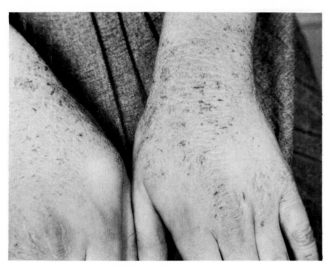

Atopic dermatitis in an adult

Eczema, Atopic Dermatitis, Neurodermatitis (In Adults)

Synonym. Tetter, seven-year itch.

Sites of predilection. Popliteal spaces, antecubital fossae, axillae, face, trunk, genitocrural area, perianal area, neck and dorsal surfaces of the hands.

Objective symptoms. The condition may become apparent at any age. In adults, the lesions are ill-defined, confluent and lichenified. This disease appears to be identical with atopic dermatitis in children except that a strong familial history of atopic diseases is lacking. (See previous section on Atopic Dermatitis in Children.)

A unique feature of the disorder is the fact that it may mimic mycosis fungoides so closely that repeated biopsies should be performed. The therapy of this disease is identical with that of the childhood form. Systemic corticosteroids should be avoided whenever possible because of their multiple side effects.

Ehlers-Danlos Syndrome

Synonym. Cutis hyperelastica.

Sites of predilection. Generalized.

Objective signs. The skin is soft and smooth without evidence of any active inflammatory process. The skin is hyperelastic and a fold may be stretched far beyond its normal attachment. When released, the fold returns to its normal appearance. Associated with this condition is hyperextensibility of joints, particularly of the fingers and toes. Following trauma, pseudotumors develop, usually over the elbows and knees. These tumors are extravasations of blood and serum which collect in the traumatized areas because of ruptured

Ehlers-Danlos syndrome

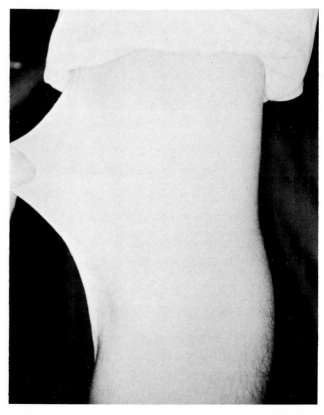

blood vessels. The lesions involute spontaneously and are replaced by scars, but recur immediately.

Subjective symptoms. None.

Etiology. Congenital. Several variants of this disease have already been described.

Histopathology. Some fragmentation of elastic fibers may be demonstrated by the use of special strains.

Diagnostic aids. History, clinical findings, biopsy, urinary hydroxyproline excretion.

Relation to systemic disease. None.

Differential diagnosis. Cutis laxa, anetoderma.

Therapy. None. Genetic counseling is advised.

Epithelioma, Intraepithelial

Synonym. Paget's disease, erythroplasia of Queyrat, Bowen's disease.

Sites of predilection. Paget's disease occurs in the areola and the nipple area of the breast or in the genital area; erythroplasia of Queyrat occurs on the glans penis; Bowen's disease occurs on the trunk and extremities.

Objective signs. *Paget's Disease.* It occurs primarily in women between the ages of 40 and 60 although men may also develop these lesions. This condition usually exhibits a well-defined, scaly, reddish, macular lesion involving the areola and nipple or groin. The margin is usually slightly raised, although this may be obscured by serous exudation and crust formation. It is usually unilateral.

Erythroplasia of Queyrat. This lesion, which is usually limited to the glans penis, is a scaly, erythematous macule which is sharply defined and covered with a slight amount of adherent dry scale. Occasionally there is some serous exudation and crust formation. It does not heal spontaneously.

Bowen's Disease. The primary lesion is a light brown, pinkish or reddish maculopapule

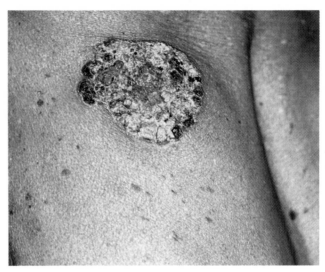

Intraepithelial epithelioma

which is covered with a thickened horny layer. The margin is sharply defined; there may be a serous crust. When the scale or crust is removed the underlying surface is reddish and may be moist. The base is granular and occasionally papillomatous in appearance.

Extramammary Paget's Disease. These lesions, which resemble erythroplasia, occur on the lips, vulva, penis, trunk, nose and extremities.

Subjective symptoms. In the early phases of the disease, pruritus may be present.

Etiology. Unknown.

Histopathology. *Paget's Disease.* Epidermal cells and large, sharply-defined, mononucleated cancer cells possessing deeply staining nuclei and faintly staining cytoplasm are present. Paget's cells occur singly and in small groups in the epidermis.

Bowen's Disease. The histologic picture is that of the classic intraepithelial epithelioma. Dyskeratotic cells and extensive individual cell keratinization are present in the epidermis.

Erythroplasia of Queyrat. The histologic picture is that of an intraepithelial epithelioma with characteristic dyskeratotic cells.

Diagnostic aids. The biopsy is a pathognomonic test.

Relation to systemic disease. It is generally believed that Paget's disease is a locally invasive carcinoma at the onset. A deeper intraductal carcinoma is usually present. In advanced cases prognosis is poor. Both Bowen's disease and erythroplasia of Queyrat are intraepithelial epitheliomas which eventually become squamous cell carcinomas.

Differential diagnosis. Infectious eczematoid dermatitis, neurodermatitis, contact dermatitis, melanoma.

Therapy. Most of these lesions will respond to treatment with topical applications of 5-fluorouracil, which produces a violent local reaction but in most instances will eradicate the lesions. If this therapy fails, then surgical excision or other destructive measures are indicated.

Epitheliomatosis, Superficial Basal Cell

Synonym. Eczematous epithelioma, erythematoid epithelioma.

Objective signs. The lesions may be few or numerous. They are well-defined, confluent and discrete, flat macules. Occasionally the lesions may be slightly elevated. There is a moderate amount of adherent dry scale. The lesions spread peripherally and vary from 1-10 cm in diameter. Each lesion is limited by a slightly raised, very thin, shiny, rolled margin. Excoriations and crusting are frequently present. The condition develops most commonly after the third decade.

Subjective symptoms. Usually none, but moderate to intense pruritus may be present.

Etiology. Unknown.

Histopathology. Characteristic of basal cell epithelioma with the tumor tissue closely applied to the under surface of the epidermis. It is not an invasive lesion.

Diagnostic aids. Biopsy.

Relation to systemic disease. None demonstrated. May be associated with a history of inorganic arsenic ingestion.

Differential diagnosis. Lupus erythematosus, eczema, psoriasis, mycotic infection, neurodermatitis.

Therapy. The options include: excision or fulguration and curettage; topical application of 5-fluorouracil ointment or cream; and low voltage roentgen ray treatment (grenz-ray treatment).

Erysipelas

Synonym. St. Anthony's fire, streptococcal cellulitis.

Sites of predilection. Face, but may appear anywhere on the body.

Objective signs. The condition begins as one or more bright red, raised macules which extend peripherally to form a well-defined, edematous, shiny, flat lesion with superficial vesicles on the surface. There is a marked increase in tenderness and local heat and the area may become hemorrhagic. The patients are usually acutely ill; The temperature may reach 40-40.5°C. There is enlargement of regional lymph nodes and the lymph vessels may be palpable. Many patients have recurrent attacks of erysipelas with the redevelopment of lesions in the original site. With succeeding attacks persistent swelling of the involved parts may develop.

Erysipelas

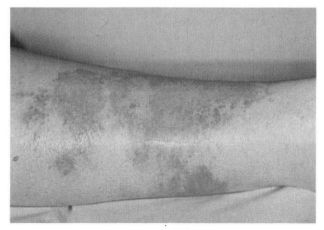

Subjective symptoms. Malaise, chills, fever and vomiting. Locally there is usually burning, pruritus and pain.

Etiology. Group A beta-hemolytic streptococcus.

Histopathology. There is superficial cellulitis in which the blood and lymph vessels are dilated, and a marked perivascular infiltrate consisting primarily of intact polymorphonuclear leukocytes.

Diagnostic aids. Culture on blood agar, serology (antihyaluronidase, anti-DNase B).

Relation to systemic disease. Erysipelas is a systemic disease which may be followed by acute glomerular nephritis, otitis media, myocarditis or bacteremia.

Differential diagnosis. Acute contact dermatitis, thrombophlebitis.

Therapy. Penicillin is the antibiotic of choice. If this infection develops on a surgical or maternity ward, or if the lesion is open, the patient should be isolated.

Erysipeloid

Synonym. None.

Sites of predilection. Hands.

Objective signs. The lesions develop at the site of trauma in people who handle crabs, oysters and other seafood. The primary lesion is a macule with a sharply defined border, and a dull red or purplish appearance. The lesions are slightly elevated and edematous and show a tendency to peripheral spread. Vesicles may develop. The patients are not usually febrile.

Subjective symptoms. Burning and pruritus.

Etiology. Erysipelothrix rhusiopathiae.

Histopathology. A superficial cellulitis with vascular dilatation and an infiltrate of polymorphonuclear leukocytes closely packed about the vessels.

Diagnostic aids. Culture, history of handling seafood, biopsy.

Relation to systemic disease. In diffuse generalized cases, the patient may develop septicemia and occasionally endocarditis. Severe and prolonged

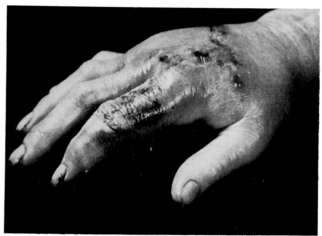
Erysipeloid

arthritis is a common sequela.

Differential diagnosis. Erysipelas and other pyodermas.

Therapy. Penicillin, sulfonamides and broad-spectrum antibiotics according to in vitro sensitivity studies.

Erythema ab Igne

Synonym. Toasted shins.

Sites of predilection. Extensor surfaces of the legs, buttocks, trunk or other areas exposed to heat.

Objective signs. The lesion begins as a reticulated, pinkish, macular eruption. Chronic lesions present a reticulated, brownish, pigmented macular network corresponding to the underlying vascular pattern.

Subjective symptoms. None.

Etiology. The condition develops because of exposure of the legs to heat from open fireplaces, ovens or oil stoves. The reticulated pattern develops because of local hemostasis. The condition may also develop from exposure to infrared lamps or constant application of hot water bags or electric pads.

Histopathology. Atrophy of the epidermis, dermal pigmentation and vascular dilatation in the upper

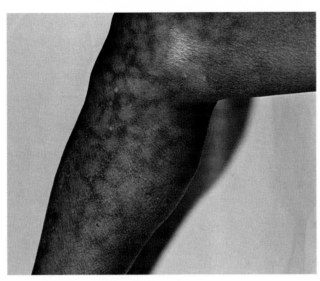

Erythema ab igne

dermis. The pigments are both melanin and hemosiderin.

Diagnostic aids. History of exposure, clinical appearance.

Relation to systemic disease. No specific relationship.

Differential diagnosis. Cutis marmorata, livedo reticularis.

Therapy. None.

Erythema Dyschromicum Perstans

Synonym. Lyme's disease, erythema chromicum, ashy dermatosis of Ramirez.

Sites of predilection. Trunk.

Objective signs. Erythematous macules which later exhibit a slate gray color surrounded by a slowly expanding active border which may or may not be elevated. Arthritis and arthralgias usually follow the eruption.

Subjective symptoms. None produced by the skin.

Etiology. Recent speculation suggests that Lyme's arthritis is due to a tick-borne rickettsiosis. This skin condition is regarded as a reaction pattern to autoimmune disease, malignancy, intestinal parasitism, food, insect bite or infections.

Histopathology. Degenerative vacuolization of the deep epidermal layers, and a mixed mononuclear cell and melanophage perivascular dermal infiltrate are present.

Diagnostic aids. Biopsy, sedimentation rate.

Relation to systemic disease. See etiology. Lyme's arthritis begins as a multijoint inflammation which later affects only one joint, usually the knee.

Differential diagnosis. Any hyperpigmented disorder: pinta, leprosy, sarcoid, lichen planus, fixed drug eruption, poikiloderma vasculare atrophicans.

Therapy. None.

Erythema Multiforme

Synonym. None.

Sites of predilection. Hands, forearms, face, lips, trunk, genitalia and feet.

Erythema multiforme

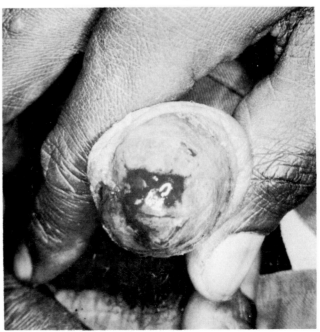

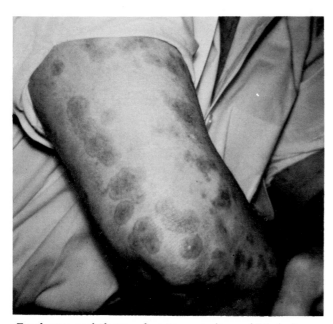

Erythema multiforme showing annular and iris lesions

Objective signs. The lesions are of various sizes and shapes, well-defined, flat macules or slightly raised, flat lesions. They may vary from 5-20 cm in diameter. The individual lesions are pink, reddish or violaceous in color and there is absence of scale. The characteristic lesion consists of concentric rings of different colors about a central small vesicle known as an iris or target lesion. Annular lesions may develop and several lesions coalesce to form a confluent or gyrate lesion. Papules and vesicles may also form part of the clinical picture. In some patients all three types of lesions may be present (see Erythema Multiforme in Chapters 15 and 16); these lesions tend to occur in the spring and fall.

Subjective symptoms. The condition is characterized by recurrence. In some individuals there is mild to moderate pruritus. Arthralgia and malaise may be symptoms.

Etiology. Unknown. This disorder may also be a reactive erythema (reaction pattern) indicative of lupus erythematosus or other connective tissue disease. Other patients develop lesions after attacks of herpes simplex or other infections. The clinical syndrome has also been produced by sensitization to penicillin, antipyrine and other drugs.

Histopathology. The collagen is edematous and there is vascular dilatation in the papillary portion of the corium. The perivascular cellular infiltrate consists of lymphocytes and polymorphonuclear leukocytes.

Diagnostic aids. Clinical examination and history. There is a subepidermal vesicle visible in skin biopsy slides. Direct and indirect immunofluorescence studies demonstrate no binding of immune globulins at the basement membrane.

Relation to systemic disease. The condition may be associated with splenomegaly, foci of infection, allergic disturbances or rheumatic fever. Erythema marginatum, commonly observed in rheumatic fever, is a variant of erythema multiforme. Other systemic infectious diseases, such as lupus erythematosus, may produce the same cutaneous picture.

Differential diagnosis. Urticaria, macular syphilid, bullous impetigo, lichen planus, "id" eruptions, systemic lupus erythematosus.

Therapy. An intensive search must be made for the cause. In severe cases, systemic corticosteroid therapy is justified. Any infection should be eliminated. If the causative factor is drug allergy, the patient should be warned not to take the same agent again.

Erythema, Toxic

Synonym. None.

Sites of predilection. Generalized.

Objective signs. The onset of this condition is acute, with the development of a profuse, symmetrical, macular eruption, consisting of numerous discrete and confluent areas. The lesions spread rapidly until the entire body is involved, presenting the ultimate picture of a bright red, confluent, occasionally mottled eruption. There is usually prominent circumorbital edema. The oral mucosa is not involved.

Exfoliation of large, thin, translucent sheets will appear while the erythema is still spreading and continue for a week or longer. The scales are fine, abundant and adherent on the scalp and in the eyebrows and beard. Glove-like exfoliation of the palms and soles may occur. The condition is recurrent.

Subjective symptoms. The onset is marked by chills, fever up to 40°C, generalized malaise and possibly nausea. Patients may have moderate to severe pruritus.

Etiology. Usually a virus infection or a drug reaction. Diphenylhydantoin may produce this picture; it can be accompanied by marked lymphadenopathy.

Histopathology. No specific picture.

Diagnostic aids. Clinical appearance and history. Elevation of relative and total eosinophil counts.

Relation to systemic disease. No specific relationship.

Differential diagnosis. Scarlet fever, severe sepsis.

Therapy. Systemic corticosteroid therapy with prednisone, 20-60 mg a day, and good nursing care.

Erythrasma

Synonym. None.

Sites of predilection. Axillae, genitocrural region.

Objective signs. Well-defined, confluent, macular lesions with round or serpiginous borders. The areas are reddish-brown and slightly infiltrated. The surface is covered with a fine furfuraceous scale.

Subjective symptoms. Mild to moderate pruritus.

Etiology. Corynebacterium minutissimum.

Histopathology. Linear threads may be demonstrated in the stratum corneum with the Hotchkiss-McManus stain.

Diagnostic aids. Culture on media containing 20% fetal bovine serum. The thin branching hyphae and spores may be demonstrated in a potassium hydroxide preparation. The lesions develop a characteristic, bright red fluorescence on exposure to the Wood light.

Relation to systemic disease. No relationship to any specific disease.

Differential diagnosis. Tinea cruris, tinea versicolor, seborrheic dermatitis, intertrigo.

Therapy. Five percent sulfur-salicylic acid ointment, 1% selenium sulfide ointment, antibacterial soaps, systemic administration of erythromycin.

Fat Necrosis of the Newborn

Synonym. Adiponecrosis subcutanea neonatorum.

Sites of predilection. Trunk, buttocks.

Objective signs. The eruption begins at birth or within the first two weeks of life as one or more nontender, indurated areas which vary in size from 2-10 cm and are scattered over the back and buttocks. The lesions may be pinkish or red only in the early phase of the disease. Although the lesions appear to be slightly elevated, the skin surface is smooth and pale. The lesions do not pit on pressure, have well-defined borders and depressed central portions. Lesions will occur on any part of the body where there is fat. The condition lasts for about two months, then gradually subsides without sequelae.

Subjective symptoms. None.

Etiology. Unknown; possibly some defect in fat metabolism.

Histopathology. There is fat necrosis with the development of needle-like crystals of fat. The infiltrate consists primarily of epithelioid and giant cells (some of which are filled with fat crystals).

Diagnostic aids. Biopsy, history and physical examination.

Relation to systemic disease. None.

Differential diagnosis. Sclerema, scleredema, scleroderma, edema neonatorum.

Therapy. None effective.

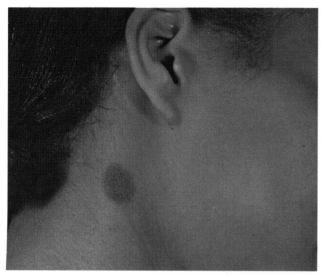

Fixed dermatitis

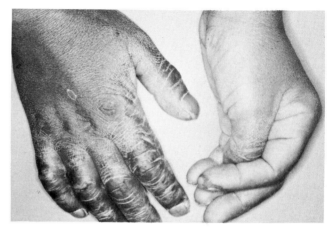

Frostbite

Fixed Drug Eruption

Synonym. Fixed Eruption.

Sites of predilection. Any part of the body.

Objective signs. The primary lesion is a hyper-pigmented macule which is light to dark brown and varies in size and shape. One or more of these lesions may be present. In the active phase the lesions are erythematous and edematous. Occasionally vesicles develop. When the active lesion subsides, areas of hyperpigmentation remain. If the offending substance is readministered systemically, the pigmented areas will reactivate and become inflamed. During the acute phase the lesions may resemble erythema multiforme. The pigmented areas which form the inactive phase are persistent.

Subjective symptoms. During the active stage the symptoms vary from moderate to severe pruritus, but there are no symptoms during the inactive or pigmented stage.

Etiology. This type of allergic reaction is produced by the systemic administration of phenolphthalein,
antipyrine and other drugs.

Histopathology. The histopathologic picture is not diagnostic.

Diagnostic aids. A careful history may reveal the drug responsible for producing the condition. To prove the diagnosis, challenge the inactive patient with a small dose of the suspected allergen.

Relation to systemic disease. This is a specific allergic reaction. The appearance of these lesions may indicate the habitual use of cathartics, coal tar antipyretics or other drugs.

Differential diagnosis. Erythema multiforme, eczema, chronic contact dermatitis.

Therapy. Discontinue use of the offending substance.

Freckles

Synonym. Ephelides, lentigines.

Sites of predilection. Face, forearms, shoulders, back, chest.

Objective signs. Variously sized, discrete, well-defined, brownish macules which range from 1 mm-1 cm in diameter. The number of lesions and the depth of pigmentation is greater in the summer months. There are few freckles found on the distal dorsal digits.

Subjective symptoms. None.

Etiology. The action of sunlight on the exposed surfaces produces these deposits of melanin in the skin. This condition may also be produced by roentgen rays.

Histopathology. An increased deposit of melanin in the basal layer of the epidermis.

Diagnostic aids. Biopsy.

Relation to systemic disease. None.

Differential diagnosis. Xeroderma pigmentosum, urticaria pigmentosa, tinea versicolor, café au lait spots, seborrheic keratosis.

Therapy. None.

Frostbite

Synonym. Chilblains, pernio.

Sites of predilection. Distal portions of the extremities, ears, nose.

Objective signs. Severity of the disorder depends on the duration of cold exposure. Mild cases are manifested initially by blanching; then ill-defined, erythematous macules become infiltrated, and eventually vary in color from dark pink to violaceous. There may be a concomitant reticulated, reddish eruption on the arms and legs. The skin surface feels cool and is somewhat edematous. The acute lesions will usually gradually subside without sequelae. If vascular occlusion occurs, gangrene may develop.

Subjective symptoms. Vary in degree from numbness, tingling, pruritus or burning to intense pain.

Etiology. The condition is common in cold damp climates and occurs as a result of repeated exposure to cold. It most commonly develops in individuals who have a circulatory defect referred to as "chilblain circulation." Alcohol injection can accelerate the process, as can contact of the affected part with a good heat conductor such as metal.

Histopathology. There is vascular dilatation in the upper portion of the cutis with round cell infiltration. Moderate acanthosis and hyperkeratosis are present. In chronic cases there is vascular occlusion and subsequent necrosis.

Diagnostic aids. Clinical appearance supported by history and biopsy.

Relation to systemic disease. Peripheral vascular disease.

Differential diagnosis. Raynaud's disease.

Therapy. In acute cases rapid warming (40-42°C) of involved areas by immersion in warm water is the therapy of choice. If vascular occlusion and gangrene occur, surgical intervention is necessary. In more chronic cases, systemic vasodilators may be of value. Caution should be employed so that the patient dresses properly and does not drink alcohol when exposed to cold.

Graft-vs-Host Reaction

Synonym. Runt disease.

Sites of predilection. None.

Objective signs. A diffuse, confluent, erythematous, nonspecific, maculopapular eruption appears 5-10 days after grafting. Bullae and alopecia may also be present. Later a chronic, mild exfoliative erythroderma occurs within several weeks after the onset of the eruption. This erythroderma may progress to dermal sclerosis, epidermal atrophy, hyperkeratosis, ulceration and reticular hyperpigmentation. There is no tendency to heal. After many weeks or months the skin becomes thin, bronzed and atrophic. Systemic symptoms such as diarrhea, colitis, hepatitis, wasting and eventually death may occur.

Subjective symptoms. Pain, discomfort, malaise.

Etiology. Graft-vs-host reactions may occur in recipients of organ transplants (bone marrow, exchange transfusions, kidney, heart). The mechanism of host cell death (directly by cellular or humoral factors) is unknown.

Histopathology. Exocytosis, discrete acantholysis, basal cell liquefaction and individual cell dyskeratosis or necrosis can be present. A "mummified" body surrounded by satellite lymphocytes in epidermal spaces is also seen in the acute eruption. The chronic pathologic alterations include hyperkeratosis, epidermal atrophy and increased dermal melanin deposition.

Diagnostic aids. History, biopsy.

Relation to systemic disease. A graft-vs-host reaction is a generalized disease.

Differential diagnosis. Seborrheic dermatitis, poikiloderma vasculare atrophicans, Leiner's disease, histiocytosis X, drug eruptions, exfoliative erythrodermas, lymphoma, toxic epidermal necrolysis, lichen planus and viral exanthem.

Therapy. Massive systemic corticosteroids, administration of antileukocyte serum or immunosuppressives. Appropriate systemic antibiotic therapy is prescribed.

Histiocytosis X

Synonym. Several disorders with varying ages of onset and prognosis are encompassed by the term histiocytosis X: Letterer-Siwe disease, Hand-Schüller-Christian disease and eosinophilic granuloma.

Sites of predilection. Scalp, intertriginous folds, trunk.

Objective signs. *Letterer-Siwe Disease.* This is an acute, generalized disease of the very young which is usually fatal. It occurs usually in males and is accompanied by a confluent, scaly, yellow-brown eruption on the scalp, face, neck and trunk. Petechiae may be visible. Other manifestations include vesiculopustules, necrotic mucous membrane ulcers and nodules which may later ulcerate.

Hand-Schüller-Christian disease. This chronic generalized disease occurs in older children and adults. A triad of cranial bone defects, diabetes insipidus and exophthalmos occurs. A chronic otitis media may produce a crusted otitis externa. The eruption is similar to that of Letterer-Siwe disease with less petechiae. Papulopustules, nodules, granulomatous lesions, xanthelasma and bronze pigmentation have been reported. Mucous membrane ulceration may be seen.

Eosinophilic granuloma. This is a benign localized process which produces osteolytic lesions with accompanying cutaneous nodules. Ulcerative or nodular mucous membrane granulomata are seen in the oral cavity or around the genitalia.

Subjective symptoms. Malaise, lassitude, occasional pain.

Etiology. Unknown proliferation of histiocytes.

Histopathology. A proliferation of histiocytes into both the dermis and epidermis is seen with a surrounding granulomatous or xanthomatous reaction. Varying amounts of other cell types may be present in the lesions.

Diagnostic aids. History, physical examination, bone X ray, biopsy.

Relation to systemic disease. Histiocytosis X is a systemic disorder with multisystem involvement.

Differential diagnosis. Letterer-Siwe disease may be confused with seborrheic dermatitis, Darier's disease, pyoderma and hermorrhagic diseases. Hand-Schüller-Christian disease may mimic xanthomas, liver disease or seborrheic dermatitis. Eosinophilic granuloma may resemble any other granuloma.

Therapy. Systemic antibiotics should be used when indicated. Vinblastine therapy is employed in Letterer-Siwe disease. Vinblastine, in addition to corticosteroids and methotrexate, is used in cases of Hand-Schüller-Christian disease and eosinophilic granuloma. Radiotherapy may also be useful in the latter disorder. Other complications such as hemorrhage or diabetes insipidus should be treated specifically.

Ichthyosis

Synonym. Fishskin disease, sauriasis, xeroderma, xerosis, congenital hyperkeratosis.

Types of Ichthyosis	Inheritance	Epidermal Granular Layer	Associated Findings
Ichthyosis vulgaris	Dominant	Absent	Keratosis, fine scales, normal flexors, corneal changes
Lamellar ichthyosis	Recessive	Increased	Ectropion
Epidermolytic hyperkeratosis	Dominant	Normal	Bullae
X-linked ichthyosis	X-linked	Prominent	Corneal damage

Sites of predilection. Trunk, extremities.

Objective signs. The condition may appear at birth or develop shortly thereafter. Confined to the skin, it is more evident on the extensor surfaces of the extremities. During warm weather, lesions almost completely disappear in the majority of patients, but become obvious as soon as cool weather returns. The skin surface in the affected areas is dry and harsh. It is covered with a profuse, adherent, dry scale which is frequently irregularly quadrilateral. The condition may exist in a latent state.

The development of small hyperkeratotic follicular papules on the lateral aspects of the extremities, known as keratosis pilaris, is frequently associated with ichthyosis vulgaris.

Occasionally the condition is so advanced at birth that death occurs immediately or soon thereafter. This condition is known as harlequin fetus: the skin lacks elasticity and large fissures are present on the trunk and at the commissures. Corneal damage and occlusion of the ear canals may be seen.

Subjective symptoms. Patients are irritated by soap and have intense pruritus following the bath. Excessive dryness caused by the extent of the lesions may also cause pruritus.

Etiology. Congenital.

Histopathology. Hyperkeratosis, acanthosis and irregular dermal papillae without any evidence of inflammatory reaction.

Diagnostic aids. History, physical examination.

Relation to systemic disease. The general health of these patients is usually not affected.

Differential diagnosis. Eczema, atopic dermatitis.

Therapy. Therapy is supportive and not curative. Topical retinoic acid is effective in many cases. Current research studies are evaluating the use of oral retinoic acid in lamellar ichthyosis.

Impetigo Neonatorum

Synonym. Ritter's disease, pemphigus neonatorum, dermatitis exfoliativa neonatorum.

Sites of predilection. Generalized.

Objective signs. The primary lesion may begin as an erythematous macule or bleb which spreads to involve the entire body. Vesicles, vesicopustules and bullae develop and spread. Pus rapidly develops in the bullae and vesicles. Exfoliation occurs in large plaques. Fissues develop at the mouth angles. Blood, serous and pus crusts form in areas of ruptured vesicles and blebs. The child may have stomatitis, rhinitis, corneal ulcers and cachexia.

Subjective symptoms. Chills, fever and loss of appetite. This is a serious illness which may terminate in death.

Etiology. Staphylococci.

Histopathology. Edema of the epidermis. Vascular dilatation is present in the papillary portion of the corium and there is a cellular infiltrate composed of polymorphonuclear leukocytes and lymphocytes.

Diagnostic aids. Culture and sensitivity tests of the exudate.

Relation to systemic disease. This condition may precede the onset of bacteremia and terminate in death. It may also be the presentation of an immune deficiency.

Differential diagnosis. Leiner's disease, scarlatina, ichthyosis, eczema, epidermolysis bullosa.

Therapy. These children should be hospitalized and

isolated. Systemic antibiotics are essential. Gently compress or sponge with warm normal saline to remove crusts and detritus.

Incontinentia Pigmenti

Synonym. Bloch-Sulzberger syndrome.

Sites of predilection. Trunk, extremities.

Objectives signs. This condition primarily occurs in female infants. Lesions may be present at birth or develop during the first 10 days of life. Although there are three clinical stages, they may or may not occur in sequential order. Clear tense bullae develop in recurrent linear groups. These lesions are followed by irregular linear groups of reddish papules and subsequent linear groups of warty lesions. The eruption may be followed by pigmentary changes which appear in whorls and swirls producing a bizarre pattern. In many patients the pigmentary changes are present at birth and the other stages do not occur. Small patches of alopecia may occur and nails may be dystrophic.

Subjective symptoms. None produced by the cutaneous lesions.

Etiology. This condition is transmitted by an autosomal dominant gene.

Histopathology. The vesicular phase is characterized by an intraepidermal vesicle containing eosinophils in the exudative fluid and the dermis. The papular phase is composed of hyperkeratotic and acanthotic lesions. Increased chromatophores full of melanin are present in the upper dermis in the final stage of the disorder.

Diagnostic aids. History, clinical appearance, biopsy.

Relation to systemic disease. Dental and ocular defects including cataracts, optic atrophy and fibrolenticular dysplasias develop. Patients may have mental retardation, epilepsy or spastic paraplegia.

Differential diagnosis. Bullous pemphigoid, epidermolysis bullosa, pemphigus vulgaris.

Therapy. No therapy is effective.

Intertrigo

Synonym. Chafing.

Sites of predilection. Occurs on apposing surfaces such as under the breasts, between the folds of the abdomen, thighs and buttocks.

Objective signs. Well-defined to partially defined, bright pink, macular lesions which are edematous, moist and macerated. The lesions may eventually become infiltrated and eroded.

Subjective symptoms. Moderate to intense pruritus. Fissures may be painful.

Etiology. The condition may be precipitated between the apposing surfaces by the irritating action of soap, deodorant, bath powder, perfume, *etc*. Intertrigo is not a specific disease, but is a symptom of maceration or occasionally of seborrheic dermatitis or psoriasis. The lesions frequently become secondarily infected by *C albicans*.

Histopathology. No specific picture.

Diagnostic aids. Culture on Mycosel® or DTM media, confirmed by cornmeal agar transfer.

Relation to systemic disease. Intertrigo often develops in obese patients; monilial infections are common in obese diabetic patients.

Therapy. The selection of the treatment method depends upon the causative factor.

Keratoderma Climactericum

Synonym. None.

Sites of predilection. Palms, soles or both.

Objective signs. These lesions occur predominantly in women between 40 and 60 years of age. They appear as circumscribed areas of keratoderma which increase in thickness over the heels and transverse arches. At first the lesions are discrete and then become confluent. The skin becomes exceptionally dry over the involved areas, and develops fissures. Similar lesions may develop on the palms. Women who are affected by this condition are usually greatly overweight. The condition is usually much worse during the winter.

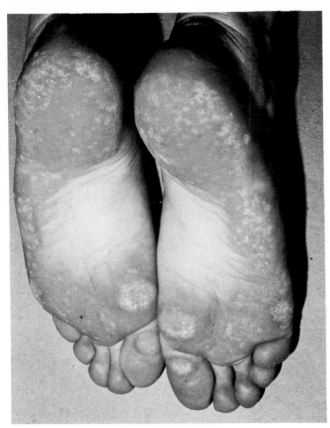

Keratoderma climactericum

Subjective symptoms. Pain and tenderness, particularly when the patient stands or walks for any length of time.

Etiology. A possible hormone dysfunction exists but no specific endocrine factor can be incriminated.

Histopathology. Dense hyperkeratosis.

Diagnostic aids. Clinical appearance and biopsy.

Relation to systemic disease. Patient should be studied for hormone dysfunction if other symptoms are present. Obesity is a concomitant finding.

Differential diagnosis. Calluses and plantar corns.

Therapy. Patient should be put on a weight reduction schedule. Topical application of 15-20% salicylic acid in petrolatum or Aquaphor.

Keratosis Palmaris et Plantaris

Synonym. Ichthyosis palmaris et plantaris.

Sites of predilection. Palms, soles.

Objective signs. This is a congenital condition in which the tissues of the palms and soles are symmetrically hyperkeratotic. The intense hyperkeratosis varies in color from a dirty gray to brown and the surface is exceptionally dry. The condition varies from slight roughness to marked thickening of the keratin layer and intensification of the surface markings. Loss of elasticity is productive of painful fissure formation.

Subjective symptoms. Discomfort caused by inability to close the hands or bend the feet; pain caused by fissure formation.

Etiology. The condition is usually hereditary as a dominant characteristic. It is occasionally associated with ichthyosis or several other congenital cutaneous abnormalities.

Histopathology. Marked hyperkeratosis and acanthosis without any evidence of inflammatory reaction.

Diagnostic aids. None specific; history and physical examination.

Relation to systemic disease. The general health is usually not involved.

Differential diagnosis. Dermatophytosis, eczema, calluses, arsenical keratoses, contact dermatitis.

Therapy. Emollients.

Leprosy

Synonym. Hansen's disease.

Leprosy is classified primarily on the basis of clinical manifestations but laboratory confirmation is mandatory. Bacterial studies, lepromin test and histopathologic examinations must be performed. The lepromatous, tuberculoid and borderline types are clinically recognized. An indeterminate group of patients exhibit benign, but usually unstable, manifestations which develop into lepromatous or tuberculoid leprosy or remain indeterminate indefinitely. The borderline or dimorphic group is the unstable malignant form in which the lepromin test is generally negative. The lesions in this type are flat, bands or nodules with regional distribution similar to that of the lepromatous type (see Chapter 15).

Leprosy, Tuberculoid

Sites of predilection. Trunk, elbows, knees, face.
Objective signs. The condition begins as reddish, variously sized macules which range from 3-10

Tuberculoid leprosy

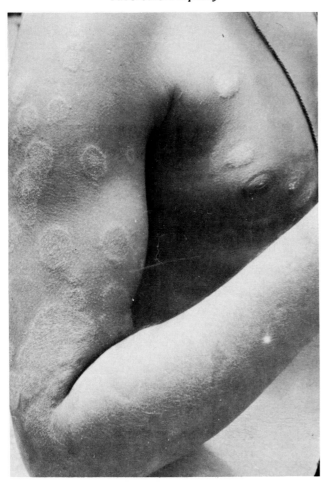

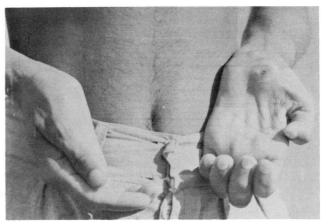

Leprosy, showing claw hand and trophic ulcer

cm or more in diameter. The lesions are well-defined and usually coalesce, forming large areas which change to a yellowish or brownish color and later become depigmented. Trophic changes may occur in the vicinity of the patches. The hair in the involved area becomes depigmented. The course of the disease is slowly progressive over many years. The large nerve trunks, particularly the ulnar and peroneal become thickened, rope-like and tender. The macular skin lesions may become anesthetic. Trophic changes including ulcers and bone resorption occur on the extremities. Alopecia, eye lesions and mucous membrane lesions may develop.

Subjective symptoms. The macular lesions are initially sensitive but later become partially anesthetic. The large nerve trunks may be tender.

Etiology. Mycobacterium leprae. The mode of transmission is unknown. Infection occurs only after prolonged and close contact.

Histopatholgy. All active leprosy lesions have a tuberculoid histologic structure. The nodules consist of masses of connective tissue cells with intermingled lymphocytes, plasma cells and mast cells.

Diagnostic aids. The lepromin test is negative in the lepromatous type. Biopsy findings are characteristic.

Relation to systemic disease. The patient with tuberculoid leprosy may live for many years.

Differential diagnosis. Syphilis, sarcoidosis, tuberculosis, syringomyelia, vitiligo, lupus erythematosus, lupus vulgaris, leukemia cutis.

Therapy. Chemotherapy with sulfones or rifampin is specific.

Leukemia Cutis

Synonym. Leukemia with cutaneous manifestations.

Sites of predilection. Generalized.

Objective signs. There is usually a widespread, confluent, erythematous, macular eruption which is pink to dark red or violaceous in color. The lesions are moderately to markedly infiltrated and lichenification may be pronounced. Occasionally the involved areas are covered with a moderate amount of adherent dry scale. Linear excoriations and blood crusts are part of the clinical picture. Other cutaneous lesions occasionally associated with the leukemias are purpura of various types, bullae, nodules and ulcerations.

Subjective symptoms. Pruritus is usually intense.

Etiology. Unknown. The development of these cutaneous lesions may precede the appearance of changes in the circulating blood.

Histopathology. There is a well-demarcated infiltrate of round cells and occasionally large lymphoblasts in the upper layers of the cutis. The infiltrate is not necessarily limited to nodules or tumors. There is some acanthosis and hyperkeratosis.

Diagnostic aids. Biopsy, blood count, bone marrow aspirate or biopsy, history and physical examination.

Relation to systemic disease. The condition is a cutaneous manifestation of a systemic disease. The appearance of the cutaneous lesions frequently precedes onset of changes in the blood picture.

Differential diagnosis. Eczema, seborrheic dermatitis, exfoliative dermatitis, atopic dermatitis, Hodgkin's disease. Diphenylhydantoin may produce an acute syndrome with lymphadenopathy, fever and an eruption similar to early stages of leukemia cutis.

Therapy. Treatment of systemic disease. Local therapy is of no value.

LUPUS ERYTHEMATOSUS

Lupus erythematosus is a constitutional disease because, regardless of the clinical type, discoid, subacute or disseminated, it extends beyond the skin and affects the entire body. Like other collagen diseases its symptoms are inconstant; however, the basic pathologic features observed in the discoid form are similar to those of the systemic form. Variations in the clinical picture correspond to the different developmental stages of the disease. The transition from discoid lupus erythematosus to the final severe picture of systemic lupus erythematosus is frequently characterized by a corresponding increase in intensity and extent of the cutaneous lesions with the development of visceral symptoms. In some patients the symptoms of systemic lupus erythematosus develop in the absence of cutaneous lesions.

Lupus erythematosus is an autoimmune disease which occurs most frequently in women between the ages of 20 and 40 years. Approximately 5% of those patients who have discoid lupus erythematosus eventually develop systemic manifestations. In systemic lupus erythematosus, hypergammaglobulinemia is a constant finding. Hematologic abnormalities include hypochromic and hemolytic anemias, leukopenia, granulocytopenia, eosinophilia, increased erythrocyte sedimentation rate, cold agglutinins, a positive direct Coombs' test, positive antinuclear (peripheral, homogenous or speckled patterns) circulating DNA complexes and antibodies to double-stranded DNA antibody test. The lupus erythematosus cell and characteristic patchy positive immunofluorescence band to IgG, IgM, as well as C1g, C3 and C4, at the epidermal basement membrane is present. Biologic false-positive serologic tests for syphilis and abnormal liver function tests may occur.

Actinic trauma may precipitate or aggravate lupus erythematosus. The sunburning spectrum is regarded as the most damaging.

Lupus Erythematosus, Discoid

Synonym. None.

Sites of predilection. Face, scalp, ears, neck; other areas may be involved.

Objective signs. There are one or more sharply defined, slightly raised macules which are usually asymmetric. The lesions are dull pink to red and are covered with a scant amount of adherent dry scale. The lesions spread peripherally. Butterfly lesions occasionally develop on the face. In older lesions the inflammatory reaction occurs primarily in the margin and the central areas are atrophic and depigmented. Telangiectases may occur. The dilated follicular orifices are filled with hyperkeratotic material (follicular plugs). Mucous membrane lesions simulating leukoplakia may develop. Inactive lesions are atrophic scars with hyperpigmented margins. When discoid lupus erythematosus (DLE) lesions involve the scalp, a scarred permanent alopecia develops.

Subjective symptoms. Mild pruritus or burning may be present. In extensive discoid lesions, the cosmetic defect may cause emotional imbalance.

Etiology. Unknown.

Histopathology. Atrophy of the epidermis and epidermal appendages, hyperkeratotic plugging, slight edema of the lower epidermal cells (liquefactive degeneration of the basal layer), and a dense, well-defined mononuclear cell infiltrate which tends to be periappendageal.

Diagnostic aids. Biopsy; the histopathologic picture is diagnostic. Positive immunofluorescence at the epidermal basement membrane is present in involved skin only. Lupus erythematosus cell

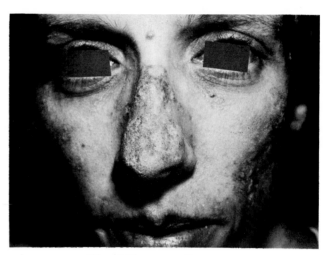

Discoid lupus erythematosus

studies, serum antinuclear antibody, hemograms, albumin-globulin ratio, urinalysis, liver function studies, X-ray examination of the chest. The presence of double-stranded DNA antibodies in the serum is regarded as a bad prognostic sign.

Relation to systemic disease. Although in the vast majority of cases, the discoid variety of lupus erythematosus runs a chronic benign course, approximately 5% of these patients eventually develop symptoms of systemic lupus erythematosus. The clinical picture of lupus erythematosus does not exclude the possibility of systemic disease. The diagnosis must be confirmed by laboratory findings in each patient. Patients with discoid LE must be checked periodically for possible development of the systemic form.

Differential diagnosis. Seborrheic dermatitis, rosacea, eczema, psoriasis, erysipelas, sarcoidosis, lupus vulgaris.

Therapy. Hydroxychloroquine, an antimalarial, is effective in treating DLE. Before using this drug the patient should have an ophthalmoscopic examination which should be repeated every 6 months. Topical corticosteroid creams under occlusive plastic dressings are effective. Avoid unnecessary exposure to sunlight. The use of sunscreens is important.

Lupus Erythematosus, Systemic

Synonym. None.

Sites of predilection. Generalized.

Objective signs. Discrete and confluent, sharply defined, pinkish, edematous macules. Telangiectases may develop and occasionally the lesions become hemorrhagic or vesicular. On the hands the distal phalanges develop a bluish-red discoloration and on the feet the lateral margins, the transverse arch and the distal phalanges develop a similar appearance. The early lesions may simulate erythema multiforme or urticaria. Older lesions on the face and trunk may become covered with adherent dry scale. Atrophic scarring is usually not present unless discoid lesions precede the systemic manifestations. Fever may be present. In many cases these lesions are symmetrically distributed.

Subjective symptoms. Generalized malaise, loss of weight, night sweats, joint pains, muscle tenderness and gastric disturbances.

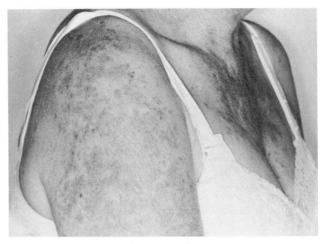

Systemic lupus erythematosus

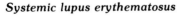

Systemic lupus erythematosus

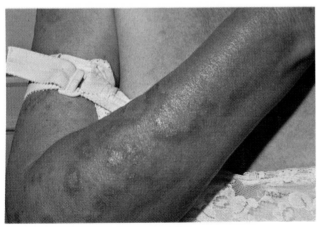

Etiology. An autoimmune tissue disease which occurs most commonly in women.

Histopathology. Atrophy of the epidermis with severe edema in the lower cells of the rete; lack of infiltrate; marked edema in the cutis. A patchy immunofluorescent band is present on the basement membrane of both involved and uninvolved skin.

Diagnostic aids. Biopsy; lupus erythematosus cell studies; immunofluorescent antinuclear antibody titers (over 1:32) with homogenous, speckled or peripheral patterns; antidouble-stranded DNA antibodies; albumin-globulin ratio; hemograms; chest X ray; liver function studies; electrocardiogram; serum protein; electrophoresis.

Relation to systemic disease. This is a systemic illness which occasionally develops in the absence of skin lesions. Clinical manifestations are frequently produced by excessive exposure to sunlight. Systemic manifestations of lupus erythematosus include: hepatitis, bronchopneumonia, pulmonary abscess, pleural effusions, verrucous endocarditis, depression of the bone marrow, polyserositis, peritonitis, nephrosis, nephritis, thrombocytopenic purpura, and central nervous system symptoms.

Differential diagnosis. The cutaneous lesions resemble those of purpura, erythema multiforme, urticaria, seborrheic dermatitis or eczema.

Therapy. Systemic corticosteroid therapy using adequate dosage of prednisone (or other corticosteroid). It may be necessary to use supplementary therapy with immunosuppressive drugs. Supportive treatment. Avoid exposure to sunlight. Systemic lupus erythematosus may run a benign course not requiring intensive corticosteroid therapy. Because many drugs either stimulate or produce reactions which simulate lupus erythematosus, all unncessary drugs should be withdrawn.

Melasma

Synonym. Liver spots.

Sites of predilection. Face, genitalia, areolae of breasts.

Objective signs. Variously sized, well-defined, non-scaly, light to dark brown macules. These lesions vary in size from 2-4 cm or larger. There is no evidence of any previously existing active inflammatory process. Intensification of normal pigment on genitalia or areolae of breasts occurs if the patient is pregnant.

Subjective symptoms. Emotional distress produced by the cosmetic defect.

Etiology. Unknown.

Histopathology. Increase in the melanin content of the basal layer.

Diagnostic aids. Biopsy findings are not specific.

Relation to systemic disease. The condition may indicate the presence of an ovarian tumor, pregnancy, liver disease, hormonal dysfunction or ingestion of exogenous estrogens.

Differential diagnosis. Postinflammatory hyperpigmentation, postradiation hyperpigmentation, argyria, Addison's disease.

Therapy. Avoidance of exposure to sunlight. The use of a bleaching preparation such as hydroquinone (3-5%) with 1% hydrocortisone in a cream or ointment base in conjunction with topical retinoic or salicylic acids.

Mole, Pigmented

Synonym. Pigmented nevus, birthmark, mole, hairy mole, bathing trunk nevus, nevus pilosus, junction nevus, nevus pigmentosus.

Sites of predilection. May occur on any part of the body. The bathing trunk nevus involves the lower trunk and upper thighs.

Objective signs. These lesions are well-defined macules which are most commonly present at birth or develop during the first few years of life. The lesions vary in size and shape from a few millimeters to large plaques many centimeters in diameter. Nevi vary in color from tan to dark brown or black. They are soft in texture, not inflamed and not elevated. Dark brown to blackish papules may appear in the larger plaque-like lesions.

The bathing trunk nevus is a medium to dark brown nevus which involves the lower trunk, the genitalia and the upper portions of the thighs. There is profuse hair growth within the confines of the lesion.

Nevus pilosus is the name applied to a macular nevus in which there is a profuse growth of hair.

Subjective symptoms. None except the embarrassment caused by the cosmetic defect.

Etiology. Congenital.

Histopathology. The nevus cells are characteristically large, pale or dark, and have oval nuclei. These cells, occurring in strands and nests, are massed in the cutis.

Diagnostic aids. Biopsy.

Relation to systemic disease. None.

Differential diagnosis. Varicosities, café au lait spots of neurofibromatosis, warts of various types.

Therapy. There is no specific treatment. The larger lesions may be removed by plastic repair. These lesions do not respond to radiation. Prophylactic removal of the lesions because of the chance of malignant transformation has to be individualized. Patients who have a family history of melanoma and who have clusters of 3-5 nevi, each with a differing morphologic pattern, may have nevi transforming to malignancy (BK syndrome). Also, large bathing trunk nevi are more apt to have a higher incidence for malignant transformation than other nevi.

Mongolian Blue Spot

Synonym. None.
Sites of predilection. Lower sacral area.
Objective signs. Variously sized and shaped, bluish or dark brown, macular lesions which range from 2-10 cm in diameter. The lesions are partially to well-defined, of normal skin texture and noninflammatory. They are more commonly seen in dark-skinned peoples. These nevoid lesions usually disappear or become less obvious after a few months.
Subjective symptoms. None.
Etiology. Congenital.
Histopathology. The spindle-shaped, pigmented nevus cells are present deep in the dermis.
Diagnostic aids. Biopsy, history and physical examination.
Relation to systemic disease. None.
Differential diagnosis. Nevus of any type.
Therapy. None. The condition is usually self-limited.

Mycosis Fungoides

Synonym. None.
Sites of predilection. Generalized.
Objective signs. This peculiar neoplastic disease begins in the skin. The cutaneous manifestations are divided into four stages: dermatitis, infiltration, tumor and ulceration.

In the first stage there are few to numerous, localized areas of dermatitis which may be discrete or confluent, ill-defined or partially defined, round or oval, and either dry or moist. The presence of any chronic lichenified eruption which does not respond to treatment should suggest the possibility of mycosis fungoides.

During the second stage, circumscribed areas of lichenified infiltrated dermatitis develop. The lesions range from 1-10 cm in diameter and may be intermingled with the plaque-like lesions described in the first stage. Scaling lesions resembling those of psoriasis may be present. Annular and gyrate lesions may develop.

The tumor phase gradually develops following the stage of infiltration. The growths vary in size and shape and usually arise from lichenified plaques. These lesions seldom cause any subjective symptoms and they may disappear spontaneously. Occasionally tumors arise in an area of skin not previously involved by the process.

During the ulcerative phase the tumors or infiltrated lesions break down, eventually developing granulomatous, mushroom-like masses.
Subjective symptoms. Pruritus during the first and second phases. During the tumor phase and the stage of ulceration the lesions may be painful.
Etiology. Unknown.
Histopathology. The well-defined cellular infiltrate in the upper layers of the cutis is polymorphous and is localized in the papillary portion. Mycosis fungoides or Sézary cells are present. There is acanthosis of the rete with both intercellular and intracellular edema. Microabscesses (Pautrier) form in the epidermis.
Diagnostic aids. Biopsy, ultramicroscopic survey of the biopsies for characteristic cells, sternal marrow puncture.
Relation to systemic disease. Other organs in the body may be involved. The prognosis is uncertain; however, once the tumor phase is reached, death may be anticipated in 5-10 years.

Differential diagnosis. In the first phase the condition may mimic parapsoriasis en plaques, poikiloderma atrophicans vasculare, mild radiodermatitis, eczema, psoriasis or lichenified dermatitis. Later stages may resemble leprosy, sarcoidosis, tuberculosis or other granulomatous diseases.

Therapy. The cutaneous lesions frequently respond to conventional X-ray or grenz-ray therapy. Topical nitrogen mustard or systemic antimetabolites, such as methotrexate or vincristine, are of value in some cases. Recent studies indicate that PUVA therapy will cause involution of some lesions.

Myringomycosis
(Ringworm of the Ear Canals)

Although this diagnosis is frequently made clinically there is no laboratory foundation for its existence. In patients with poor hygiene heavy wax deposits are formed in the ear canal, and opportunistic fungi will form a surface growth.

What is thought to be a mycotic infection is usually seborrheic dermatitis or neurodermatitis. The intensity of the lesions varies from mild erythema to lichenification with scaling and fissure formation. Occasionally, secondary pyogenic infection develops. Associated with this condition, in the presence of secondary pyogenic infection, is the eruption known as infectious eczematoid dermatitis.

Myxedema, Generalized

Synonym. Hypothyroidism.

Sites of predilection. Generalized.

Objective signs. The skin is dry, yellowish and edematous but does not pit on pressure. The lips and nose are thickened and the eyelids droop, forming the mask-like, expressionless facies characteristic of the condition. There is irregular hyperpigmentation on exposed surfaces. The nails become fragile and there is thinning of hair in the frontotemporal areas and in the lateral third of the eyebrows. Hyperkeratoses may develop on the palms and soles. The patient is subnormal mentally, moves sluggishly, is apathetic, and his hearing and speech are affected.

Subjective symptoms. The cutaneous lesions are not productive of subjective symptoms.

Etiology. Hypothyroidism. The condition may develop following thyroidectomy.

Histopathology. Mucinous infiltration of the dermis with development of immature connective tissue cells. PAS staining material may be found around the sweat glands.

Diagnostic aids. History and physical examination, thyroxin blood levels, serum carotene determination, skin biopsy, pituitary function test.

Relation to systemic disease. Myxedema is caused by primary thyroid disease or secondary thyroid hypofunction due to pituitary failure.

Differential diagnosis. Scleroderma, scleredema, elephantiasis.

Therapy. Thyroid hormone replacement.

Myxedema, Localized Pretibial

Synonym. Pretibial myxedema.

Sites of predilection. Extensor surfaces of the legs.

Objective signs. The lesions are variously sized, irregular plaques of non-pitting edema. Small papules may be present on the surface of the lesions. The follicular orifices are greatly dilated. The color of the skin in the involved area varies from pale yellow to light reddish-brown.

Subjective symptoms. The cutaneous lesions are asymptomatic.

Etiology. The mechanism of production of localized myxedema in the presence of hyperthyroidism is unknown. It has been theorized that the mechanism of production of localized myxedema is the same as that responsible for the production of exophthalmos. The relationship of pretibial myxedema with long-acting thyroid stimulating hormone (LATS) is unclear. The lesions may develop following thyroidectomy, radiation therapy

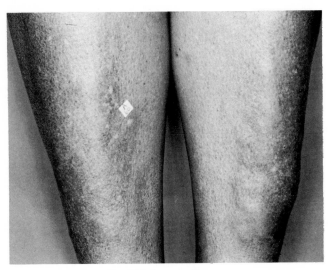

Pretibial myxedema

of hyperactive thyroid or chemotherapy of hyperthyroidism.

Histopathology. There is mucinous infiltration in the dermis and immature connective tissue cells are present.

Diagnostic aids. History and physical examination, biopsy of skin lesions, thyroxin blood levels, thyroid scan.

Relation to systemic disease. Associated with localized myxedema, there are usually signs of hyperthyroidism, including exophthalmos, but in rare instances the thyroid function may be normal or depressed.

Differential diagnosis. Elephantiasis, scleroderma.

Therapy. There is no specific therapy for the cutaneous lesion. Some improvement may be obtained by using fluorinated corticosteroid creams under occlusion.

Nevus, Anemic

Synonym. Nevus anemicus.

Sites of predilection. Chest, face, back and other areas of the body.

Objective signs. The lesions, which vary in size and shape from 2-5 cm in diameter, are depigmented macules. The borders are sharply defined and the surrounding skin is normal in color. There is no change in skin texture.

Subjective symptoms. None.

Etiology. Congenital.

Histopathology. There is a lack of blood vessels in the involved areas. Elastic fibers are normal in amount. The epidermis is unchanged.

Diagnostic aids. History and physical examination, biopsy.

Relation to systemic disease. Often found in patients with von Recklinghausen's disease.

Differential diagnosis. Vitiligo.

Therapy. None.

Nevus, Comedo

Synonym. Follicular nevus, nevus comedonicus.

Sites of predilection. Face, trunk.

Objective signs. A unilateral, circumscribed area which varies in size and is irregularly shaped, and in which there are numerous lesions resembling comedones. These comedo-like lesions are dilated follicles filled with keratin. Cystic lesions and acneform lesions may develop.

Subjective symptoms. None.

Etiology. Congenital.

Histopathology. Cystic cavities in the follicle are lined with fat cells, and atrophic or proliferating stratified hyperkeratotic epithelium. The sweat and sebaceous glands in the region of the nevus are distorted. Usually no hair shaft is seen.

Diagnostic aids. Biopsy.

Relation to systemic disease. None.

Differential diagnosis. Chloracne, tattoo.

Therapy. Excision and plastic repair.

Nevus Flammeus

Synonym. Vascular nevus, port-wine stain.

Sites of predilection. Any part of the body.

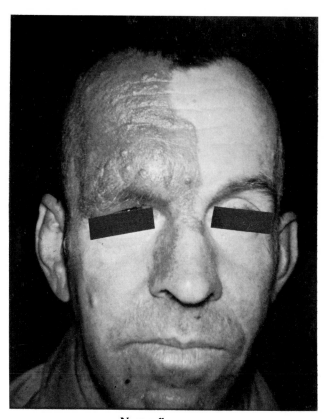

Nevus flammeus

Subjective symptoms. None except the embarrassment caused by the cosmetic defect.

Etiology. Congenital.

Histopathology. This varies with the extent and severity of the lesion and may be manifested as simple acanthosis with vascular dilatation in the upper dermis.

Diagnostic aids. Clinical appearance, biopsy.

Relation to systemic disease. May be associated with the Sturge-Weber syndrome.

Differential diagnosis. Clinical appearance is diagnostic.

Therapy. Small lesions may be obliterated by the use of carbon dioxide snow. The use of a covering cosmetic is helpful in improving the appearance of the lesion.

Nevus, Halo

Synonym. Sutton's nevus, leukoderma acquisitum centrifugum.

Sites of predilection. Trunk.

Objective signs. The lesion is a depigmented macule which varies from 1-3 cm in diameter. In the center of the vitiliginous area there is a small brown maculopapule.

Halo nevus

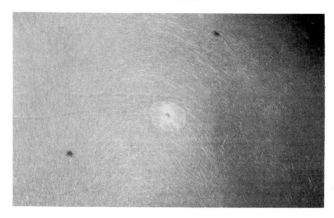

Objective signs. These well-defined, red to purplish-red, macular lesions vary from 1-20 cm or more in diameter. The lesions may be slightly raised, presenting a plaque-like appearance, with few to numerous dark papules or nodules scattered over the surface.

A variant of this nevus is the irregularly shaped, reddish, macular lesion which frequently occurs on the back of the neck, just below the external occipital protuberance and makes its appearance at birth. This type of lesion may frequently disappear spontaneously within the first 10 years of life or be persistent.

Subjective symptoms. None.

Etiology. Congenital.

Histopathology. The central nevus consists of an intradermal mass of melanophores. Arrest of melanosome maturation is present in the halo. Halo nevi are rarely malignant in behavior, yet there is some speculation that these lesions are resolving melanomas.

Diagnostic aids. Biopsy.

Relation to systemic disease. None.

Differential diagnosis. Vitiligo.

Therapy. None. The condition is self-limited. Lesions disappear spontaneously.

Nevus, Spider

Synonym. Spider mole, nevus araneus.

Sites of predilection. Face, trunk, extremities.

Objective signs. This common vascular nevus consists of a tiny, central, red spot from which numerous, tortuous, minute vessels radiate for a short distance. The central point may be slightly elevated. The lesion may pulsate. In children these lesions are frequently self-limited; in adults, they are persistent.

Subjective symptoms. None.

Etiology. Exact cause unknown. Increased estrogens at the skin level may play a role.

Histopathology. The microscopic picture is not diagnostic.

Diagnostic aids. Clinical appearance.

Relation to systemic disease. These lesions are also associated with chronic alchoholism, estrogen hormone therapy, pregnancy and liver disease.

Differential diagnosis. Telangiectases from any cause.

Therapy. In young children or pregnant women the lesions are usually self-limited and no treatment is indicated. In adults the lesions may be obliterated by the use of electrolysis or high frequency current. The needle must be inserted into the central vessel before the current is turned on.

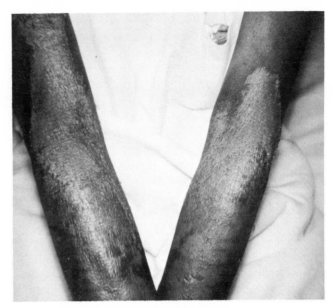

Pellagra

Pellagra

Synonym. None.

Sites of predilection. Dorsal surfaces of the hands, wrists and forearms; the face, neck and exposed portion of the chest; the feet and legs. Mucous membranes are also involved.

Objective signs. The cutaneous lesions begin as erythematous macules simulating sunburn. As the eruption develops the lesions become dark red and hyperpigmented. The skin in the involved areas is edematous and exfoliation occurs in large flakes or plaques. The eruption is usually sharply demarcated at the distal thirds of the forearms and the legs, producing the so-called "glove and stocking" appearance. In intervals between attacks, the skin retains its hyperpigmentation, but with repeated attacks, hyperkeratotic lesions may develop on the exposed surfaces. Chronic lesions present a "scalded" appearance.

Associated with the cutaneous lesions is fissure formation at the commissures of the lips (perlèche), and a beefy, red appearance of the tongue and buccal mucosa.

Severe systemic symptoms are associated with the cutaneous and mucous membrane lesions.

Sunlight aggravates the eruption.

Subjective symptoms. Cutaneous lesions itch or burn. Other symptoms vary in severity with the degree of systemic involvement.

Etiology. Deficiency in the vitamin B complex, particularly nicotinic acid. Dietary inadequacy.

Histopathology. Nonspecific. There is irregular hyperkeratosis, atrophy of the epidermis and an inflammatory infiltrate in the upper layers of the cutis.

Diagnostic aids. History and physical examination.

Relation to systemic disease. The cutaneous lesions are important as diagnostic factors only. This is a specific avitaminosis. The classic "four D's," dermatitis, diarrhea, dementia and death, indicate the degrees of severity.

Neurologic manifestations include polyneuritis and paresthesias. Psychotic symptoms may be mild or severe. Gastrointestinal symptoms vary from mild, digestive disturbances to severe, watery diarrhea. Secondary monilial infection may occur in the mouth or about the genitalia. Emaciation and weakness may be extreme.

Although this condition predominates in people of the lower economic strata and the elderly, the condition also occurs in chronic alcoholics, patients with bowel resection or mentally defective individuals who refuse to eat proper foods.

Differential diagnosis. Eczema, sunburn, seborrheic dermatitis, contact dermatitis, Hartnup disease.

Therapy. Nicotinic acid by mouth or by injection; vitamin B complex by mouth or by injection; adequately balanced diet containing large amounts of protein; restriction of alcohol intake and solar exposure.

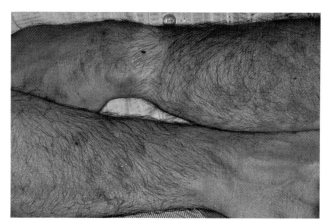

Photosensitivity

Photosensitivity

Photosensitivity is an abnormal skin reaction to exposure to light. It may be an exaggeration of a normal sunburn response or an allergic reaction. Light-induced eruptions may be classified as either phototoxic or photoallergic. The phototoxic eruptions involve the majority of people and develop within a few hours after exposure. They may be provoked by intense light or light-sensitive chemicals. The pathology is predominantly in the epidermis. These patients develop a uniform erythematous eruption confined to the exposed areas. Photopatch testing may reveal a positive reaction in most of the population.

Photoallergic reactions affect relatively few people and do not occur with the initial exposure to the drug. The incubation period may be delayed and the lesions can be induced by short exposures to light. Although the predominant eruption occurs on the exposed areas, other sites of the body may be involved. These patients have an allergic response to a photopatch test.

Photosensitivity eruptions may be produced by many drugs including the sulfonamides, antibiotics, phenothiazines, antihistamines, barbiturates, and antimalarials.

Included among the light-sensitive dermatoses are the congenital poikilodermas, phenylketonuria, albinism, pellagra, porphyrias, lupus erythematosus and eruptions produced by the contact photosensitizing agent.

Pigmentary Dermatosis, Progressive

Synonym. Schamberg's disease, hemosiderosis.
Sites of predilection. Lower extremities.
Objective signs. The eruption begins with the development of minute, pinpoint, reddish, macular lesions which spread peripherally to form irregular confluent areas. The reddish spots (cayenne pepper spots) eventually disappear, leaving confluent, brownish or reddish brown pigmented areas which may be persistent or slowly fade. Lichenification and scaling may develop as secondary manifestations. Purpura annularis telangiectodes (Majocchi's disease) and pigmented purpuric lichenoid dermatitis present a similar appearance and are probably variants of the same pathologic process.
Subjective symptoms. None.
Etiology. Unknown.
Histopathology. The epidermis may be normal or hyperkeratotic and hyperpigmented. The cellular infiltrate in the cutis consists of connective tissue cells and polymorphonuclear leukocytes, some of which contain iron pigment granules. When the inflammatory reaction subsides there is a deposit of hemosiderin.
Diagnostic aids. Biopsy. Platelet count should be normal.
Relation to systemic disease. None has been determined. This is a purpuric eruption; therefore, laboratory studies must be performed to rule out any systemic disease.
Differential diagnosis. Stasis dermatitis, idiopathic thrombocytopenic purpura.
Therapy. None of value.

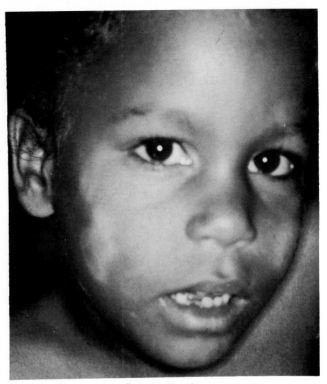

Pityriasis alba

Pityriasis Alba

Synonym. None.
Sites of predilection. Face, chest, upper extremities.
Objective signs. The lesions are ill-defined or partially defined, slightly scaly, partially depigmented macules. It occurs most commonly in infants and young children. It may begin as an erythematous macule which is slightly scaly, and when the erythema subsides, the depigmentation remains. This condition occurs in all races. It may be a variant of seborrheic dermatitis.
Subjective symptoms. None as a general rule. Slight pruritus may be present.
Etiology. Unknown.

Histopathology. Slight hyperkeratosis and acanthosis with a nonspecific cellular infiltrate in the upper layer of the cutis.

Diagnostic aids. Clinical appearance.

Relation to systemic disease. None.

Differential diagnosis. Vitiligo, eczema, tinea circinata, tinea versicolor.

Therapy. The condition is usually self-limited, but several months may be required for its resolution. An ointment containing 2.5% salicylic acid and precipitated sulfur in petrolatum is usually satisfactory. Topical corticosteroids may be useful.

Pityriasis Rosea

Synonym. None.

Sites of predilection. Trunk, neck, thighs, arms. Lesions seldom appear on the face.

Objective signs. A herald patch may precede the onset of the generalized eruption by 1-3 weeks. This patch is a single large, round or oval, slightly scaly, annular lesion which may be located anywhere on the body. The herald patch is not always present. The generalized eruption consists of numerous discrete, pinkish, oval or round, macular or papular, well-defined lesions. Central involution may occur, forming annular lesions which vary in color from dull red to pink. Scale formation may be central or marginal, but it usually peels toward the margin. The long axes of the oval lesions parallel the lines of cleavage. In adults, these lesions spare the palms, soles and central face. Some patients may have only a few lesions which may be restricted to the shoulders or hips.

Because of overzealous treatment or local irritation, the eruption may become eczematized, and the lesions lose their sharp definition. Children may have lesions which are only papular or follicular.

The eruption is self-limited, disappearing spontaneously in 8-16 weeks. It is nonconta-

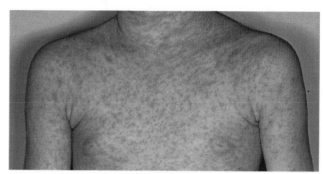

Pityriasis rosea

gious and recurrences are rare.

Subjective symptoms. None to severe pruritus.

Etiology. Unknown. It may be infectious in origin. The highest incidence of the eruption is during the late fall and spring months.

Histopathology. Not diagnostic. There is vascular dilatation of the capillaries in the papillae with a mild inflammatory infiltrate consisting of lymphocytes and plasma cells.

Diagnostic aids. Clinical appearance; rule out fungus infection by scraping and culture; rule out syphilis by STS.

Relation to systemic disease. No specific relationship.

Differential diagnosis. Macular syphilis, tinea circinata, seborrheic dermatitis, eczema.

Therapy. Emollient baths and antihistamines may relieve the pruritus.

Poikiloderma Atrophicans Vasculare

Synonym. Poikiloderma atrophicans vasculare of Jacobi.

Sites of predilection. Axillary folds, inguinal regions and other parts of the body. Rarely on the face.

Objective signs. The eruption begins as circumscribed macular lesions which generally spread to involve the entire body. The lesions are well-defined to partially defined, confluent areas of reddish-

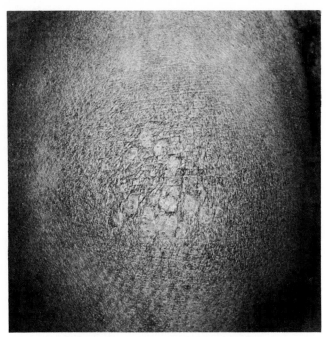

*Poikiloderma atrophicans vasculare
eventuating in mycosis fungoides*

brown macules in which there is telangiectasis, capillary hemorrhages and areas of depigmentation. The surface is dry, wrinkled and atrophic; the clinical appearance resembles that of radiodermatitis.

Subjective symptoms. Mild to moderate pruritus or burning.

Etiology. Unknown.

Histopathology. There is atrophy of the epidermis, perivascular round cell infiltration, degeneration of collagen and diminution to disappearance of the elastic tissue.

Diagnostic aids. Biopsy.

Relation to systemic disease. This condition may be the first sign of mycosis fungoides or a connective tissue disease.

Differential diagnosis. Radiodermatitis, lupus erythematosus, mycosis fungoides, scleroderma, Riehl's melanosis.

Therapy. Topical nitrogen mustard if biopsy confirms the diagnosis of mycosis fungoides. Topical corticosteroids are effective only in the minority of cases.

Poikiloderma of Civatte

Synonym. Riehl's melanosis.

Sites of predilection. Face, forehead, sides of the neck, chest.

Objective signs. The onset is gradual. The earliest lesions are erythematous macules with follicular hyperkeratosis and scaling. The eventual picture is that of a moderately extensive macular eruption consisting of discrete and confluent, well-defined, light to dark brown, reticulated lesions. The pigmentation is permanent. The skin under the jaw is normal.

Subjective symptoms. Usually free of subjective symptoms. Early in the course there may be slight pruritus.

Etiology. Probably due to chronic actinic exposure.

Histopathology. The microscopic picture is not diagnostic.

Diagnostic aids. History and physical examination.

Relation to systemic disease. Poikiloderma atrophicans vasculare, actinic dermatitis, contact dermatitis, chloasma.

Therapy. None of value.

Polymorphous Light Eruption

Synonym. None.

Sites of predilection. The light-exposed areas of the body.

Objective signs. Erythema, edema and occasional vesiculation can be observed on the exposed areas, with sharp demarcation in areas protected by clothing. Urticarial or erythematous lesions may develop on the light-protected skin surfaces.

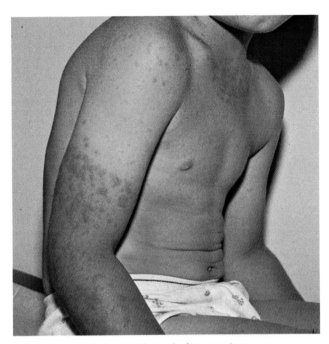

Polymorphous light eruption

Subjective symptoms. Moderate to severe pruritus.

Etiology. No apparent cause exists for this disorder. In a susceptible person the eruption may be produced by exposure to natural sunlight or appropriate artificial lights.

Histopathology. There is edema of the epidermis and vascular dilatation in the papillary portion of the corium. Vessels are surrounded by a mild inflammatory infiltrate.

Diagnostic aids. Photopatch testing to rule out patients who have ingested or applied topical photoactive agents. Quantitative urinary porphyrin excretions to rule out porphyria.

Relation to systemic disease. None apparent.

Differential diagnosis. Photosensitivity is a symptom of pellagra, Hartnup disease, porphyria, lupus erythematosus and drug ingestion. The cutaneous lesions may mimic toxic erythema, sunburn, contact sensitivity or cellulitis.

Therapy. Search for and eliminate the cause of photosensitivity. Avoidance of sunlight exposure. Use of sunscreens.

Pruritus Ani

Synonym. Itching anus.

Sites of predilection. Anus and perianal region.

Objective signs. Objective evidence varies from none to chronic lichenified dermatitis with fissure formation. If an eruption is present it begins as a reddish, edematous, macular lesion which encircles the anus and extends toward the coccyx and the perineum. The surface is excoriated and blood crusting may be present. In the chronic stage the skin in the involved area becomes thickened and lichenified. Fissures develop in the gluteal cleft, over the coccyx and in the perineum.

Pruritus ani which develops following systemic antibiotic therapy presents an eczematous appearance and is usually complicated by monilial infection. In these patients the surface of the lesion is macerated and is covered with a moist, whitish film.

Subjective symptoms. Moderate to intense pruritus. Loss of sleep and emotional distress may result.

Etiology. Where objective symptoms are present, emotional tension, diabetes, food allergy or other systemic illness may be the responsible agent.

Systemic antibiotic therapy is a frequent cause of this condition. Fungus infection and contact sensitization, as well as intestinal tumors, foreign bodies, pinworms and colitis, may also cause pruritus ani.

Histopathology. The microscopic picture is nonspecific.

Diagnostic aids. Adequate history and physical examination, urinalysis, scrapings and culture for fungi or parasite ova, proctoscopic examination.

Relation to systemic disease. Diabetes mellitus, Hodgkin's disease, rectal malignancies, systemic infection, mental illness and allergic disturbances are among the underlying systemic diseases responsible for the production of pruritus ani.

Differential diagnosis. Fungus infection, parasitic diseases, eczema.

Therapy. Treatment of the underlying systemic disease. Adequate sedation, local application of hydrocortisone ointment or lotion, or other corticosteroid preparations.

Pruritus Vulvae

Synonym. Itching vulva.

Sites of predilection. Female genital area.

Objective signs. Objective findings may be absent. The lesions vary in appearance according to the causative factors. The eruption may involve a single, localized area on one labium majus or it may be generalized, involving both labia, the mons pubis, the perineum and the labia minora. In the early stages the lesions are pinkish macules but, as the eruption becomes persistent, the skin becomes thickened and lichenified. Excoriations are present. Furuncles may develop. If secondary monilial infection occurs the involved areas may be covered with a whitish film. The eruption may extend across the perineum to surround the anus.

Subjective symptoms. Moderate to intense pruritus.

Etiology. Pruritus vulvae, like pruritus ani, is a symptom and not a disease. It may be due to fungus infection, *Trichomonas vaginalis,* emotional tension, contact dermatitis, parasitic infestation or various systemic diseases.

Histopathology. The microscopic picture is not diagnostic.

Diagnostic aids. Urinalysis, history and physical examination, vaginal examination, cultures for fungi, smears for *Trichomonas vaginalis.*

Relation to systemic disease. This condition can be associated with diabetes mellitus, carcinoma, gynecological disease, malignancies, systemic infection and senescence.

Therapy. The elimination of local causative factors. One percent hydrocortisone ointment or other topical corticosteroid preparations are of value.

Adequate sedation is usually necessary. Clotrimazole or nystatin creams are indicated in the treatment of monilial infections.

Pseudoxanthoma Elasticum

Synonym. Grönblad-Strandberg syndrome.

Sites of predilection. Sides of the neck, the axillary folds, groin, umbilical region.

Objective signs. This condition, which is usually limited to adults, develops as discrete and confluent, small, yellowish-white maculopapules which coalesce to form plaques. The skin in the involved areas is soft and velvety. Occasionally calcification develops in the lesions. On ophthalmoscopic examination angioid streaks may be seen in the retina.

Subjective symptoms. None.

Etiology. Unknown.

Histopathology. There is fragmentation and clumping of the elastic tissue which takes a basic stain.

Diagnostic aids. Biopsy.

Relation to systemic disease. The elastic tissue of any or all of the blood vessels in the body may be involved. The condition may occur in association with scleroderma or lupus erythematosus. Severe gastric or uterine hemorrhage, hypertension, aneurysms and calcification of the vessels of the lower extremities have been reported in the various subtypes of this disease. Elastosis perforans, an unusual cutaneous disease, may coexist with this disease.

Differential diagnosis. The clinical appearance is characteristic.

Therapy. None effective.

Purpura Annularis Telangiectodes

Synonym. Majocchi's disease.

Sites of predilection. Lower extremities.

Objective signs. Lesions are sharply defined, bright pink to red macules, distributed over the thighs, legs and feet and occasionally upwards on the

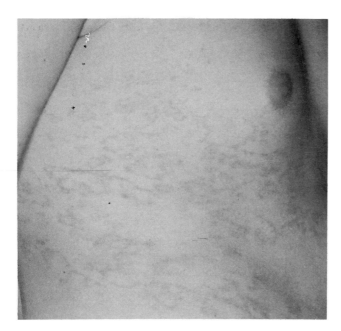

Purpura annularis telangiectodes

upper extremities and trunk. The lesions are well-defined, round or irregular, annular macules. Brownish pigmentation suggestive of hemosiderosis appears about the periphery of the annular lesions. Telangiectasia in the form of tiny red spots (cayenne pepper spots) develops throughout the lesions. Although the clinical picture is different, the basic pathologic process is the same as that of Schamberg's progressive pigmentary dermatosis and Gougerot-Blum pigmented purpuric lichenoid dermatosis.

Subjective symptoms. Mild pruritus may be present.

Etiology. The cutaneous lesions may be a manifestation of some underlying systemic disease.

Histopathology. The epidermis is not involved. There are vascular dilatations, perivascular round cell infiltrations and iron pigment deposits in the cutis.

Diagnostic aids. Biopsy, general physical examination, bleeding and clotting times, complete blood count.

Relation to systemic disease. This cutaneous lesion may be a manifestation of cardiovascular disease, endocrine disturbances or other constitutional illnesses.

Differential diagnosis. Schamberg's disease, pigmented purpuric lichenoid dermatitis, eczema, leukemia and other bleeding disorders.

Therapy. Treatment of systemic illness if present.

Purpura, Nonthrombocytopenic

Synonym. Purpura simplex, Henoch-Schönlein purpura, symptomatic purpura.

Sites of predilection. May be generalized. Extent of lesions varies with type and severity.

Objective signs. Purpura simplex is manifested by an eruption of variously sized, red to purplish, macular lesions which do not blanch on pressure. The condition is characterized by relapses and remissions. Occasionally urticaria or erythema multiforme may accompany the attacks.

Henoch's purpura usually occurs in childhood. Urticaria or erythema multiforme may occur concurrently with the development of the purpuric lesions. The condition is frequently accompanied by hematemesis, abdominal discomfort and tarry stools.

Schönlein's purpura is purpura simplex associated with arthritis or rheumatic fever. The hemorrhagic type of erythema multiforme may develop.

Subjective symptoms. The cutaneous lesions are usually asymptomatic. Urticarial lesions may cause pruritus. Other subjective symptoms are those related to the systemic disease causing the eruption.

Etiology. Penicillin, coal tar antipyretics, tetanus antitoxin, smallpox vaccine, other drugs and food allergens are frequently responsible for the production of these lesions. Ingestion of alcohol may produce purpura simplex. Henoch's purpura may be caused by bacterial infection, food or drug allergies. Schönlein's purpura is associated with rheumatic fever. Not all the causes of this disorder are known.

Histopathology. Vascular dilatation with hemorrhaging into the cutis.

Diagnostic aids. History, physical examination, complete blood picture, bleeding and clotting time, tourniquet test, prothrombin time.

Relation to systemic disease. The condition may indicate some underlying allergic disease, rheumatic fever, vitamin deficiency, kidney damage, liver damage, systemic infections and endocrine disorders.

Differential diagnosis. Thrombocytopenic purpura.

Therapy. Treatment of the underlying disease. Local therapy is of no value.

Purpura, Thrombocytopenic

Synonym. Primary idiopathic purpura, purpura hemorrhagica.

Sites of predilection. Extremities, mucous membranes; occasionally generalized.

Objective signs. This is a severe, frequently fatal condition characterized by extensive hemorrhaging into the skin, mucous membranes and viscera. The cutaneous lesions are discrete and confluent, nonblanching small and large, red, bluish-red or dark purplish areas. Frequently hemorrhage appears from the mucous membranes of the nose and mouth, with the formation of blood crusts on the lips. The gums are soft and spongy, and bleed on slight trauma. Splenomegaly may develop.

Subjective symptoms. Weakness, anorexia.

Etiology. The symptoms are produced by platelet destruction or dysfunction. The platelets may be altered by drugs, collagen diseases or lymphoma.

Histopathology. Capillary fragility with hemorrhaging into the cutis.

Diagnostic aids. History and physical examination, complete blood count, bleeding and clotting time, platelet count, prothrombin time.

Relation to systemic disease. Condition may be associated with congenital hemolytic anemia, primary pancytopenia and aplastic anemia. It can be the first manifestation of lupus erythematosus or a myeloproliferative disease.

Differential diagnosis. Purpura simplex.

Therapy. Transfusions, vitamin K, splenectomy, systemic corticosteroid therapy. Local therapy is of no value. Removal of all drugs is essential.

Radiation Dermatitis

Synonym. X-ray burn, radium burn.

Sites of predilection. Any area exposed to ionizing radiation.

Objective signs. There are three types of cutaneous postradiation damage.

1. Hyperpigmentation, freckling, mild hypertrichosis and skin dryness may occur during or after a course of fractional X-ray treatment for acne vulgaris or other benign conditions. The intensive radiation therapy used for the treatment of epitheliomas usually produces an inflammatory reaction with edema, and a deeply

Radiation dermatitis

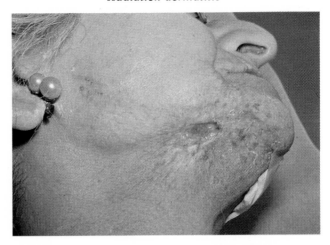

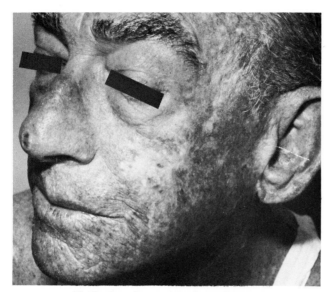

Radiation dermatitis, late changes

pigmented area which outlines the site of therapy. If the dose has not been excessive the reaction subsides without sequelae.

2. After a period of months or years following excessive radiation therapy (radium or X-ray), atrophic scarring, telangiectasia and permanent hair loss develop. Keratoses may form.

3. Another delayed reaction to excessive radiation is the development of indolent ulcers and squamous cell epitheliomas in the areas of atrophic scar formation.

Subjective symptoms. Moderate to severe discomfort may accompany radiodermatitis.

Etiology. Excessive radiation therapy or careless use of diagnostic X-ray equipment by untrained personnel.

Histopathology. Atrophy of the epidermis, dilatation of vessels, degeneration of collagenous tissue and absence of appendages. Dyskeratotic cells, karyorrhexis, epitheliomatous degeneration and squamous cell carcinoma are seen in the later stages of radiation dermatitis.

Diagnostic aids. History and physical examination, biopsy.

Relation to systemic disease. None.

Differential diagnosis. Sailor's skin, xeroderma pigmentosum, poikiloderma atrophicans vasculare, telangiectasia, mycosis fungoides.

Therapy. Excision of small areas; corticosteroid ointments may be of value in treatment of the acute phase; operative removal of carcinomas.

Raynaud's Disease

Synonym. None.

Sites of predilection. Extremities.

Objective signs. The condition begins gradually as intermittent episodes during which the fingers and toes become pale with a marked decrease of the skin temperature. The symptoms are more severe in cold weather. Eventually the affected parts become persistently cyanotic. Gangrene develops when the vasospasm is complicated by thrombosis. The fingers, toes or both may be equally affected. Scarring and atrophy of the fingertips will eventually develop.

Subjective symptoms. Numbness, tingling and pain. Exposure to cold produces pain.

Etiology. Unknown. This condition occurs more commonly in women before the age of 40. Associated factors are heredity, trauma, psychogenic stimuli and endocrine imbalance. Use of tobacco may be a factor.

Histopathology. The microscopic picture is not diagnostic.

Diagnostic aids. History and physical examination, peripheral vasodilatation induced by drugs, skin temperature studies.

Relation to systemic disease. The condition is associated with scleroderma, other collagen diseases, emotional tension and hereditary vascular defects.

Differential diagnosis. Thromboangiitis obliterans, arteriosclerotic gangrene.

Therapy. Vasodilator drugs are rarely of value.

Physiotherapy, rest, restriction of the use of tobacco and avoidance of cold. Sympathectomy may be necessary in severe cases.

Rosacea

Synonym. Rum blossom, rum nose.
Sites of predilection. Nose, cheeks.
Objective signs. The condition begins insidiously as ill-defined, bright red, transient areas involving the nose and the contiguous portions of the cheeks. This transient hyperemia may last for a few days and disappear completely. The lesions recur frequently. The hyperemia eventually becomes persistent, and the involved areas are dull red to bright red. Small dilated blood vessels are present over the alae of the nose and the flush areas of the cheeks. The affected skin is comparatively cool. Migraine headaches and keratitis may be associated with the disease.

The ultimate picture, known as rhinophyma, is one of tissue proliferation. The skin of the nose and the nasolabial folds become thickened with dilated follicles over the surface. Dilated and tortuous blood vessels are also present on the surface. The nose becomes bulbous in appearance.

Follicular papules and pustules frequently occur in any of the stages previously described. Because of sebaceous hyperactivity, the skin surface is exceptionally oily. Seborrheic dermatitis is frequently present.

Subjective symptoms. Slight pruritus and pain. Emotional imbalance because of the disfigured appearance.

Etiology. The cause is unknown. Dietary indiscretions, alcoholism, emotional tension and foci of infection are commonly incriminated as causative factors although conclusive evidence is lacking.

Rosacea

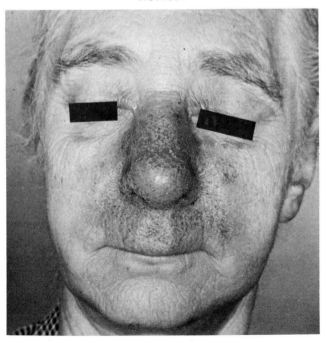

Rhinophyma

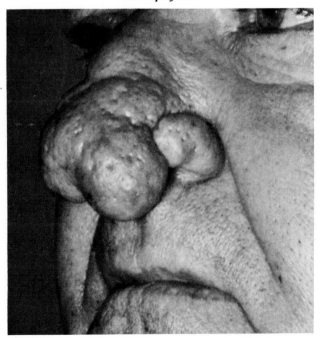

Histopathology. There is hypertrophy of sebaceous glands. A round cell and plasma cell infiltrate occurs in the cutis. Occasionally a tuberculoid architecture is seen in chronic cases.

Diagnostic aids. History and physical examination.

Relation to systemic disease. Achlorhydria, hormonal imbalance, emotional instability, alcoholism.

Differential diagnosis. Eczema, tuberculosis cutis, acne vulgaris, bromide acne, lupus erythematosus.

Therapy. Tetracycline (250 mg, 1-3 times daily) is the drug of choice. Topical applications of colloidal sulfur lotions may be of value. Dilated vessels may be obliterated with high frequency current. Rhinophyma may be treated surgically to repair the cosmetic defect.

Rubella

Synonym. German measles, three-day measles.

Sites of predilection. Generalized.

Objective signs. The condition begins with mild prodromal symptoms. The eruption first appears on the face, then spreads to the neck and chest. The lesions are numerous, discrete, partially to well-defined, pinkish macules or maculopapules with absence of scale. The lesions may be numerous and so closely grouped that the condition simulates scarlatina. Associated with the eruption is enlargement of the postcervical, postauricular and suboccipital lymph nodes. The patient's temperature seldom exceeds 37.7°C. The lesions fade in from 3-5 days without perceptible exfoliation. The incubation period is from 14-21 days. One attack confers immunity.

Subjective symptoms. Slight malaise.

Etiology. A virus.

Histopathology. The microscopic picture is not diagnostic.

Diagnostic aids. History and physical examination. Viral isolation from blood, sputum or urine; neutralizing antibody titer may be obtained.

Relation to systemic disease. The cutaneous lesions are evidence of a systemic virus infection. Rubella, complicating pregnancy, may produce congenital defects in the fetus. A newborn infant with this disease may excrete virus for years.

Differential diagnosis. Measles, macular syphilid, drug eruptions, scarlatina, erythema simplex.

Therapy. Bed rest, aspirin.

Rubeola

Synonym. Measles, red measles, 14-day measles.

Sites of predilection. Generalized.

Objective signs. After an incubation period of 10-15 days the eruption may begin in the buccal mucosa with reddened fauces, coated tongue and reddish lesions with central, whitish points (Koplik's spots) opposite the molars. The cutaneous lesions first appear on the face and spread to involve the neck and then the rest of the body. The lesions are numerous, variously sized small macules and papules which range from 2 mm-1 cm in diameter. The larger lesions are oval or crescent-shaped, ill-defined and reddish, and appear primarily on the trunk. After 4-6 days the eruption fades and a fine furfuraceous exfoliation occurs. Koplik's spots disappear when the cutaneous lesions develop.

Upper respiratory symptoms include rhinitis, laryngitis and stomatitis. Palpebral conjunctivitis is the major ocular symptom. At the height of the disease the temperature ranges from 38.3-40°C. The eruption lasts from 5-10 days.

Subjective symptoms. Malaise, photophobia, chills and fever, and slight pruritus.

Etiology. Virus.

Histopathology. The microscopic picture is not diagnostic. Giant cells may occasionally be seen in biopsies of the lesions.

Diagnostic aids. History and physical examination; tissue culture of blood, sputum or urine; hemagglutinin studies; viral neutralization antibody determination.

Relation to systemic disease. Measles is frequently productive of sequelae such as pneumonia and encephalitis. Measles may depress the tuberculin reaction and exacerbate tuberculosis.

Differential diagnosis. Rubella, scarlatina, macular syphilid, pityriasis rosea, erythema simplex, drug eruptions, Rocky Mountain spotted fever.

Therapy. Bed rest, supportive treatment. Prevention of the disease can be achieved by the use of gamma globulin.

Scarlet Fever

Synonym. Scarlatina.

Sites of predilection. Generalized.

Objective signs. The condition is manifested by a sudden onset of a macular eruption which quickly involves the entire body. The lesions are closely aggregated, discrete, minute, bright red macules which give the body surface a scarlet hue. There is usually circumoral pallor. The bright red color temporarily disappears on light pressure. When the acute phase subsides, between the seventh and tenth days, exfoliation begins in small flakes or in large plaques and is profuse. "Glove and stocking" exfoliation occurs and occasionally the nail plates are lost.

The buccal mucosa is usually bright red and the tonsils and uvula are swollen and present red puncta. There is a characteristic "strawberry tongue" which is at first coated and then red, glazed and covered with enlarged papillae. The cervical nodes are enlarged.

Subjective symptoms. The patient is acutely ill with sore throat, headache, vomiting, chills and fever (40-40.5°C), and occasionally convulsions.

Etiology. Group A beta-hemolytic streptococcus.

Histopathology. The microscopic picture is not diagnostic.

Diagnostic aids. History and physical examination, throat culture, antistreptolysin O titer.

Relation to systemic disease. Complications include mastoiditis, otitis media, nephritis, arthritis and septicemia.

Differential diagnosis. Rubeola, rubella, drug eruptions, toxic dermatitis, erythema scarlatiniform, mucocutaneous lymph node syndrome.

Therapy. Penicillin or erythromycin systemically.

Scleredema

Synonym. Scleredema adultorum of Buschke.

Sites of predilection. Head, neck, upper thorax.

Objective signs. This condidtion begins with an ill-defined pinkish macular eruption, which is followed by spreading induration and swelling of the skin and subcutaneous tissues. The thickening usually begins on the back of the neck and spreads over the scalp, face and neck to the upper trunk. Although there is thickening and apparent edema, the surface does not pit on pressure. Gross inflammatory changes are absent, and there is no hair loss, atrophy or pigmentation. The condition occurs primarily in adults.

Subjective symptoms. There are usually no sensory changes. Some discomfort is experienced because of the swelling. Dysphagia due to swelling of the tongue can be seen.

Etiology. This condition usually develops following some infectious disease.

Histopathology. There is noninflammatory swelling of the collagen. Mucin is present between the collagen fibers, about the vessels and the epidermal appendages.

Diagnostic aids. Biopsy.

Relation to systemic disease. Hypoproteinemia, hyperlipemia, pleural and pericardial effusions may occur. Skin involvement is self-limited, usually involuting within a year.

Differential diagnosis. Scleroderma, sclerema, edema.

Therapy. None specific. This condition is self-limited.

Sclerema

Synonym. Sclerema neonatorum, sclerema adiposum.

Sites of predilection. Generalized except the palms, soles and scrotum.

Objective signs. This condition, which usually appears at birth or during the first few weeks of life, is most commonly seen in premature infants. The skin lesions first appear on the calves or other portions of the lower extremities, and rapidly extend upward to involve the entire body with the exception of the palms, soles and scrotum. The surface is cold, dry, solid and has a waxy, whitish color. The induration and rigidity may be severe enough to immobilize the joints and present difficulties in feeding. The prognosis is poor except in those cases with small localized lesions. Severe diarrhea, dehydration and malnutrition may be associated symptoms.

Subjective symptoms. Difficulty in moving, inability to eat properly and diarrhea.

Etiology. Unknown; possibly defective fat metabolism.

Histopathology. Fat necrosis and needle-like crystals of fat are present.

Diagnostic aids. Biopsy.

Relation to systemic disease. In advanced cases there is probably involvement of the visceral fat as well.

Differential diagnosis. Scleroderma, edema neonatorum, scleredema, aplasia cutis.

Therapy. Systemic corticosteroids may be of value. Patient must be kept in a warm environment.

Scleroderma

Synonym. Hidebound disease.

Sites of predilection. Any area of the body.

Objective signs. The circumscribed or localized type of scleroderma is morphea which develops as one or more, discrete or confluent, sharply defined, round or oval macular lesions ranging from 1-10 cm in diameter. The surface is whitish or ivory, greatly thickened and usually surrounded by a pinkish or violaceous halo. The surface becomes atrophic and loses its normal topography. In the form known as morphea guttata, small lesions may develop. These lesions usually involute

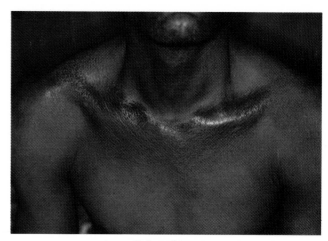

Scleroderma

spontaneously.

A localized linear form of scleroderma involving the forehead and scalp is called scleroderma en coup de sabre.

Diffuse scleroderma, or systemic sclerosis, may begin as areas of infiltration or edema but, when fully developed, presents large confluent areas involving a portion of an extremity, an entire extremity, the trunk or the entire body. The skin is like leather, inflexible, yellowish, whitish or waxy in appearance, and there is loss of the normal topography and loss of hair. In advanced cases there is restriction of joint movement, diminution of thoracic excursion, loss of facial expression and inability to open the mouth to chew food. Muscular atrophy may develop. Ulcerations occur at pressure points (elbows, knees, *etc*).

Acrosclerosis is a syndrome which combines the features of scleroderma and Raynaud's disease. The fingers become fixed (claw-like) and the skin becomes hidebound. This is called sclerodactyly. There is intermittent blanching of the fingers, and the hands become cyanotic. Occasionally ulcerations develop on the distal phalanges. Facial sclerosis is often associated with acrosclerosis and sclerodactyly.

Subjective symptoms. The extent of the condition in the areas involved determines the subjective symptoms. Stiffness of the extremities, inability to move because of the hidebound involvement of the skin over the joints, pain, dysphagia and hypersensitivity to cold may occur.

Etiology. Unknown.

Histopathology. There is atrophy of the epidermis and the collagen fibers are hyalinized, homogeneous and eosinophilic. Atrophy of striated muscle fibers and vascular occlusion are present. Hair follicles and sweat glands are obliterated.

Diagnostic aids. History and physical examination, biopsy, chest X ray, gastrointestinal (GI) series, antinuclear antibody test with speckled or nucleolar immunofluorescence patterns.

Relation to systemic disease. Scleroderma is a systemic disease. There is decreased peristalsis and rigidity of the esophagus. The entire gastrointestinal tract may be involved. Lung changes occur. The kidneys may be affected and myocardial damage may develop.

Differential diagnosis. Vitiligo, scars, keloids, dermatomyositis, scleredema.

Therapy. There is no satisfactory treatment.

SEBORRHEIC CONDITIONS

Seborrheic dermatitis, seborrhea oleosa, seborrhea sicca, pityriasis alba, rosacea and acne vulgaris are included in this group.

Oily Skin

Synonym. Seborrhea oleosa.

Sites of predilection. Scalp, face, chest, back.

Objective signs. The skin in the involved areas is excessively oily because of an overabundant secretion of sebum. The hair becomes very oily and sometimes matted. The skin surface is shiny over the face, nose and forehead. The follicular orifices over the nose and the nasolabial folds are patulous.

Subjective symptoms. Embarrassment caused by the cosmetic defect.

Etiology. The exact cause is unknown. Pubertal hormone secretion may stimulate excess sebaceous gland function. Emotional tension may be important.

Histopathology. There is hypertrophy of the sebaceous glands but no infiltrate in the cutis. Slight hyperkeratosis is present.

Diagnostic aids. History and clinical appearance, biopsy.

Relation to systemic disease. Parkinson's disease and constitutional illnesses such as acromegaly, hyperthyroidism or other hormone dysfunctions may be responsible for this condition.

Differential diagnosis. The clinical appearance is typical.

Therapy. The hair and scalp should be washed each week with an antiseborrheic shampoo. The face may be cleansed with sulfur-containing soap or simple bland soaps. Topically applied colloidal sulfur lotions give temporary relief.

Seborrheic Dermatitis

Synonym. Seborrheic eczema.

Sites of predilection. Scalp, face, retroauricular area, ear canals, presternal area, interscapular area,

Seborrheic dermatitis

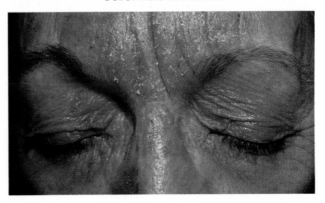

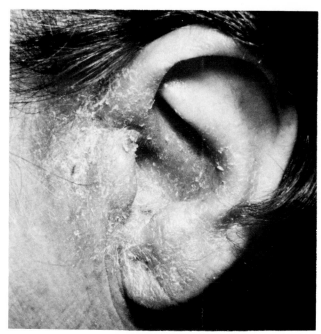

*Seborrheic dermatitis
involving the ear*

inframammary folds, pubic area.

Objective signs. In the scalp the lesions may develop as few to numerous, partially or well-defined, discrete or confluent, scaly areas. The eruption may involve the entire scalp and extend onto the forehead as well-defined, reddish, slightly infiltrated, festooned lesions.

The lesions may appear in the external auditory canals as slight scaling, or ill-defined, slightly infiltrated, scaly macules which are covered with adherent scale or blood crust. Secondary infection may develop with the formation of pus crusts. Occasionally the entire auricle is involved. Well-defined, lichenified, infiltrated lesions frequently develop behind the ears. The reddish areas are covered with adherent dry scale and eventually extend into the scalp and onto the back of the neck. Fissures develop in the sulcus between the ears and the scalp. The lesions which develop within the ear canal are frequently misdiagnosed as fungus infection.

The festooned lesions on the forehead may be pinkish in color or depigmented and are covered with a scant or profuse amount of adherent oily scale. Well-defined, scaly, macular lesions may develop anterior to the ears and in each nasolabial fold. On the anterior chest wall or between the scapulae the lesions develop as well-defined, discrete or confluent, pinkish-yellow macules covered with an adherent dry scale. Similar lesions may develop within the pubic area, extending over the genitalia, perineum and perianal area. Scaling may be absent in moist areas.

Annular lesions may form. At times the scaling is so profuse that differentiation from psoriasis is difficult. The lesions in the scalp may cause temporary alopecia from the presence of very thick scales or from trauma due to rubbing.

Subjective symptoms. Moderate to marked pruritus.

Etiology. Unknown. A contributing factor is emotional tension. The condition has also been associated with debilitating diseases.

Histopathology. There is slight acanthosis and parakeratosis. Some vascular dilatation is present in the papillary bodies. The picture is not specific.

Diagnostic aids. History and physical examination; biopsy is nonspecific.

Relation to systemic disease. The condition is frequently associated with emotional tension and occasionally with debilitating diseases.

Differential diagnosis. Psoriasis, fungus infections, lupus erythematosus, eczema, pityriasis rosea.

Therapy. An ointment containing 2-5% sulfur and salicylic acid in petrolatum is of value in the treatment of areas where scaling is profuse. One percent hydrocortisone ointment or other corticosteroid preparations are effective in local therapy. If secondary pyogenic infection is present, it should be treated independently.

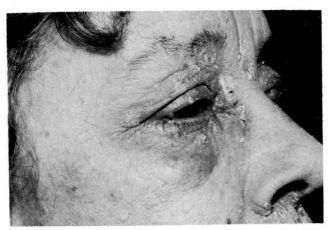

Seborrheic dermatitis

Seborrheic Dermatitis of Infancy

Synonym. Leiner's disease, erythroderma desquamativum, cradle cap.

Sites of predilection. Generalized.

Objective signs. This condition, which occurs in infants, may begin on the scalp as a profuse, scaling, macular eruption with an erythematous base. The lesions extend over the face, neck, ears, trunk, extremities and genital area. There may be some maceration on the folds of the neck or groin and monilial infection may be superimposed. The clinical picture is that of extensive seborrheic dermatitis.

Subjective symptoms. Children are usually anorectic and restless because of severe pruritus.

Etiology. Unknown. The character of the lesion is frequently altered by overzealous topical therapy.

Histopathology. The microscopic picture is nonspecific.

Diagnostic aids. Biopsy to rule out histiocytosis X.

Relation to systemic disease. The prognosis is fairly good with proper care. However, some of these patients are severely cachectic and may die.

Differential diagnosis. Ritter's disease, atopic dermatitis, scarlatina, histiocytosis X.

Therapy. Emollient baths, proper diet, good hygiene and application of sulfur-salicylic acid ointment (2-5%). Topical hydrocortisone can be utilized in severe cases.

Septicemia, Bacterial

Synonym. Bacteremia.

Sites of predilection. None.

Objective signs. Splinter hemorrhages, Osler's nodes and Janeway's lesions are seen in many bacteremias, especially those due to endocarditis. Janeway's lesions are erythematous, edematous patches on the fleshy volar surface of the digits or the palms. Osler's nodes are small painful erythematous, sometimes necrotic spots appearing on the palms. Other bacteremias may cause cutaneous infarcts, ecchymosis, pustules, bullae, hemorrhagic bullae and petechiae. Disseminated gonococcemia can be accompanied by gray necrotic pustules on erythematous bases. Meningococcemia produces a purpuric petechial eruption which at times may be locally gangrenous.

Subjective symptoms. None to severe pain and fever.

Etiology. Invasion of the bloodstream by bacteria. This event may be preceded by manipulation of a prior cutaneous lesion, dental extraction, surgical operation, wound infection, heroin injection or abortion. The patient may have been previously healthy or immunosuppressed.

Histopathology. Bacteria may be demonstrated in the lesion by immunofluorescent techniques. The specimen will exhibit the changes of acute inflammation, thrombosis, infarction or abscess formation.

Diagnostic aids. Smear and culture of the local lesion, blood cultures, urinalysis for erythrocytes, cardiac auscultation for murmurs.

Relation to systemic disease. Bacteremias are a generalized disease. The possibility of endotoxin release, disseminated intravascular coagulation or concomitant adrenal failure must be considered.

Differential diagnosis. Drug eruptions, rickettsioses, leukemias.

Therapy. Specific systemic antibiotic therapy and supportive care.

Stasis Dermatitis

Synonym. Varicose eczema.

Objective signs. This eruption usually develops in the lower third of the legs. The skin involved in the area becomes dusky pink in color. Due to manipulation and excoriation the involved areas become lichenified and hyperpigmented. Following a break in the skin due to excoriation or other types of trauma, ulcers may develop which are usually chronic lesions varying from 1-5 cm or more in diameter. The lesions usually develop just above the malleolus and spread peripherally. The margins are rolled and show little tendency to heal. The base of the ulcer usually contains a grayish to green slough. Surrounding the eczematous area there may be extensive brownish pigmentation due to the hemosiderin deposit. Varicose veins may or may not be present nearby.

Subjective symptoms. Variable. Patients who have no ulceration suffer moderate to severe pruritus, and those with ulceration have pain.

Etiology. The cause of the basic dermatitis is obscure. Although it has been attributed to vascular insufficiency, this defect is not always clinically evident. Trauma and bacterial infection play a large role.

Histopathology. The pathologic picture will be determined by the presence or absence of ulceration. If ulceration is not present, there is acanthosis with some edema of the epidermis and the underlying dermis. There is vascular dilatation with a perivascular infiltrate of round cells and polymorphonuclear leukocytes. The histopathologic picture of a stasis ulcer is that of a nonspecific chronic ulcer.

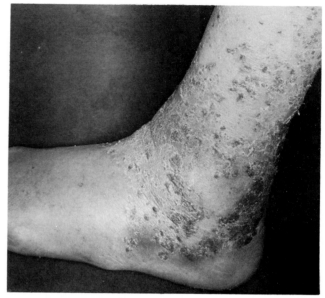

Stasis dermatitis

Relation to systemic disease. Usually none.

Differential diagnosis. Bromoderma, contact dermatitis, cellulitis, thrombophlebitis. If an ulcer is present, the possibility of gumma or sickle cell ulcers must be considered.

Therapy. The peripheral dermatitis may be treated with topical corticosteroid preparations whereas the central ulceration, if present, can be compressed. An occlusive zinc oxide gel cast is effective if no infection or exudate is present. Vascular insufficiency should be corrected. Bed rest is often necessary to reduce edema and promote healing.

Striae

Synonym. Striae gravidarum, striae atrophicae, striae distensae.

Sites of predilection. Trunk, thighs.

Objective signs. These lesions may begin as purplish,

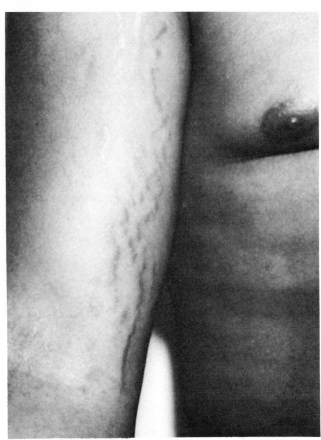

Striae

linear, irregular or band-like streaks. Later they appear as white, smooth or wrinkled, slightly depressed, atrophic scars.

Subjective symptoms. None.

Etiology. Lesions result from distention and stretching of the skin associated with pregnancy, obesity, Cushing's disease and prolonged corticosteroid therapy. Plastic film occlusion with topical corticosteroid creams will frequently produce striae in prepubescent children. Excessive exercise such as weight lifting may produce striae over large muscle groups.

Histopathology. Fragmentation of elastic tissue and scar formation.

Relation to systemic disease. Pituitary adenomas, obesity. Topical or extensive parenteral corticosteroid therapy may produce striae. Striae also occur in pregnant women.

Diagnostic aids. None.

Differential diagnosis. Clinical picture is characteristic.

Therapy. None.

Sunburn

Synonym. None.

Sites of predilection. Exposed parts of the body.

Objective signs. Large, bright red, well-defined, macular lesions. The configuration of the lesion is determined by the exposed area. The intensity of the color varies with the severity of the exposure and the complexion of the individual. The surface may be covered with numerous small vesicles. When the acute erythema subsides, exfoliation occurs.

Subjective symptoms. Pain. When exfoliation begins, pruritus occurs.

Etiology. Direct action of the actinic rays of the sun. The reaction to exposure varies with the pigmentation of the skin.

Histopathology. Acanthosis, hyperkeratosis and edema of the epidermis. There is vascular dilatation and perivascular cellular infiltration in the papillary portion of the cutis.

Diagnostic aids. Clinical appearance and history.

Relation to systemic disease. In extensive cases, secondary pyogenic infection may develop. Acute nephritis may complicate extensive sunburn. Topically applied substances containing benzocaine may cause a contact dermatitis.

Differential diagnosis. Toxic erythema, pellagra.

Therapy. Sunbathing should be forbidden. Use of sunscreen preparations containing para-aminobenzoic acid as a preventive measure. Topical corticosteroids are effective in reducing inflammation. Cooling baths may give relief. Systemic corticosteroids are occasionally indicated. Thiazide diuretics to relieve symptomatic edema may be necessary as a temporary measure.

Syphilis, Secondary

Synonym. Macular manifestation of secondary syphilis.

Sites of predilection. Trunk, extremities.

Objective signs. The eruption consists of numerous, ill-defined, nonscaly, monomorphic, dull pinkish macules which present a splotchy appearance. The lesions are generalized, symmetrically distributed and are best seen at a distance of 5-6 feet from the patient, with the light reflected against the skin at an angle. Macular lesions are rarely annular. The eruption appears quickly over a few days, but may last 2-3 weeks.

The chancre or the scar of the initial lesions may still be present. Associated with macular syphilid are erosive lesions on the mucous membranes, condylomata lata, "moth-eaten" alopecia, generalized lymphadenopathy, iritis, coryza and other secondary manifestations.

Subjective symptoms. Cutaneous lesions seldom provoke any subjective symptoms. Lesions in the mucous membranes may produce discomfort.

Etiology. Treponema pallidum (see Chapter 9).

Histopathology. Basic pathology of all syphilitic lesions is that of a perivascular round cell and plasma cell infiltrate.

Diagnostic aids. Demonstration of the *T pallidum* on darkfield examination. A positive darkfield examination may be obtained from macular or papular lesions by abrasion of the lesion to produce a moist surface. Darkfield examination may also be performed by gland puncture. Serologic tests for syphilis must be done as part of the diagnostic routine.

Relation to systemic disease. Syphilis is always a systemic disease.

Differential diagnosis. Erythema multiforme, pityriasis rosea, rubella, rubeola, dermatitis medicamentosa, toxic dermatitis.

Therapy. See Chapter 9.

Tattoo

Synonym. None.

Sites of predilection. Intentional tattoo marks are usually produced on the upper extremities or trunk. Accidental tattoo marks produced by foreign bodies occur at sites of trauma.

Objective signs. The intentional tattoo marks are produced by injections into the skin of various pigments to form patterns such as pictures, roses, names, *etc.* The colors are blue, red, black or green, depending on the type of ink. For several weeks after the tattoo has been performed the treated area is crusted, edematous and erythematous. The pigmentation remains after the acute inflammatory symptoms subside.

Morphine addicts frequently develop bluish spots at the site of injection, caused by carbon from the alcohol lamp used to sterilize their equipment or by impurities in the drug. These lesions usually occur on the extremities or sides of the trunk.

Gunpowder or dirt may also be tattooed into the skin and remain as a permanent foreign body.

Subjective symptoms. None.

Histopathology. Biopsy shows the presence of pigment in the dermis.

Diagnostic aids. The clinical appearance is characteristic; history is important in accidental cases and in narcotic addiction.

Relation to systemic disease. None, except in narcotic addicts.

Differential diagnosis. Clinical appearance is characteristic.

Therapy. The small lesions may be removed surgically. Dermabrasion or salabrasion is of limited value. Laser therapy and superimposed tattooing with flesh colored dyes are not cosmetically acceptable.

Telangiectasia, Hereditary Familial

Synonym. Osler's disease, Osler-Weber-Rendu disease.

Sites of predilection. Skin and mucous membranes.

Objective signs. There are reddish or purplish, small telangiectases on the lips, tongue and buccal mucosa. Small groups of dilated blood vessels and small, bright red angiomas are present over the face, trunk and extremities. Purpuric spots develop on distal ends of the tongue, fingers and toes.

Subjective symptoms. The cutaneous lesions are asymptomatic. Malaise and weakness may develop if bleeding is profuse.

Etiology. Congenital.

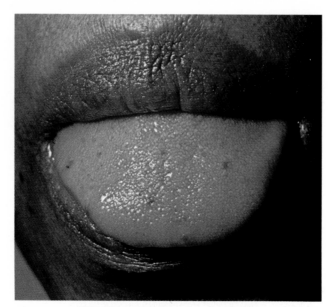

Hereditary familial telangiectasia

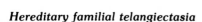

Hereditary familial telangiectasia

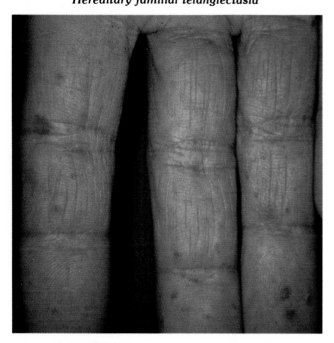

Histopathology. There are telangiectases in the cutis with a diminution in elastic tissue.

Diagnostic aids. History, physical examination, biopsy.

Relation to systemic disease. Angiomas and telangiectases may also develop in internal organs. Bleeding from the nose, rectum or other mucous membranes may be the initial symptom. Cutaneous lesions do not usually appear before puberty.

Differential diagnosis. Rosacea, nevus araneus, senile angioma.

Therapy. None effective. Transfusions may be necessary if bleeding is profuse. Genetic counseling is advised.

Tinea Circinata

Synonym. Ringworm.

Sites of predilection. Face, neck, trunk, extremities.

Objective signs. The lesions caused by *Microsporum*

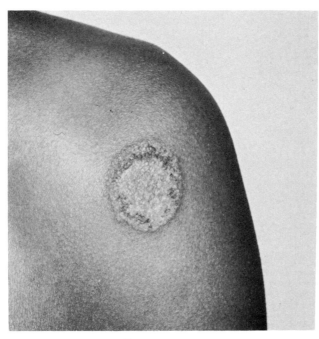

Tinea circinata

audouini are single or multiple, well-defined, round or oval, pinkish or reddish, scaly macules. They vary in size from 1-5 cm in diameter and may be discrete or confluent. The lesions spread peripherally with a tendency towards central clearing to form annular lesions. Concentric rings may develop. The advancing peripheral margin may be vesicular or papular. Blood crusts may be present on the surface. Lesions caused by *Microsporum canis* present a similar appearance; however, the lesions have a more acute inflammatory appearance and frequently a superimposed bacterial infection.

Subjective symptoms. Mild to moderate pruritus.

Etiology. This contagious disease is caused by *M audouini* (the human type of *Microsporum*) or *M canis* (the animal type of *Microsporum* which is transmitted to humans from cats, dogs and monkeys).

Histopathology. Fungi may be demonstrated in the stratum corneum with the Hotchkiss-McManus stain.

Diagnostic aids. The causative organisms may be demonstrated from skin scrapings treated with the potassium hydroxide method. Specific identification of the organism is made by culture on Sabouraud's medium.

Relation to systemic disease. None.

Differential diagnosis. Seborrheic dermatitis, pityriasis rosea, psoriasis, eczema.

Therapy. Topically applied clotrimazole, miconazole or tolnaftate creams are the therapy of choice for limited lesions. Extensive disease is best treated with systemic griseofulvin. Keratolytic ointments containing 3-6% salicylic acid may also also be of value.

Tinea Corporis

Synonym. *Trichophyton rubrum* infection, Trichophytosis corporis.

Sites of predilection. Trunk, extremities.

Objective signs. This noncontagious fungus infection may be limited to one or more fingernails or toenails, one or both palms, one or both soles, extensive plaques involving large portions of the trunk, or a single small area involving one buttock, one thigh, *etc.* The condition rarely involves both hands and both feet simultaneously.

Involvement of the nails produces distortion, increased fragility, pit formation and thickening of the nail plate. If the palms or soles are involved, the lesions are excessively dry, dull red, scantily scaly and fissured. On the trunk or extremities, the plaques are sharply defined, dull red, scantily scaly and resemble the lesions of seborrheic dermatitis or psoriasis. Blood crusted excoriations are usually present. The sharply defined border may be slightly elevated.

Subjective symptoms. The lesions cause intense pruritus.

Etiology. *T rubrum.*

Histopathology. The fungus may be demonstrated by the PAS stain in the stratum corneum.

Diagnostic aids. Culture on Sabouraud's medium is necessary for identification of the organism. Microscopic examination of skin scrapings or particles of nail by use of potassium hydroxide solution is an immediate diagnostic measure.

Relation to systemic disease. None.

Differential diagnosis. Eczema, seborrheic dermatitis, psoriasis.

Therapy. Griseofulvin, systemically administered, will effectively clear skin lesions and is the only satisfactory treatment for nail involvement and extensive cutaneous infection. Clotrimazole cream or solution will clear skin lesions and give prompt relief from pruritus.

Tinea Cruris

Synonym. Eczema marginatum, jock itch, ringworm of the groin.

Sites of predilection. Inner sides of the thighs, buttocks. Occurs more frequently in men.

Objective signs. There is usually one confluent, sharply defined, reddish macule on the inner aspect of one or both thighs, extending into the groin and involving the scrotum. The eruption frequently extends across the perineum to the buttocks. The areas are moderately infiltrated and scaly. The border is slightly elevated. Occasionally the surface is macerated and moist. The condition is usually worse in warm weather.

Subjective symptoms. Moderate to severe pruritus.

Etiology. *Trichophyton mentagrophytes, Epidermophyton floccosum* or *Trichophyton rubrum* are the organisms most frequently causative of tinea cruris. The cutaneous lesions produced by these organisms are similar although the eruption produced by *T rubrum* is the most chronic.

Histopathology. The fungi may be demonstrated in the stratum corneum by the use of PAS or methenamine stains.

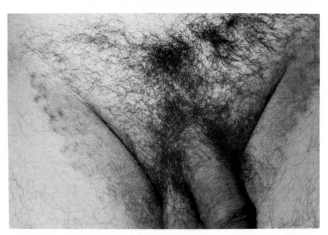

Tinea cruris

Diagnostic aids. Fungi may be demonstrated by direct examination of skin scrapings treated with silver potassium hydroxide. The organism may be identified by culture on Sabouraud's medium.

Relation to systemic disease. None.

Differential diagnosis. Seborrheic dermatitis, eczema, psoriasis.

Therapy. Topically applied clotrimazole, miconazole or tolnaftate creams are the therapy of choice for limited lesions. Extensive disease is best treated with systemic griseofulvin. Keratolytic ointments containing 5-10% salicylic acid may also be of value.

Tinea Versicolor

Synonym. Pityriasis versicolor.

Sites of predilection. Chest, back. The lesions, which rarely involve the face, may extend onto the neck, arms, abdomen and thighs.

Objective signs. This macular eruption is characterized by the development of discrete and confluent, small to large areas which tend to involve the major portion of the chest and back. The lesions are dry, well-defined, and noninfiltrated. The color may be light tan (fawn colored), pink, brown or depigmented. Very fine scaling may be

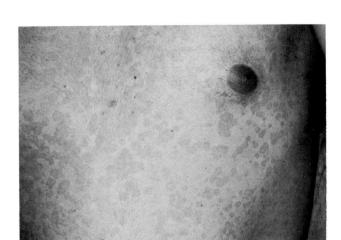

Tinea versicolor

present in some cases. In reflected light there is slight, apparent elevation of the lesion, and the surface appears to be covered with a slightly wrinkled film. The lesions become more prominent during the summer months when the patient is exposed to sunlight. The areas involved by the disease fail to tan on exposure to sunlight.

If this disease is ever contagious, the evidence must be extremely rare. Attempts at experimental inoculation have consistently failed.

Subjective symptoms. None. Mild pruritus with excessive perspiration.

Etiology. *Pityrosporon orbiculare.*

Histopathology. The fungi may be demonstrated in the stratum corneum by use of the PAS stain.

Diagnostic aids. The short hyphae and clusters of spores of *P orbiculare* may be easily demonstrated in scales treated with potassium hydroxide.

Relation to systemic disease. None.

Differential diagnosis. Melasma, vitiligo, seborrheic dermatitis, pityriasis rosea, pityriasis alba.

Therapy. Clotrimazole cream is very effective. Other effective medications are saturated solution of sodium thiosulfate and selenium sulfide shampoos.

Vitiligo; Leukoderma

Synonym. Vitiligo is idiopathic depigmentation; leukoderma is acquired depigmentation. These terms are frequently used synonymously.

Sites of predilection. Any part of the body.

Objective signs. There are variously sized and shaped, discrete and confluent, sharply defined areas of total loss of pigment. The lesions tend to be symmetrical and to spread peripherally. Hyperpigmentation may develop at the margin between the area of depigmentation and the normal skin. If the condition is persistent, the hair in the involved area also loses its pigment. The depigmented areas become bright red on slight exposure to sunlight, but do not tan. Spontaneous remissions may occur.

Subjective symptoms. None caused by the cutaneous lesions. The condition may cause emotional im-

Vitiligo

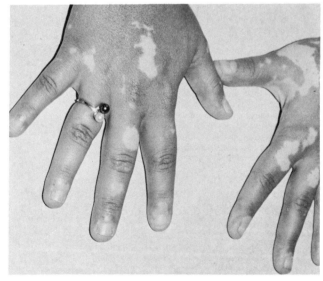

balance due to the cosmetic defect.

Etiology. Vitiligo is idiopathic depigmentation. Leukoderma may develop following contact with phenols, quinones or agerite alba, or may follow some inflammatory condition such as psoriasis, herpes zoster and eczema. Leukoderma may also be a sequela of exfoliative dermatitis.

Histopathology. There is absence of melanin and melanocyte in the basal layer.

Diagnostic aids. History and physical examination biopsy.

Relation to systemic disease. Vitiligo can be associated with atopic diseases, collagen vascular diseases, autoimmune diseases (pernicious anemia, Addison's disease, thyrotoxicosis) and melanoma.

Differential diagnosis. Pinta, morphea, leprosy (macular depigmented lesions), tinea versicolor.

Therapy. Psoralens given orally and exposure to ultraviolet rays (UVA).

CHAPTER 15

Papular Eruptions

Acanthosis Nigricans

Synonym. Keratosis nigricans.

Sites of predilection. Axillae, inframammary areas, genitocrural region, neck.

Objective signs. Reddish-brown to black hyperpigmentation is usually the first sign. The areas become lichenified and later develop discrete, grouped or confluent, soft, papillomatous projections and vegetating masses. Loss of scalp hair and eyebrows may be associated. The palms and soles are frequently hyperkeratotic.

Subjective symptoms. None.

Etiology. Unknown.

Histopathology. Hyperkeratosis, acanthosis and atrophy of the epidermis over the dermal pegs are the chief features. Little or no inflammatory reaction is seen. Hyperpigmentation is present.

Diagnostic aids. History and physical examination, biopsy, roentgen studies, 17-ketosteroids, blood sugar, CBC, SMA$_{12}$.

Relation to systemic disease. The adult or malignant type is associated with visceral malignancy in

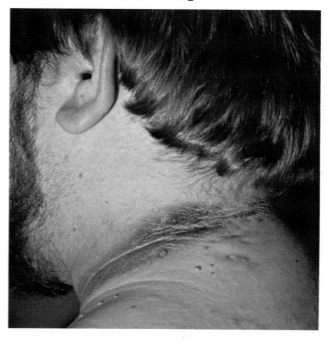

Acanthosis nigricans

over 90% of cases. The juvenile or benign type may be a familial disorder, a complication of endocrine dysfunction (*eg,* insulin resistant diabetes), or associated with obesity (also called pseudoacanthosis nigricans).

Differential diagnosis. Fox-Fordyce disease, keratosis follicularis, eczematous eruptions of the axillae, Ehlers-Danlos syndrome.

Therapy. There is no effective specific therapy for the cutaneous lesions. In the adult type, operable malignancies should be removed. In the juvenile type, reduction of weight produces involution of lesions.

Acne, Halogen

Synonym. Bromide acne, iodide acne.

Sites of predilection. Face, chest, back. Lesions often involve the extremities and lower portion of the trunk. (Acne vulgaris is usually limited to the upper back and chest.)

Objective signs. Follicular papules, papulopustules and pustules develop. The condition resembles acne vulgaris. The lesions may be brownish and coalesce to form groups with a serpiginous border. The inflammatory element may be pronounced. Granulomatous lesions may develop.

Subjective symptoms. Usually none, except the emotional reaction to the cosmetic defect.

Etiology. Ingestion of bromides or iodides (frequently contained in commercial headache remedies).

Histopathology. Leukocytes, plasma cells and foreign body giant cells form an infiltrate in and about the pilosebaceous apparatus.

Diagnostic aids. History and physical examination, blood bromide determinations.

Relation to systemic disease. The underlying condition which necessitates bromide ingestion.

Differential diagnosis. Acne vulgaris, rosacea.

Therapy. Bromide medication should be discontinued, and large doses of sodium chloride administered daily. Local therapy is of little value.

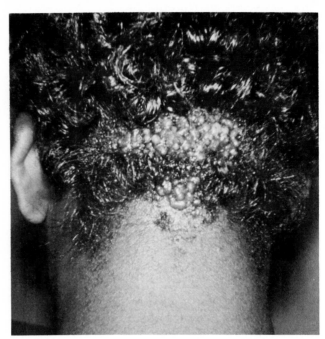

Acne keloid

Acne Keloid

Synonym. Dermatitis papillaris capillitii, folliculitis cheloidalis.

Sites of predilection. Back of neck, chest, back.

Objective signs. The lesions begin as follicular papules or papulopustules. As the acute inflammatory phase subsides, the lesions develop into keloids which may remain discrete or become confluent.

Subjective symptoms. Slight to severe pruritus.

Etiology. Scar formation in acne lesions.

Histopathology. Dense fibrous tissue (keloid). A chronic granuloma which contains many plasma cells.

Diagnostic aids. Biopsy.

Relation to systemic disease. None usually.

Differential diagnosis. The condition is characteristic.

Therapy. Sublesional injections of triamcinolone diacetate are occasionally beneficial, as are liquid nitrogen and carbon dioxide "slush." Systemic tetracyclines may counteract new lesions but will not affect the keloid. Treatment is generally unsatisfactory.

Acne Rosacea

Rosacea has been described in Chapter 14: Macular Eruptions. When the disease is complicated by the presence of papules or papulopustules, it has been called acne rosacea. Rosacea is now the preferred term.

Acne Vulgaris

Synonym. Pimples, acne.
Sites of predilection. Face, chest, back.
Objective signs. The primary lesion is a follicular papule, papulopustule or comedo (blackhead). Secondary lesions are crusts, excoriations and scars. The papules vary from red to blue-red in color and are conical or rounded. The individual lesions may be superficial papules or deep nodules (indurated acne). Occasionally the lesions form subcutaneous burrows filled with thick pus. The lesions vary in size from a few millimeters to 2 cm or more in diameter. The burrows may be 4 cm or more in length.

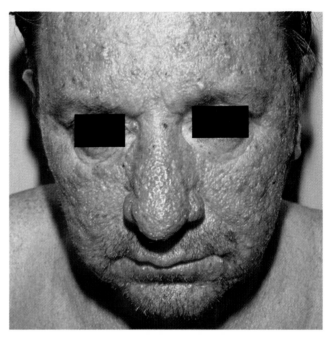

Acne rosacea

Scars result from spontaneous rupture, self-inflicted trauma (picking), surgical procedures or healing of the deep-seated burrowing lesion

Acne vulgaris

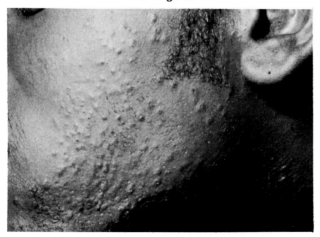

Acne conglobata

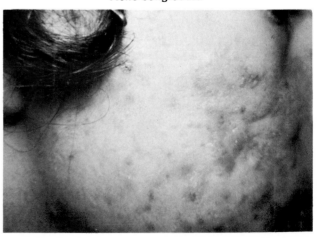

(acne conglobata). Scars may be shallow and broad, deeply pitted or have an overhanging edge. Patients usually have more than one type of lesion present. The involved areas are oily. Seborrheic dermatitis may also be present.

Subjective symptoms. Subjective symptoms are usually minimal. Pruritus may be present. The larger and cystic lesions are painful. The cosmetic defect caused by acne or its sequelae may produce emotional problems.

Etiology. The cause of acne is unknown. It may be associated with endocrine imbalance and usually begins about the time of puberty.

    The role played by the surface flora or acne bacillus is obscure. Secondary infection with staphylococci can occur. Dietary factors may play a role in some cases of acne.

Histopathology. Lymphocytic and plasma cell infiltration surround a comedo-filled hair follicle. Abscesses may form due to secondary infection. Giant cells are occasionally seen. The black color of a comedo is caused by melanin.

Diagnostic aids. Clinical acumen is usually sufficient. Biopsy is rarely necessary. Cultural studies are indicated if secondary bacterial infection is present.

Relation to systemic disease. The course of acne is influenced by endocrine imbalance. Excessive corticosteroid administration increases severity. There is a hereditary tendency to develop acne.

Differential diagnosis. Halogen acne, papular and pustular secondary syphilis, impetigo contagiosa, rosacea, verruca plana, adenoma sebaceum, acnitis (tuberculid).

Therapy. Treatment must be individualized for each patient. Avoid unnecessary trauma or picking. Gentle cleansing is preferred. Observe dietary restrictions when indicated. Benzoyl peroxide or retinoic acid in cream or gel will effectively remove comedones. Clindamycin in propylene glycol-alcohol suspensions is an effective topical preparation. Colloidal sulfur lotions are useful in treatment when the skin is excessively oily. Systemic tetracycline is the drug of choice in reducing pustule formation. Incision and drainage of fluctuant lesions is frequently necessary.

Actinomycosis

Synonym. Lumpy jaw.

Sites of predilection. Face, neck.

Objective signs. Deep-seated nodules or subcutaneous masses which develop slowly and become soft and fluctuant over a period of several weeks to months. The overlying tissues slough and the ensuing purulent discharge contains small masses called "sulfur granules." Sinus tracts and chronic subcutaneous abscesses form.

Subjective symptoms. Local pain.

Etiology. Actinomyces bovis.

Histopathology. Fungi can be demonstrated by a biopsy taken near the edge of a lesion. They are surrounded by a zone of polymorphonuclear leukocytic infiltration and, in the periphery, plasma cells, giant cells and epithelioid cells.

Diagnostic aids. Biopsy; demonstration of the fungus in "sulfur granules" usually found in pus or sputum; culture of the organism on Sabouraud's media; skin tests are of no value.

Relation to systemic disease. Primary actinomycosis of the skin is rare. Gastrointestinal tract infection is common. Involvement of the lungs is usually by extension through tissues or secondary to other visceral infection.

Differential diagnosis. Scrofuloderma, peridontal sinuses, syphilis (gumma), malignancies, other deep mycoses.

Therapy. Systemically administered penicillin in adequate dosage over a period of 3-4 months is the therapy of choice.

Adenoma Sebaceum, Balzer Type

Synonym. Trichoepithelioma.

    See Trichoepithelioma for full description.

Adenoma, Senile Sebaceous

Synonym. Hypertrophic sebaceous glands, senile sebaceous nevus.

Sites of predilection. Face.

Objective signs. One or more yellowish, flat, umbilicated papules, varying from 2-5 mm in diameter. The skin is usually oily, and there may be associated folliculitis or rosacea.

Subjective symptoms. None.

Etiology. Unknown.

Histopathology. Large numbers of normal-appearing, mature or nearly mature, sebaceous glands.

Diagnostic aids. Biopsy.

Relation to systemic disease. None. Other senile changes are present.

Differential diagnosis. Epithelioma, seborrheic keratoses.

Therapy. Excision or destruction by electrodesiccation.

Angiokeratoma

Synonym. Telangiectatic warts, angioma of the scrotum.

Sites of predilection. Scrotum, extremities.

Objective signs. Few to numerous, pinpoint to splitpea sized, reddish or purplish, warty papules on the extremities (Mibelli type). On the scrotum the lesions appear as purplish papules which may or may not be grossly keratotic (Fordyce type). Angiokeratomas can be seen on the trunk and leg of patients with a sex-linked recessive disorder (Fabry's disease). In this disorder there is a deficiency of ceramide trihexosidase. The extra cutaneous symptoms which include abdominal pain and renal failure are presumably related to increased deposits of ceramide trihexoside.

Solitary or group angiokeratomas may appear on the legs where they may simulate melanoma.

Subjective symptoms. None.

Etiology. Unknown.

Histopathology. Variable chronic infiltrate, vascular dilatation and thickening of the stratum corneum. The telangiectatic vessels appear to course within the epidermis.

Diagnostic aids. History and physical examination, biopsy.

Relation to systemic disease. May be related to chilblains and to hereditary telangiectasia (Rendu-Osler-Weber). (See Fabry's disease above.)

Differential diagnosis. Verruca vulgaris, melanoma, pyogenic granuloma.

Therapy. Destruction of individual lesions by desiccation or cryotherapy.

Atopic Dermatitis, Papular

Synonym. Papular eczema, neurodermatitis.

Sites of predilection. Face, neck, trunk, flexural aspects of the extremities.

Objective signs. Usually confluent patches of small erythematous papules, with discrete lesions noted in the periphery of the ill-defined areas. The individual lesions may develop as follicular papules or be miliary papules not associated with hair follicles. The eruption may be localized or generalized. This type of atopic dermatitis is usually associated with other forms of the condition. Excoriations are a prominent feature, and secondary pyogenic infection frequently occurs.

Subjective symptoms. Moderate to severe pruritus.

See Atopic Dermatitis in Chapter 14: Macular Eruptions, for etiology, histopathology, diagnostic aids and relation to systemic disease.

Differential diagnosis. Papular urticaria, folliculitis, lichen planus.

Therapy. See Atopic Dermatitis in Chapter 14.

Basal Cell Nevus Syndrome

Synonym. None.

Sites of predilection. Face, scalp, neck, chest.

Objective signs. Same as multiple benign cystic epithelioma. Patients may also have jaw cysts, bifid ribs, mental deficiency, hypertelorism and palmar dyskeratoses, as well as other skeletal and nervous system defects.

Subjective symptoms. None.

Etiology. An inherent defect.

Histopathology. See Benign Cystic Epithelioma.

Diagnostic aids. Biopsy, jaw and rib X ray.

Relation to systemic disease. None.

Differential diagnosis. None.

Therapy. Surgical excision or radiation therapy of any malignant lesion.

Blastomycosis

Synonym. North American blastomycosis, Gilchrist's disease.

Sites of predilection. Face, upper extremities; any area may become involved.

Objective signs. The primary cutaneous lesion is a papulopustule which spreads peripherally, form-

Blastomycosis

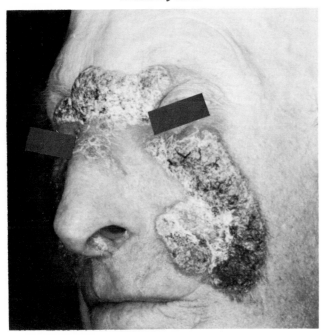

ing an elevated plaque. The lesions grow slowly and present a verrucous surface which is usually crusted. The border of the lesion is smooth, purplish-red in color, and may present numerous tiny abscesses from which the *Blastomyces dermatitidis* may be demonstrated. Cutaneous granulomatous lesions may develop along the course of the lymphatics, draining the primary affected areas.

Subjective symptoms. Usually absent but there may be slight pain in areas which are secondarily infected.

Etiology. *B dermatitidis*.

Histopathology. Miliary abscesses and a dense infiltrate of leukocytes, epithelioid and plasma cells. Giant cells are present, and usually contain the organism. *B dermatitidis* is a round, oval or slightly irregular body with a double-contoured capsule. Budding forms are seen, but mycelia have not been demonstrated in tissues.

Diagnostic aids. History and physical examination, biopsy, culture.

Relation to systemic disease. Any organ or tissue in the body may be attacked. The lungs are affected in over 90% of the cases of systemic disease. The kidneys, bone and central nervous system may become involved.

Differential diagnosis. Tuberculosis cutis, epitheliomas, nodular syphiloderm.

Therapy. Stilbamidine, 2-hydroxystilbamidine and amphotericin B are effective.

Callus

Synonym. Callosity, callositas.

Sites of predilection. Palmar and plantar surfaces.

Objective signs. Calluses occur on areas of the body which are subject to chronic trauma. They may develop as an industrial dermatosis among tool handlers, musicians or shoemakers. They are slightly raised, whitish or grayish-white in color, with a smooth hyperkeratotic surface. The edges merge gradually into the normal skin. The fingerprint or footprint patterns are intact.

Subjective symptoms. None to considerable discomfort.

Etiology. Chronic trauma.

Histopathology. Thickening of the stratum corneum and stratum granulosum.

Diagnostic aids. Clinical appearance is characteristic.

Relation to systemic disease. None.

Differential diagnosis. Plantar warts and arsenical keratoses.

Therapy. None necessary unless the lesion becomes painful. The lesions may be pared with a sharp blade or treated with 20-40% salicylic acid plasters. Remove the cause. Properly fitting shoes are important for this condition.

Carcinoma, Squamous Cell

Synonym. Prickle cell cancer, malignant acanthoma, epidermoid carcinoma.

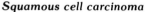

Squamous cell carcinoma

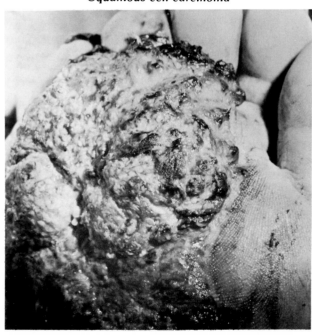

Sites of predilection. Exposed surfaces of the body. Occurs frequently on the lower part of the face, lower lip or the dorsal surfaces of the hands.

Objective signs. These malignant lesions may begin as small, hard, whitish or yellowish nodules, or may arise from leukoplakic lesions, senile keratoses or chronic ulcers. The base is firm and usually telangiectatic. The lesions grow rapidly in size compared to the growth of a basal cell epithelioma. Ulceration may occur and offers a rough index of the degree of malignancy; the more highly differentiated tumors usually have an intact surface. The ulcers usually have a wide, rolled, pearly border, although rapidly growing lesions may be fungoid in appearance. The lesions vary from 1-5 cm or more in diameter.

Squamous cell cancers of the lower lip may resemble small papillomas with intact surfaces (relatively benign), or begin as fissures, which rapidly break down and form early metastases.

Subjective symptoms. Little or no pain is present unless the lesion is large or has metastasized.

Etiology. Unknown.

Histopathology. The histologic picture varies with the grade of malignancy. In low-grade malignancies the degree of anaplasia is small and the cancer cell has little ability to penetrate the corium. As the cancer becomes more malignant, the degree of anaplasia increases (amount of mitosis, abnormal rete cells and disorderly appearance). In low-grade malignancy, pearl formation predominates, but in the very malignant form there is complete lack of adhesiveness and an increase in the ability of cells to penetrate the corium.

Diagnostic aids. Biopsy findings are characteristic.

Relation to systemic disease. None unless the lesion has metastasized.

Differential diagnosis. Verrucae, pyogenic granuloma, gumma, tuberculosis cutis, lupus vulgaris, other types of epitheliomas, chronic granulomas, keratoacanthoma.

Therapy. Wide excision of the lesion, followed by

radiation therapy. These lesions are radio-sensitive but require a somewhat higher dose of X-ray than do basal cell epitheliomas.

Chloracne

Synonym. Tar acne, paraffin acne.

Sites of predilection. Arms, legs, face, chest, back.

Objective signs. Follicular papules, papulopustules and comedo-like lesions resembling acne vulgaris, develop on surfaces that come in contact with oily substances. Comedones occur in patches on the extensor surfaces of the upper extremities and are concentrated about the elbows. The lesions are chronically inflamed. The comedones in this condition are hard, keratinous plugs which are difficult to remove by expression. There may be an associated contact dermatitis of the hands.

Subjective symptoms. Moderate to intense pruritus.

Etiology. Industrial handling of tar, grease, paraffin and oil, with resultant follicular irritation and mechanical plugging of the follicular orifices.

Histopathology. Infiltration of leukocytes, plasma cells and foreign body giant cells in and about the pilosebaceous apparatus.

Diagnostic aids. History and physical examination.

Relation to systemic disease. None.

Differential diagnosis. Acne vulgaris, steroid acne.

Therapy. Wear protective clothing when working with oil; avoid contact with oil; use 5-10% salicylic acid in 95% alcohol locally. Do not use oily ointment bases when treating this condition.

Corn

Synonym. Clavus.

Sites of predilection. Areas of the foot, *eg,* the dorsal surface of the fifth toe, on which greatest pressure is exerted by shoes. Plantar corns also occur most frequently over the heads of the first or fifth metatarsal.

Objective signs. One or more small (3 mm-1 cm), rounded, raised, yellowish-gray, callus-like lesions. The lesions appear to be formed of layers of horny material. The summit is usually rough. Plantar corns are frequently confused with plantar warts. The plantar corn is formed of an avascular plug of keratin surrounded by a dense zone of hyperkeratosis. They are almost always adjacent to a bony prominence such as the heads of the distal metatarsals.

Subjective symptoms. Moderate to severe pain.

Etiology. Chronic intermittent pressure of shoes.

Histopathology. Hyperkeratosis.

Diagnostic aids. None usually necessary.

Relation to systemic disease. None.

Differential diagnosis. Callus, keratoses, warts.

Therapy. Use of 20-40% salicylic acid plasters offers temporary relief. Properly fitting shoes may eliminate the lesions. Surgical removal should be avoided.

Cylindroma

Synonym. Turban tumor, nevus epitheliomatocylindromatosus, endothelioma capitis, sarcoma capitis.

Sites of predilection. Scalp.

Objective signs. This condition is characterized by the development of slow-growing, flesh-colored to red tumors which vary from 1-8 cm in diameter. The lesions may cover the entire scalp, and smaller lesions may appear on the face, chest and back.

Subjective symptoms. None.

Etiology. Unknown; probably congenital.

Histopathology. The microscopic picture is characterized by masses of basal cells, surrounded by connective tissue membranes. The peripheral cells are palisaded, whereas the central portion shows hyaline degeneration and cyst formation.

Diagnostic aids. Biopsy.

Relation to systemic disease. None.

Differential diagnosis. The disease is characteristic in appearance. Isolated lesions may resemble basal cell cancers, sebaceous cysts or metastatic tumors.

Therapy. Excision.

Cyst, Benign Synovial

Synonym. Periarticular cyst.

Sites of predilection. Phalangeal joints, usually the distal one.

Objective signs. One or more rounded, papular, cystic lesions, usually less than 1 cm in diameter. The summit is frequently umbilicated. The lesions may be smooth and shiny, or may have a roughened surface, varying from flesh-colored to purplish. When the lesion is incised, a thick, viscid fluid exudes. Synovial cysts occur more frequently in women.

Subjective symptoms. Pain.

Etiology. Unknown.

Histopathology. The corium and epidermis are atrophic. The lesion is a degenerative cyst whose wall is composed of flat, connective tissue cells.

Diagnostic aids. None is usually necessary, although the lesions frequently resemble verrucae. Puncture may help differentiate the cyst from a solid lesion.

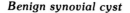

Benign synovial cyst

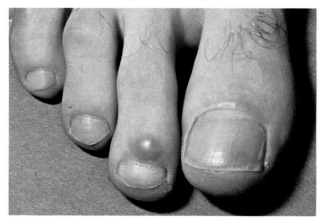

Relation to systemic disease. None usually.

Differential diagnosis. Verruca vulgaris.

Therapy. The lesions are easily emptied by incision and expression of the fluid; however, when the incision heals, the cyst rapidly refills. Surgical treatment is usually unsuccessful. The most satisfactory results are obtained by injection of depository corticosteroids, even though many attempts may prove necessary. Cryotherapy with a carbon dioxide snow pencil or liquid nitrogen has also been reported as successful treatment.

Cyst, Dermoid

Synonym. None.

Sites of predilection. Head, neck; generally overlying suture lines of the bones or the branchial arches.

Objective signs. Dermoid cysts are noninflammatory, subcutaneous tumors which are not attached to epidermal structures. They vary in size from a few millimeters to several centimeters in diameter.

Subjective symptoms. Usually none.

Etiology. Dermoid cysts are congenital in origin and may appear at any time in life.

Histopathology. The lining of the cyst is stratified squamous epithelium and all dermal elements may be present, including sebaceous glands, hair, sweat glands and teeth. Sometimes the lesions are teratomas.

Diagnostic aids. Biopsy.

Relation to systemic disease. There may be other evidences of faulty development. Dermoid cysts may be found in internal organs, chiefly the ovaries and testes.

Differential diagnosis. Other tumors of the skin.

Therapy. Surgical excision is necessary, since squamous cell carcinomatous degeneration frequently occurs.

Cyst, Sebaceous

Synonym. Steatoma, wen, epidermal cyst.

Sites of predilection. Face, scalp, back, scrotum.

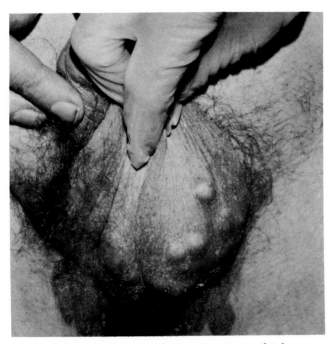

Sebaceous cysts with tinea cruris on thighs

Objective signs. These slowly growing, benign, cystic lesions are attached to the skin but not to the subcutaneous tissues. They are usually firm in consistency, but may become soft due to secondary infection. They are filled with a caseous, foul-smelling material. The wall of the cyst is a fibrous capsule. When inflamed, the contents become much more fluid and the capsule adheres more closely to the surrounding tissues. The lesions may be solitary or multiple, and vary from 1-10 cm in diameter. The condition may be associated with acne.

Subjective symptoms. Usually none unless the lesions become secondarily infected.

Etiology. Plug formation in sebaceous duct orifices and hyperactivity of the gland.

Histopathology. The wall is composed of nonkeratinized epithelial cells. The peripheral layer shows palisading. The cysts are filled with amorphous material.

Diagnostic aids. Biopsy.

Relation to systemic disease. None.

Differential diagnosis. Lipoma, fibroma, acne cysts, other tumors, abscess (if inflamed).

Therapy. Surgical excision; the entire capsule must be removed in order to prevent recurrence.

Cyst, Traumatic Epithelial

Synonym. Epidermoid cyst.

Sites of predilection. Palmar surfaces, scars.

Objective signs. Usually solitary and less than 1 cm in diameter, these subcutaneous, noninflamed lesions occur on the palms of mechanics and other individuals whose hands are subjected to trauma. If ruptured, they exude a thick fluid. They may become secondarily infected.

Subjective symptoms. None, unless infection is present.

Etiology. Unknown.

Histopathology. Noninflammatory cystic lesion with a wall composed of stratified epithelium with a thick, inner, horny layer. No sebaceous gland elements are present, since the lesions usually appear on the palms.

Diagnostic aids. Biopsy to differentiate from sebaceous cysts.

Relation to systemic disease. None.

Differential diagnosis. Sebaceous cyst, fibroma.

Therapy. Excision.

Dermatosis Papulosa Nigra

Synonym. Seborrheic keratosis of the Negro.

Sites of predilection. Face, chiefly about the nose and cheeks.

Objective signs. Few to numerous discrete, brown to black, flat or slightly rounded lesions, measuring 1-5 mm in diameter. These benign lesions occur only in blacks.

Subjective symptoms. None.

Etiology. Unknown.

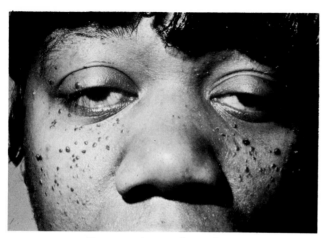

Dermatosis papulosa nigra

Histopathology. Identical with the changes observed in seborrheic keratoses.

Diagnostic aids. Biopsy.

Relation to systemic disease. None.

Differential diagnosis. Adenoma sebaceum, verruca plana juvenilis, moles, trichoepithelioma.

Therapy. None indicated or necessary. Surgical removal may be followed by keloid formation. Electrodesiccation can be effective.

Ear Corn

Synonym. Chronic painful nodule of the ear, chondrodermatitis nodularis chronica helicis.

Sites of predilection. Rim of the ear.

Objective signs. Well-defined, hard, round or oval lesions, varying in size from 3-8 mm. The lesions are usually whitish or yellowish with a central crusted depression. Ulcerations may occur. They may be single or multiple and are attached to the underlying cartilage. They occur more frequently in men.

Subjective symptoms. Slight discomfort to severe pain, particularly when the ear is in contact with the pillow or telephone.

Etiology. Unknown.

Histopathology. Edema, collagen degeneration and vascular proliferation in the corium with the inflammatory process involving the cartilage. Moderate acanthosis is present.

Diagnostic aids. Biopsy.

Relation to systemic disease. None.

Differential diagnosis. Epithelioma, keratoses, tophi.

Therapy. Excision or destruction of the lesion may only be of temporary value. Recurrences are frequent.

Edema, Familial Angioneurotic

Synonym. Hereditary angioedema.

Sites of predilection. Any area may be affected.

Objective signs. The lesion is a generalized swelling of an entire part of the body. Difficulty in breathing can be caused by a laryngeal edema. Urticarial wheals rarely, if ever, appear in this disease.

Subjective symptoms. Pruritic, painless swelling is the usual rule. Some mild discomfort may occur.

Etiology. This is a dominant genetic disease with 85% having a blood deficiency of C1-esterase inhibitor. The remainder of the patients have normal levels of the compound, but it functions abnormally. Histamine levels are normal. The disease may be induced by kinins released by the complement and bradykinin systems.

Histopathology. Dermal and subcutaneous fatty tissue edema with some dermal mononuclear cellular infiltration.

Diagnostic aids. Serum C1, C2, and C4 levels.

Relation to systemic disease. None.

Differential diagnosis. Malignancy. The C1 levels are depressed in patients with malignancies.

Therapy. Administration of epsilon aminocaproic acid is the current therapy of choice. Tracheotomy is lifesaving for laryngeal edema. Recent experiments with danazol, an androgen compound, have shown promising results.

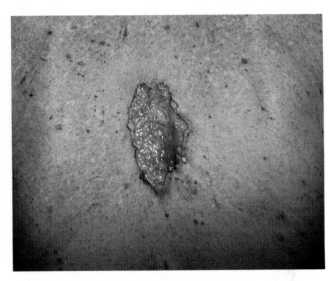

Superficial basal cell epithelioma

Epithelioma, Basal Cell

Synonym. Basal cell cancer, rodent ulcer, basal cell
carcinoma.

Sites of predilection. Usually the upper portion of the
face, although basal cell epitheliomas may appear
on any part of the body.

Objective signs. These slowly growing, malignant
tumors first appear as small keratoses or shiny,
solid, whitish or pinkish papules with telangiectasia. The lesions may vary from 2 mm to several
centimeters in diameter. They may remain as
intact papules, which do not increase in size, or
the lesions may ulcerate and spread peripherally
after varying periods of several weeks to several
months or years. The borders are "rolled,"
pearly and telangiectatic. If the central crust is
removed by "picking," or other trauma, bleeding
occurs. Eventually a crust fails to form and a
chronic indolent ulcer results.

Subjective symptoms. Usually none. The area may
become tender if ulceration develops. There may
be emotional trauma because of the cosmetic
defect. Occasionally, fear of cancer may prevent

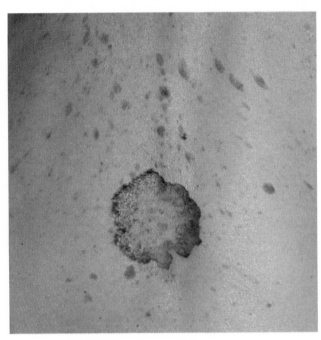

Superficial basal cell epithelioma

the patient from seeking treatment, or even produce a psychosis.

Etiology. Unknown. Prolonged and repeated exposure to the sun, trauma or chronic irritation
from other sources are factors associated with the

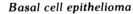

Basal cell epithelioma

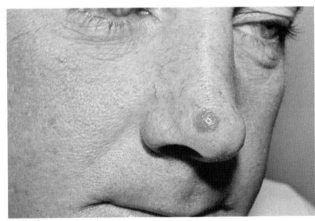

production of basal cell epitheliomas. Genetic factors are important as some families have a very high incidence of epitheliomas.

Histopathology. Differentiated basal cell carcinomas show epithelial structures such as sebaceous glands, apocrine glands, hair follicles, *etc.* The undifferentiated type is characterized by large oval or elongated, deeply staining, basophilic nuclei, usually surrounded by a small, ill-defined zone of cytoplasm. Many basal cell cancers are a mixed type and show both differentiated and undifferentiated types of structures in the same tumor.

Diagnostic aids. Biopsy.

Relation to systemic disease. None.

Differential diagnosis. Other types of epitheliomas, senile and seborrheic keratoses, verrucae, benign nevi, leukoplakia.

Therapy. Basal cell epitheliomas may be treated by surgical excision, radiation (conventional or grenz), radium therapy or a combination of surgery and radiation. Topical 5-fluorouracil and immunotherapy are experimental procedures.

These lesions are relatively benign. Because of the mental distress frequently suffered when the patient is told the diagnosis is "cancer," a careful explanation of the nature of the lesions and the good prognosis attendant on proper therapy is mandatory.

Epithelioma, Multiple Benign Cystic

Synonym. Multiple trichoepithelioma.

Sites of predilection. Face, scalp, neck, chest.

Objective signs. Few to numerous, rounded, translucent, sessile papules which are pinkish to bluish-white in color. These tumors frequently have a slight central depression. The lesions vary in size from 2-5 mm. The larger lesions may be telangiectatic.

Subjective symptoms. None.

Etiology. Unknown. There may be a familial tendency. Some experts consider this entity to be a variant of the basal cell nevus syndrome.

Histopathology. Keratin cysts, intermingled with solid strands or nests of basal cells.

Diagnostic aids. Biopsy.

Relation to systemic disease. None.

Differential diagnosis. Epithelioma of other types, adenoma sebaceum, molluscum contagiosum.

Therapy. Excision, curettage or desiccation.

Erythema Induratum

Synonym. Bazin's disease, tuberculosis cutis indurativa.

Sites of predilection. Calves.

Objective signs. One or more deep-seated nodules are located in the subcutaneous tissues. These lesions, which vary from 1-4 cm, gradually enlarge and undergo necrosis, forming ulcers which heal with depressed scars. The skin over the

Erythema induratum

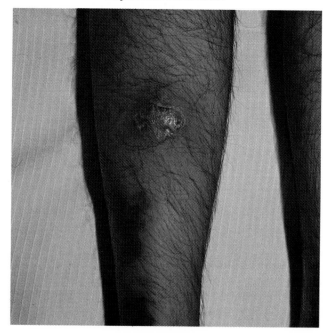

lesions is usually dull reddish to bluish-red in color.

The lesions tend to heal spontaneously, but recur. They most frequently occur in young women.

Subjective symptoms. The intact lesions are slightly tender. When ulceration occurs they may be very painful.

Etiology. This eruption is a tuberculid or cutaneous reaction to a distant tuberculous focus.

Histopathology. Numerous discrete tubercles form around the blood vessels in the subcutis. The vessel walls are thickened and the vessels are destroyed. There is marked inflammatory reaction in the subcutaneous tissue.

Diagnostic aids. History and physical examination, biopsy, chest X ray, studies for tuberculosis.

Relation to systemic disease. Active pulmonary or visceral tuberculosis may be associated.

Differential diagnosis. Gumma, erythema nodosum, nodular vasculitis, periarteritis nodosa.

Therapy. Streptomycin, isoniazid and para-aminosalicylic acid.

Erythema Multiforme

Synonym. None.

Sites of predilection. Flexor surfaces of the extremities, palmar and plantar surfaces, lips.

Objective signs. Usually numerous, pink to violaceous, nonscaly papules, varying in size from a few millimeters to 2 cm or more in diameter. The lesions vary in shape from nummular to gyrate. They are well-defined and may form annular or iris (target) lesions. The vermilion borders of the lips are usually crusted and edematous. Macules and vesicles may also be present in the same patient. The patient may be acutely ill.

Subjective symptoms. Generalized malaise, sore throat, arthralgias and a burning sensation in the eyes may be present. Patient may be febrile.

Etiology. Unknown. Erythema multiforme is a cutaneous reaction to foci of infection, drug administration, vaccines or immune sera. Herpes simplex is a common precursor. Hebra's disease is the seasonal type.

Histopathology. See Erythema Multiforme in Chapter 14: Macular Eruptions.

Diagnostic aids. History and physical examination; hemogram; direct or indirect immunofluorescence to rule out fluorescence at the basement membrane. Serologic examination for herpes simplex infections.

Relation to systemic disease. Erythema multiforme is a systemic disease; the diagnosis is usually made by observation of the cutaneous symptoms. The patient may be seriously ill.

Differential diagnosis. Chronic urticaria, secondary syphilis, drug reaction.

Therapy. See Erythema Multiforme in Chapter 14.

Erythema Nodosum

Synonym. Dermatitis contusiformis.

Sites of predilection. Extensor surfaces of the legs and thighs; lesions occasionally appear on the upper extremities.

Objective signs. The lesions may be few to numerous, usually varying from 1-3 cm in diameter. They are pink to bluish-red in color and appear in crops. They are usually firm. Lesions may become soft, but do not ulcerate. Hyperpigmentation may follow involution of the lesions. Recurrences are frequent.

Subjective symptoms. The lesions are tender and painful. There may be generalized malaise, arthralgia or gastrointestinal symptoms.

Etiology. Unknown. Erythema nodosum has been regarded as a variant of erythema multiforme. It may be associated with chronic foci of infection, rheumatic fever, tuberculosis, syphilis, sarcoidosis, other chronic granulomas and drug sensitivity.

Histopathology. Vascular dilatation of the cutis, perivascular round cell infiltration and thrombosis of small blood vessels.

Diagnostic aids. History and physical examination, biopsy, hemogram, serologic examination for streptococcal infection, throat culture, chest X ray.

Relation to systemic disease. Erythema nodosum may be associated with chronic tonsillitis, gastrointestinal disturbances, genitourinary disturbances, rheumatic fever, tuberculosis, drug reaction, birth control pills, sarcoidosis, coccidioidomycosis, and many other granulomatous diseases.

Differential diagnosis. Erythema induratum, gumma, chronic nonsuppurative panniculitis, periostitis, periarteritis nodosa, nodular vasculitis.

Therapy. Eliminate foci of infection or any suspected allergies. Enteric coated sodium salicylate, 0.5 gm, 3-4 times daily, may help. Systemic corticosteroid therapy will cause the lesions to disappear, but when the drug is discontinued, the lesions usually recur. Cure is achieved only when the cause is determined and eliminated.

Follicular Mucinosis

Synonym. Alopecia mucinosa.

Sites of predilection. Scalp, trunk, extremities.

Objective signs. Circumscribed infiltrated plaques develop in which there is some scale formation and loss of hair. The individual plaques are composed of small follicular papules which are surmounted by an adherent dry scale.

Two main types occur. The first group includes children and young adults in whom the lesions are few and self-limited. The second group is made up of older patients in whom the lesions are more extensive and 20% of these are associated with a reticulosis.

Subjective symptoms. None to moderate pruritus.

Etiology. Unknown.

Histopathology. Edema of the outer root sheath. Cystic spaces which contain mucin form. Inflammatory changes, which eventually become granulomatous, develop in the dermis.

Diagnostic aids. Biopsy.

Relation to systemic disease. Approximately 20% of older patients develop malignant reticuloendothelial changes.

Differential diagnosis. Atopic dermatitis, seborrheic dermatitis, lichen simplex, tinea capitis.

Therapy. None is specific.

Glomus Tumor

Synonym. Glomangioma.

Sites of predilection. Extremities, usually under nails.

Objective signs. The lesions are single, soft, small bluish or bluish-red tumors, 2 mm-1 cm in diameter. The lesions never become very large. Occasionally multiple lesions develop.

Subjective symptoms. Moderate to intense pain.

Etiology. Unknown.

Histopathology. The lesion is composed of an arterial element, Sucquet-Hoyer canals, and a venous element. The canal is lined by endothelium, surrounded by a thick mantle of glomus cells which resemble epithelioid cells, and has an eosinophilic cytoplasm and large oval nuclei. A rich network of nonmyelinated nerve fibrils can be demonstrated by special stains.

Diagnostic aids. Biopsy.

Relation to systemic disease. None usually, but may be associated with hypoplasia and osteoporosis of the bones of the forearm.

Differential diagnosis. Neuroma, angiosarcoma, verrucae.

Therapy. Surgical excision.

Gout

Synonym. None.

Sites of predilection. Rim of the external ear, fingers, toes.

Objective signs. Deposits of uric acid and urates under the skin, known as tophi. These papular lesions have smooth surfaces and are usually less than 1 cm in size, but may grow to 2 cm or more in diameter. They are whitish or cream colored. When ruptured the contents are gritty and whitish (uric acid and urates).

Subjective symptoms. Pain in the lesions, as well as generalized symptoms.

Etiology. Faulty uric acid metabolism.

Histopathology. A foreign body reaction with a variable number of foreign body giant cells and closely packed, needle-shaped crystals of sodium biurate.

Diagnostic aids. History and physical examination, uric acid hemoconcentration, urinalysis, biopsy of lesions.

Relation to systemic disease. Gout is a systemic disease.

Differential diagnosis. Basal cell epithelioma, chronic painful nodule of the ear.

Therapy. Colchicine is the drug of choice in acute attacks. Allopurinol or probenecid are uricosuric agents used to prevent further acute attacks by lowering the blood uric acid concentration.

Granuloma Annulare

Synonym. Ringed eruption, lichen annularis.

Sites of predilection. Localized lesions occur on distal portions of extremities over bony prominences. Generalized lesions may occur on any part of the trunk or extremities.

Objective signs. The primary lesion is a whitish, bluish or pinkish, deep-seated papule or ring of closely grouped papules, which usually forms an annular or serpiginous lesion. The lesions are firm and nonscaly with elevated borders. Annular configuration rarely occurs in the generalized form. The papules are firm, rounded and do not scale. They are skin colored and shiny.

The lesions tend to involute spontaneously but, in long-standing lesions, the central portion may be atrophic.

The condition commonly occurs in young children but lesions may appear at any age.

Subjective symptoms. None.

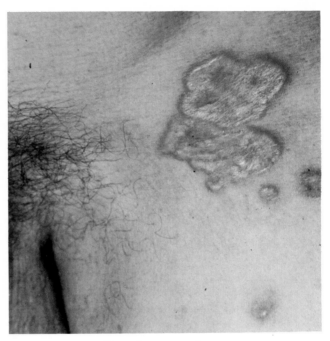

Granuloma annulare

Etiology. Unknown.

Histopathology. Moderately well-defined areas of altered collagen (necrobiosis) surrounded by epithelioid cells which may form palisading borders. Many small mononuclear cells form the perivascular infiltrate and also surround the epithelioid cells.

Diagnostic aids. Biopsy.

Relation to systemic disease. None has been established.

Differential diagnosis. Epithelioma, lichen planus, xanthoma tuberosum, erythema multiforme.

Therapy. Nonspecific. Surgical excision of a portion of the lesion for biopsy may result in complete involution.

Granuloma, Pyogenic

Synonym. Granuloma pyogenicum, botryomycosis hominis, telangiectatic granuloma.

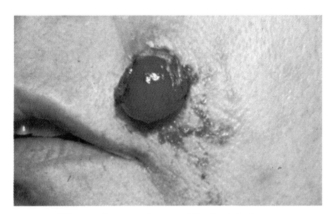

Pyogenic granuloma with dental sinus

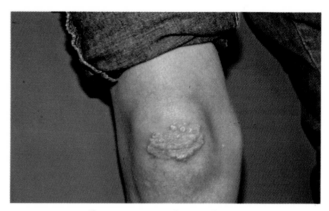

Swimming pool granuloma

Sites of predilection. Usually the face or extremities. Any area may be involved.

Objective signs. These papular lesions are single, small, pedunculated or sessile, vascular granulomas occurring at the sites of injuries. They frequently complicate an ingrown toenail or a dental sinus tract. The lesions vary from 2 mm-1 cm in diameter and are bluish-red to black. They may be covered with a thin blood or serous crust and tend to bleed profusely on slight trauma. Lymphangitic satellites have rarely been reported.

Subjective symptoms. Tenderness.

Etiology. Low-grade pyogenic infection causes formation of the granuloma.

Histopathology. The tumor is composed of numerous, newly formed and dilated capillaries, with a variable amount of endothelial proliferation. Histologically this lesion resembles a hemangioma.

Diagnostic aids. Biopsy.

Relation to systemic disease. None has been established.

Differential diagnosis. Verrucae, malignant melanoma, nevus, foreign body granuloma.

Therapy. Excision or destruction of the lesion by electrodesiccation.

Granuloma, Swimming Pool

Synonym. None.

Sites of predilection. Elbows, knees.

Objective signs. Lesion begins insidiously with a small, hyperkeratotic papule which gradually enlarges and is surrounded by a zone of dusky erythema. As the lesion enlarges, the surface becomes definitely verrucous.

Subjective symptoms. Usually none.

Etiology. Mycobacterium balnei. Patient traumatizes elbows or knees while swimming in infested water.

Histopathology. Hyperkeratosis and acanthosis. Marked cellular infiltration with tubercle formation.

Diagnostic aids. Culture on acid-fast medium, biopsy skin test for atypical mycobacteria.

Relation to systemic disease. None.

Differential diagnosis. Tuberculosis verrucosa cutis.

Therapy. Some lesions are self-limited. Excision of small lesions is curative. Cryotherapy is effective. Local heat to the lesion is an aid. Rifampin, tetracycline or a sulfamethoxazole-trimethapsin combination has been used effectively. Grenz-ray therapy has also been used successfully.

Hemangioma

Synonym. Nevus vasculosus, vascular nevus, strawberry nevus, birthmark.

Sites of predilection. Face, head, neck, trunk, extremities.

Objective signs. The lesions of simple hemangiomas are present at birth or begin shortly thereafter. They are round or irregular, slightly to moderately raised, bright reddish to purplish papules which vary in size from 2 mm to several centimeters in diameter. The lesions may be superficial or extend into the deep tissues. They may pulsate. They are usually single but may be multiple. Ulceration is followed by formation of a whitish scar. Simple hemangiomas tend to involute spontaneously.

The cavernous type, which is connected to the deep venous channels, is a soft, doughy tumor which has a smooth, light to dark blue surface and measures 1-5 cm. Simple hemangiomas may be present on the surface of these deeper lesions.

Hemangioma

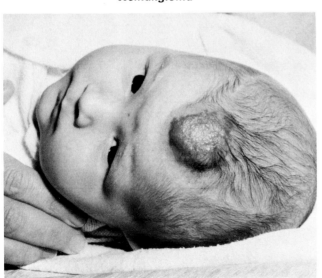

Subjective symptoms. None usually, although pain may occur with ulceration.

Etiology. Congenital.

Histopathology. There is dilatation of preexisting vessels and proliferation of new vessels, as well as connective tissue proliferation.

Diagnostic aids. History and physical examination, biopsy.

Relation to systemic disease. None usually.

Differential diagnosis. Pyogenic granuloma.

Therapy. The smaller lesions usually involute spontaneously over a period of several years. If the lesion grows out of proportion to the child's growth, it should be removed surgically. Large pulsating lesions must be excised. If these cavernous hemangiomas occlude the airway, large doses of prednisone systemically may be necessary to shrink their size so that other surgical procedures can be initiated. There is no justification for the use of ionizing radiation in the treatment of angiomas.

Histiocytoma

Synonym. Dermatofibroma lenticulare, fibroma simplex, sclerosing hemangioma.

Sites of predilection. Distal portions of the extremities, although they may appear anywhere.

Objective signs. The lesions, which occur most frequently in women, are usually single, and appear as firm, dull reddish to purplish nodules, 3 mm-1 cm in diameter. These benign lesions are hard,

Histiocytoma

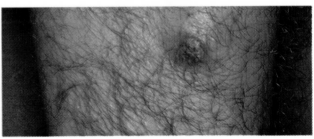

fixed in the skin, sharply defined and slow-growing. The nodules are attached to the skin but not to the underlying subcutaneous tissue.

Subjective symptoms. Usually none.

Etiology. Unknown.

Histopathology. The circumscribed tumor is composed of mature fibrous tissue. The nuclei are small.

Diagnostic aids. Biopsy.

Relation to systemic disease. None has been established.

Differential diagnosis. Keloid, nevus, wart.

Therapy. Excision.

Horn, Cutaneous

Synonym. Cornu cutaneum.

Sites of predilection. Most frequently occur on the face and hands.

Cutaneous horn

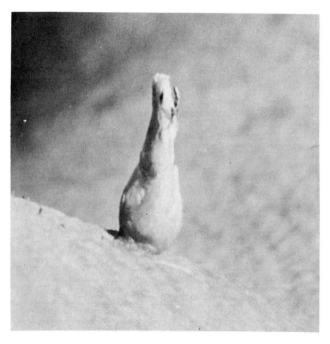

Objective signs. Usually single, these lesions are composed of horny material, projecting a few millimeters to several centimeters above the skin. The noninflamed base may have a rolled edge, and range from a few millimeters to 1.5 cm in diameter. The lesions have graduated projections of keratin as each distal segment of the horn has a smaller diameter. The horns vary from flesh colored to dark brown or black, and may be smooth, curved or twisted. They may be of such size as to suggest an animal horn, although they are not connected to underlying bony structures. The bases may undergo malignant degeneration to squamous cell carcinomas.

These lesions are usually associated with other senile changes in the skin such as actinic keratoses, and are frequently in sailor's skin.

Subjective symptoms. Usually none except the cosmetic defect.

Etiology. Unknown.

Histopathology. Hyperkeratosis with papillomatous changes of the rete. In the rete the cells are disorderly and show early signs of dyskeratosis. Low-grade squamous cell carcinoma may be present.

Diagnostic aids. Biopsy.

Relation to systemic disease. None usually.

Differential diagnosis. Verrucae.

Therapy. Excision or electrodesiccation.

Ichthyosis Hystrix

Synonym. Nevus unius lateris.

Sites of predilection. Trunk, extremities.

Objective signs. This is a peculiar type of papular nevus which frequently assumes a linear arrangement and may involve large areas of the body. The lesions are groups of thick, pointed or spine-like projections. The color varies from dark gray to brown. The condition is noninflammatory. Other congenital ectodermal defects may be present.

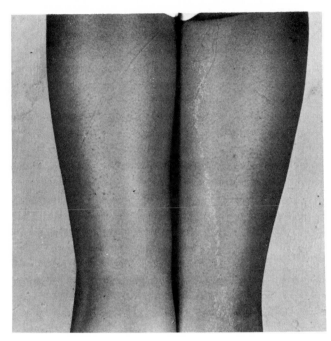

Ichthyosis hystrix

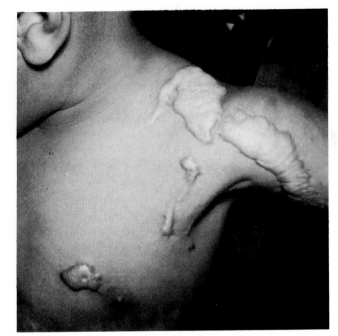

Keloids

Subjective symptoms. None.

Etiology. Congenital.

Histopathology. A variable amount of acanthosis and hyperkeratosis.

Diagnostic aids. Biopsy.

Relation to systemic disease. None. Other congenital ectodermal defects may be present.

Differential diagnosis. Ichthyosis.

Therapy. In extensive lesions treatment is of little value. Smaller lesions may be surgically excised. Topical tretinoin under occlusive dressings may be helpful.

Keloid

Synonym. Cheloid.

Sites of predilection. Any area of the body.

Objective signs. Keloids are hard, variously sized (1-10 cm), fibrous growths which develop at the site of trauma or in a scar. The lesions grow out of proportion to the original injury. Blacks have a predilection to develop these lesions following very slight injury such as pin scratch, punctured ear lobes or vaccination. The lesions are whitish, orange or reddish. They usually have smooth flat surfaces but may be pedunculated or have edges with pseudopodia. Lesions rarely ulcerate or undergo malignant change.

Subjective symptoms. Usually none, although the lesions may itch or be painful.

Etiology. Unknown. The tendency toward keloid formation is probably inherited. It is an individual tissue reaction to trauma.

Histopathology. Large homogeneous, connective tissue fibers, interspersed with connective tissue cells with small, intensely staining nuclei. The epidermis is atrophic.

Diagnostic aids. History and physical examination, biopsy.

Relation to systemic disease. None has been established.

Differential diagnosis. Epithelioma, xanthoma, gumma.

Therapy. Surgical excision, preceded and followed by radiation therapy. Very early lesions may respond to intralesional injections of triamcinolone diacetate.

Keratoacanthoma

Synonym. Self-healing epithelioma, molluscum sebaceum.

Sites of predilection. Face, hands.

Objective signs. Usually a single, rapidly growing, hemispherical, flesh-colored, firm papule. There is a central depression filled with a verrucous crust. The surface may be telangiectatic but the base is not inflammatory. The lesions vary from 2 mm-1 cm or more in diameter. Many of these lesions tend to undergo spontaneous involution.

Subjective symptoms. Usually none.

Keratoacanthoma

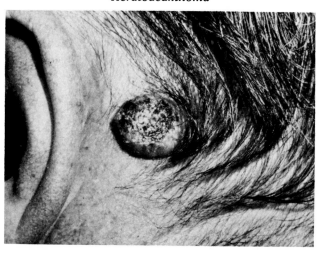

Etiology. Unknown.

Histopathology. A large central keratotic plug, with some parakeratosis is surrounded by a hyperacanthotic rete which shows a minimum of individual cell keratinization and anaplasia. Acute or subacute inflammation is present.

Diagnostic aids. Biopsy.

Relation to systemic disease. None.

Differential diagnosis. Squamous cell carcinoma.

Therapy. Excision of entire lesion and microscopic study of serial sections to rule out malignancy. Fulguration of base after excision.

Keratosis, Actinic

Synonym. Senile keratosis.

Sites of predilection. Face, neck, ears, dorsal surfaces of the hands.

Objective signs. These premalignant lesions appear in persons who have a history of exposure to sunlight over a period of years. The skin in the exposed areas is excessively dry. Wrinkling about the eyes and mouth are part of the syndrome known as sailor's skin. The individual keratoses vary from 2 mm-1 cm or more in diameter. The lesions are characterized by an adherent dry scale, removal of which causes bleeding. Some lesions may develop superficial ulcerations. Mottled to extensive freckling may occur.

Subjective symptoms. None.

Etiology. Unknown.

Histopathology. The histopathologic picture varies from benign acanthosis and hyperkeratosis to epithelioma in situ.

Diagnostic aids. Biopsy.

Relation to systemic disease. None.

Differential diagnosis. Seborrheic keratosis, epithelioma.

Therapy. One to five percent 5-fluorouracil in cream or solution will cause a violent reaction but will remove the lesions. Cryotherapy or fulguration may also be used.

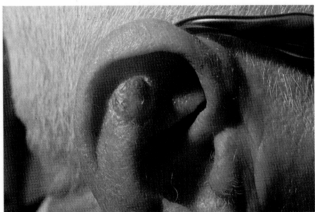

Actinic keratosis

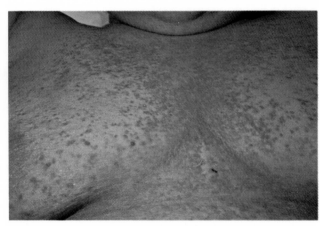

Keratosis follicularis

Keratosis Follicularis

Synonym. Darier's disease, White's disease.

Sites of predilection. Head, face, trunk, extremities.

Objective signs. The lesions begin as tiny, flesh colored or grayish-brown, follicular papules, which are hard and conical, and become topped with an oily crust. Removal of the crust reveals a small depression on the top of the papule. The lesions increase in size, become darker in color and coalesce into greasy plaques. Small dark brown tumors and papillomatous growths gradually form, and the lesions frequently emit an offensive odor. Unilateral linear lesions may occur. The papillomatous growths which develop in the axillae and crural areas may undergo malignant change.

Subjective symptoms. Mild pruritus.

Etiology. Unknown. The condition has been associated with vitamin A deficiency.

Histopathology. Flattening or elongation of the papillary bodies with acanthosis. Lacunae form between the basal and prickle cell layers or in the lower portion of the prickle cell layer. The cells bordering on the lacunae become partially keratinized and are called "corps ronds." De-

generative cells called "grains" are seen in the lacunae.

Diagnostic aids. History and physical examination, biopsy.

Relation to systemic disease. None has been definitely established.

Differential diagnosis. Acanthosis nigricans, pityriasis rubra pilaris, follicular papular syphilid.

Therapy. Localized areas will show temporary response to treatment with retinoic acid creams or gel (.05-.1%).

Keratosis Pilaris

Synonym. Keratosis suprafollicularis.

Sites of predilection. Extremities, trunk.

Objective signs. Numerous tiny, discrete, keratotic, follicular papules, pinkish to grayish in color, are topped by a tiny scale and frequently pierced by a hair. Occasionally a hair may be found curled inside the papule. The areas resemble cutis anserina or "goose flesh," and produce a feeling suggestive of the surface of a nutmeg grater. The condition is associated with dry skin and is most pronounced during the cold months of the year.

Subjective symptoms. Mild pruritus, especially after bathing in soapy water.

Etiology. Congenital.

Histopathology. Follicular hyperkeratosis with a mild, inflammatory reaction in the cutis.

Diagnostic aids. Biopsy.

Relation to systemic disease. None has been established.

Differential diagnosis. Keratosis follicularis, ichthyosis, pityriasis rubra pilaris, lichen nitidus, lichen spinulosus.

Therapy. Avoid exposure to cold; use 3-5% salicylic acid in an oily ointment base. Therapy is palliative, not curative.

Keratosis, Seborrheic

Synonym. Senile wart, seborrheic wart, acanthotic nevus, liver spot.

Sites of predilection. Face, neck, trunk, upper extremities.

Objective signs. These benign, slowly growing lesions appear during or after the fourth decade of life, as few to numerous, slightly raised, superficial papules, which vary from flesh colored to dark brown or black. They vary from 2 mm-2 cm or more in diameter and may be only slightly raised and flat or verrucous in appearance, with a heavily piled up, greasy, friable scale. Some lesions contain comedones. There is usually no inflammatory reaction about the base of the lesion.

Subjective symptoms. None except for the cosmetic defect.

Etiology. Unknown. Seborrheic keratoses are epithelial nevi which appear later in life. There is a familial tendency to develop these lesions.

Histopathology. Keratinous cysts, which are not related to hair follicle or sebaceous glands, invaginate the epidermis. There is little or no inflammatory reaction in the cutis but marked melanin production by the basal cells. This is a superficial lesion which primarily involves the epidermis.

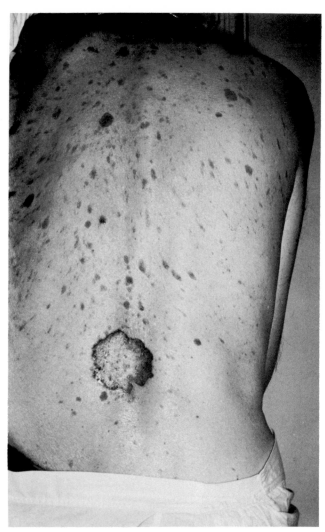

Multiple seborrheic keratoses with large superficial epithelioma

Diagnostic aids. Biopsy.

Relation to systemic disease. None.

Differential diagnosis. Verrucae, nevi, actinic keratoses, epithelioma, melanoma.

Therapy. The lesions are easily removed by light electrodesiccation, liquid nitrogen or curettage.

Larva Migrans

Synonym. Creeping eruption, myiasis linearis.

Sites of predilection. Palms, soles, buttocks, genitalia or other areas.

Objective signs. This condition first appears as a small papule at the site of infestation. A thin, red, tortuous line extends from the papule, marking the line of migration of the larva in its burrow. The larva may remain quiescent for varying periods up to several weeks, although the usual rate of migration is 2-6 cm daily. Secondary infection may occur due to excoriation.

Subjective symptoms. Moderate to intense pruritus.

Etiology. Larva migrans may be caused by a variety of helminth or botfly larvae. Larvae of the feline and canine hookworm, *Ancylostoma braziliense*, enter the skin from soil contaminated by animal excreta. This condition is common in the southeastern United States. In the Middle and North Atlantic states, lesions develop only in those persons who have visited the southern beaches. Larvae of the *Strongyloides* penetrate the perianal skin from infected feces. Two genera of fly larvae, *Hypoderma* and *Gasterophilus* have also been reported as causative organisms.

Larva migrans

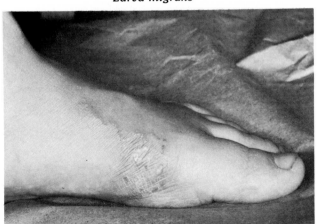

Histopathology. It is difficult to recover the helminth larvae in a biopsy specimen. Changes in the burrow wall are not characteristic. In infections produced by botfly larvae, the eggs can be visualized in the suppurative lesion.

Diagnostic aids. The clinical picture is characteristic.

Relation to systemic disease. Eosinophilia may be present in long-standing cases. Systemic disease does not follow cutaneous infection.

Differential diagnosis. The condition is characteristic.

Therapy. In helminth larva migrans the actively spreading edge of the burrow and surrounding area, about 3 cm in diameter, is frozen with liquid nitrogen, ethyl chloride or solid carbon dioxide. Thiabendazole is effective on systemic administration.

Incision of the lesions and extraction of the larva is the only effective treatment for botfly larva migrans.

Leprosy (Lepromatous Type)

Synonym. Hansen's disease.

Sites of predilection. Face, trunk, extremities.

Objective signs. Papular lesions in leprosy may so closely resemble sarcoid that clinical differentiation is impossible. Such lesions are small, reddish-brown sessile papules that do not scale

Lepromatous leprosy

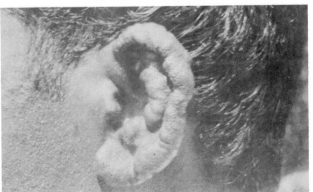

and range from 5 mm-1 cm in diameter. The lesions may begin as ill-defined, light yellowish-brown infiltrations. These gradually become well-defined, darker in color and of firm consistency. They may be discrete or confluent. The facial features may be deformed by numerous nodules which give rise to the "leonine facies." Nodules may involute spontaneously or may form plaques and ulcerate.

For more details see Leprosy in Chapter 14: Macular Eruptions.

Subjective symptoms. See Chapter 14.

Etiology. *Mycobacterium leprae.*

Histopathology. Characteristic foam cells containing *M leprae* are found in the dermis with acid-fast stain.

Diagnostic aids. Biopsy, scraping, lepromin test.

Relation to systemic disease. Leprosy is a systemic disease. Secondary amyloidosis is a common complication. Amyloid nephrosis and sepsis are the most common causes of death.

Differential diagnosis. Sarcoid, late cutaneous syphilis, cutaneous tuberculosis.

Therapy. See Leprosy in Chapter 14.

Lichen Nitidus

Synonym. None.

Sites of predilection. Flexor aspects of the wrists and forearms, the lower abdomen, inner surfaces of the thighs, penis.

Objective signs. These tiny hypopigmented papules (1-2 mm in diameter) may form a slight eruption limited to small areas or an extensive eruption covering most of the body. Linear grouping (Koebner's phenomenon) may occur.

The condition is chronic and subject to

*Lepromatous leprosy with
leonine facies and ulceration*

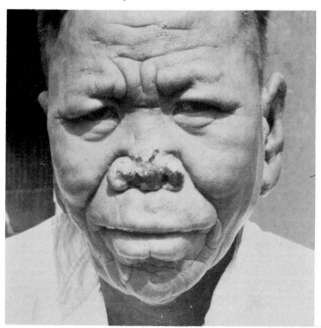

Lichen nitidus

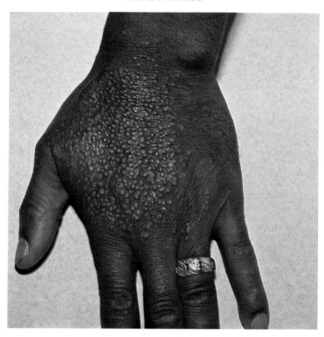

spontaneous remissions and exacerbations.

Subjective symptoms. None.

Etiology. Unknown.

Histopathology. Resembles lichen planus. Sharply defined infiltrate of lymphocytes, epithelioid cells and giant cells is limited to the papillary layer of the cutis.

Diagnostic aids. Biopsy.

Relation to systemic disease. None.

Differential diagnosis. Flat warts, lichen planus.

Therapy. Although temporary involution will follow systemic corticosteroid therapy, this form of therapy is not recommended.

Lichen Planus

Synonym. Lichen ruber planus.

Sites of predilection. Flexor surfaces of the upper extremities, trunk, buccal mucosa, male genitalia. The lower extremities are frequently involved.

Objective signs. The characteristic lesions are discrete, flat, angular or polygonal, violaceous papules which are shiny in reflected light and vary from 1-4 mm in diameter. There is a tendency to central umbilication. Lines or streaks (Wickham's striae) may be observed. There is a scant adherent scale. The lesions may be annular and tend to form linear groups (Koebner's phenomenon) or confluent areas.

The onset may be acute with a widespread eruption; individual lesions are reddish in color. However, lichen planus may be of the chronic localized variety, in which one or two areas of the body are involved with the typical angular, violaceous, flat-topped papules.

The lesions may be atrophic and whitish or ivory in color (atrophic lichen planus). On the lower extremities the lesions become large, hyperpigmented and verrucous (hypertrophic or verrucous lichen planus). The characteristic papules may be seen in the periphery of these hypertrophic lesions.

On the buccal surface, tongue or vulva the lesions appear as a retiform leukoplakia or sharply defined, white streaks.

Subjective symptoms. Moderate to severe pruritus.

Etiology. Unknown. Chronic emotional tension may be associated.

Histopathology. The microscopic picture is diagnostic. There is moderate hyperkeratosis and acanthosis, thickening of the granular layer and liquefaction of the basal layer. The lymphocytic infiltrate is sharply limited to the upper cutis. The

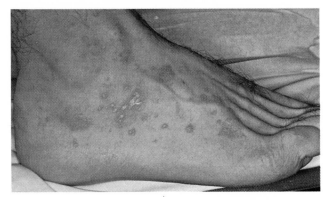

Lichen planus

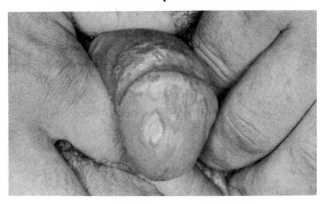

Lichen planus

mucous membrane changes are similar to those seen in cutaneous lesions.

Diagnostic aids. History and physical examination, biopsy.

Relation to systemic disease. Associated with emotional tension. Some drugs, such as quinacrine, produce either lichen planus or eruptions which closely mimic the disease. A few patients have concomitant clinical and serologic evidence of lupus erythematosus.

Differential diagnosis. Papular secondary syphilis, psoriasis, lupus erythematosus, erythema multiforme. The acute forms may be mistaken for papular pityriasis rosea or eczematous eruptions.

Therapy. In acute cases systemic corticosteroids will cause temporary involution of lesions. All unnecessary medication should be withdrawn. Emotional factors should be controlled. Tranquilizers or sedatives are good adjunctive therapy. Local antipruritics may be of value. Sublesional injections of triamcinolone diacetate may be of value in treatment of hypertrophic lesions. Occlusive dressings with plastic film and fluorinated corticosteroid creams are useful in treatment of chronic localized lesions.

Lichen Sclerosus et Atrophicus

Synonym. Lichen albus, white spot disease, kraurosis vulvae, kraurosis penis.

Sites of predilection. Trunk, genitalia; any part of the body may be involved. Occurs more commonly in women.

Objective signs. This chronic condition begins as angular, flat whitish papules that become shiny, flat atrophic lesions which are usually discrete but may become confluent. A pinkish halo is usually present about the large patches. Keratinous plug formation is frequently present in follicular orifices (dell formation). When the female genitalia is involved, there is a progressive atrophic change in the labia majora and minora which leads to disappearance of the labia minora, pre-

puce and clitoris, and gradual loss of the labia majora. These changes cause narrowing of the vaginal orifice (kraurosis vulvae). The tissues become smooth, shiny, dry, and develop a yellowish, waxy appearance. Leukoplakia may develop on the mucous membrane. In the male genitalia, chronic progressive atrophic changes may take place on the glans penis (kraurosis penis). The alterations in the mucous membranes are similar to those described in women. This is an atrophic condition in which frequent follow-up is essential in order to detect precancerous changes. It is not regarded as a premalignant disease and should not be treated with radical surgery. Lesions in prepubescent children involute spontaneously.

Subjective symptoms. Intense pruritus. Burning on urination is a common symptom.

Etiology. The cause of the condition is unknown but hormone imbalance or aging are thought to play important roles in older patients.

Histopathology. The histopathologic changes are characteristic. In the epidermis there is hyperkeratosis, follicular plugging and general epidermal atrophy with flattening of the rete pegs. There is liquefaction degeneration of the basal layer with edema in the upper cutis. The infiltrate in the midcutis consists of plasma cells and round cells.

Diagnostic aids. Biopsy.

Relation to systemic disease. It may indicate endocrine imbalance.

Differential diagnosis. Senile atrophy.

Therapy. Topical estrogens or 1% testosterone may be of temporary value. If malignant changes develop, vulvectomy must be performed. In the man, dilatation of the urethral orifice is frequently necessary. Lesions in prepubescent children require no treatment.

Lichen Spinulosus

Synonym. Keratosis follicularis spinulosa, lichen pilaris

seu spinulosus.

Sites of predilection. Trunk, extremities.

Objective signs. This is an uncommon condition found usually in children. The eruption consists of groups of minute follicular papules, each projecting a small spine. The surface feels like a nutmeg grater.

Subjective symptoms. Mild to moderate pruritus.

Etiology. Unknown.

Histopathology. The microscopic picture is not diagnostic.

Diagnostic aids. History and physical examination.

Relation to systemic disease. None has been established.

Differential diagnosis. Keratosis follicularis, keratosis pilaris.

Therapy. None specific. Local applications of 3-5% salicylic acid ointment may be beneficial.

Lichenoid Eruption of the Axillae

Synonym. Fox-Fordyce disease.

Sites of predilection. Axillae, pubes and areolae of the nipples.

Objective signs. This rare condition occurs most commonly in young women after puberty. It is characterized by an eruption of persistent, non-scaly, discrete, flat papules, varying from 1-3 mm in diameter. The lesions are located at the orifices of the hair follicles. The color varies from pink to violaceous. The papules may be closely aggregated but remain discrete. Excoriations and blood crusts, followed by hyperpigmentation, are prominent features.

Subjective symptoms. Intense pruritus.

Etiology. Unknown.

Histopathology. Surface epithelium shows changes similar to those seen in chronic lichenoid eczema. There is keratotic plugging of the duct orifices, and a variable subacute inflammatory reaction about the apocrine glands.

Diagnostic aids. Biopsy.

Relation to systemic disease. None.

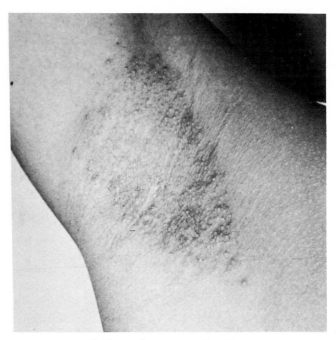

Lichenoid eruption of axillae

Differential diagnosis. Contact dermatitis, chronic lichenoid eczema (neurodermatitis).

Therapy. Topical applications are without value. Systemic administration of estrogens or estrogen-containing contraceptive pills may be of benefit. Plastic surgery may be necessary to produce relief from symptoms.

Lipoidoses

Diseases of lipid metabolism with cutaneous manifestations include not only the xanthomas but also some less common entities.

Gaucher's disease is characterized by hepatomegaly with retention of cerebrosides, rarefaction of the long bones and a distinctive brown color of the skin. Xanthomatous tumors are not present. The condition occurs most commonly in Jews. Both adult and pediatric forms of the disease exist.

Niemann-Pick disease occurs chiefly in Jewish infants. Hepatosplenomegaly, yellow skin and xanthomatous tumors characterize the condition which is associated with retention of sphingomyelin. This disease is progressive with fatal termination.

Glycogen storage disease (von Gierke's disease) is a group of disorders characterized by hypercholesterolemia and is associated with faulty glycogen metabolism. Xanthomatous tumors may be present.

Extracellular cholesterosis is a disease of cholesterol metabolism, in which lesions of the skin and mucous membrane form crops of firm, waxy nodules.

In *lipoid proteinosis* (hyalinosis cutis et mucosae) the mucous membranes and tongue become almost board-like in hardness and thickened with yellowish plaques. The skin may exhibit impetigo-like vesicular lesions which form morphea-like, atrophic, small plaques or scars. Infiltrated or single, flesh-colored papules are often seen about the face and neck. Hyperkeratotic nodules may appear on pressure areas (*eg,* elbows and knees). Alopecia, poliosis and dental abnormalities may be associated with this disease.

Lipoma

Synonym. Fatty tumor.
Sites of predilection. Any area of the body.
Objective signs. One to numerous, variously sized, subcutaneous tumors covered with normal skin, may be present. The lesions are soft and may be lobulated; they are not attached to the skin.
Subjective symptoms. A tumor located over a pressure point may cause discomfort.
Etiology. Unknown.
Histopathology. Groups of large fat cells, held together by trabeculae to form lobulated masses are enclosed within a fibrous capsule.
Differential diagnosis. Subcutaneous fibromas, sebaceous cysts.
Diagnostic aids. Biopsy.
Relation to systemic disease. There is a tendency to familial occurence.
Therapy. Excision.

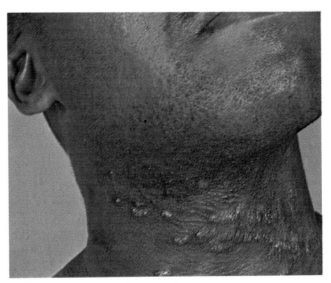

Lupus vulgaris

Lupus Vulgaris

Synonym. Tuberculosis cutis luposa.
Sites of predilection. Nose and contiguous portions of the face. Any part of the body may be involved.
Objective signs. This condition begins as one or more small, soft, yellowish-red or reddish-brown nodules that gradually increase in number and coalesce, forming plaques. If a heavy glass slide (diascope) is pressed onto the lesion, the individual translucent nodules, with their characteristic reddish-brown color, may be seen. The lesions may become hypertrophic and local edema may be present. There may be telangiectasia and regional lymphadenopathy. As the central portion of the lesion heals, a thin scar resembling crumpled tissue or cigarette paper forms. Ulceration and scar tissue may cause severe cosmetic deformity.
Subjective symptoms. None except for the cosmetic defect.
Differential diagnosis. Sarcoid, discoid lesions of lupus erythematosus, epitheliomas.

Etiology. Mycobacterium tuberculosis.

Histopathology. Tubercle formation in the mid and upper cutis, with little tendency to caseous necrosis. The early lesions have a heavy lymphocytic infiltrate, which is replaced by epithelioid and giant cells. Dermal appendages are atrophied.

Relation to systemic disease. Associated with visceral tuberculosis.

Diagnostic aids. History and physical examination, biopsy, chest X ray, culture of skin for tuberculosis.

Therapy. Streptomycin, isoniazid, para-aminosalicylic acid, rifampin.

Macular Atrophy

Synonym. Anetoderma (Schweninger and Buzzi), primary macular atrophy.

Sites of predilection. Trunk, extremities.

Objective signs. This rare condition is characterized by the development of few to numerous bluish-white, small (0.3-1 cm in diameter), smooth, soft, circumscribed, bladder-like pseudotumors. These can be inverted by slight pressure into a hollow in the underlying tissue. The lesions develop slowly and are not associated with any previous inflammatory process.

Subjective symptoms. None.

Etiology. Unknown.

Histopathology. In the early stages there is a mild inflammatory reaction which eventually tends to disappear with a loss of elastic tissue.

Diagnostic aids. History and physical examination, biopsy.

Relation to systemic disease. None has been demonstrated.

Differential diagnosis. Other macular atrophic lesions, scars.

Therapy. None effective.

Maduromycosis

Synonym. Madura foot, mycetoma, podelkoma. For details see Chapter 6: Mycology.

Mastocytosis

Synonym. Xanthelasmoidea, urticaria pigmentosa.

Sites of predilection. Trunk, upper extremities; any area of the body may be involved.

Objective signs. The condition usually develops in early infancy as wheals, papules and infiltrated macules. Bullous lesions may develop. When the lesions involute, they leave a reddish-brown or yellowish-brown color in the involved area. When irritated, these pigmented lesions urticate (Darier's sign). If the lesions occur after puberty, the lesions are persistent. This chronic disorder can be subclassified into three types: single, multiple or generalized. The first two types spontaneously involute at puberty.

Subjective symptoms. Pruritus.

Etiology. Unknown.

Histopathology. The microscopic picture is character-

Mastocytosis, bullous type

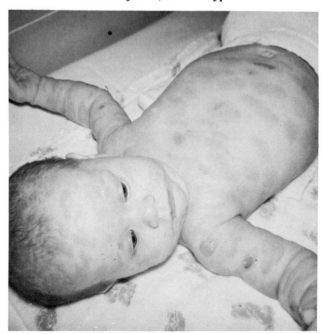

istic. Large numbers of mast cells in the cutis distend the papillary bodies. A narrow band of normal connective tissue frequently separates the corium and the epidermis. The collagen bundles are separated.

Diagnostic aids. History and physical examination, biopsy, hemograms, X ray of the long bones, urinary histamine.

Relation to systemic disease. Lytic bone lesions due to mast cell infiltration may appear. Histamine crises may occur, especially after alcohol injection.

Differential diagnosis. The lesions are characteristic in appearance.

Therapy. There is no effective therapy. Antihistamines may give relief from pruritus.

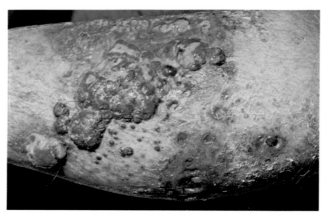

Malignant melanoma

Melanoma

Synonym. Malignant melanoma, melanocarcinoma, nevocarcinoma, malignant mole, melanoblastoma.

Sites of predilection. Any area of the body may become involved. Men are more apt to develop melanomas on their upper backs and women on their legs or backs. Melanomas rarely develop on the areas protected by a bathing suit.

Objective signs. Four types of melanoma are now recognized. *Malignant lentigo* (melanotic freckle of Hutchison) is a brown-black macule usually appearing on the face in elderly people. It slowly expands peripherally and requires many years before it begins to invade the dermis. Ten percent of melanomas are of this variety.

Superficial spreading melanoma accounts for 70% of all melanomas. This lesion begins as a brown, tan, red, blue or black macule located anywhere on the body. These lesions have a variegated color and a convoluted border. They usually spread laterally up to a size of 7-10 mm before deep dermal invasion occurs. Superficial ulceration of the epidermis is a late sign.

Nodular melanomas are blue-black or black. They invade deeply into the dermis very early in their course. *Acrolentiginous melanomas*

Malignant melanoma

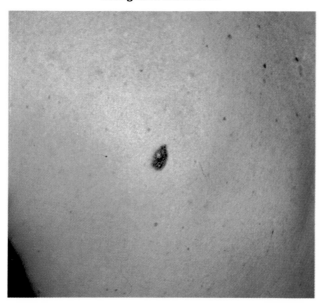

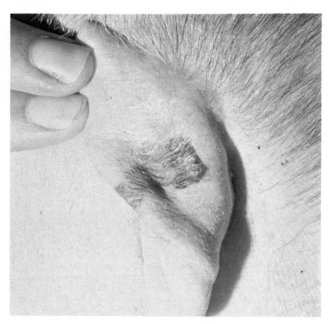

Melanotic freckle

occur on the palms, soles or mucous membranes. They are variegated in color and may ulcerate and resemble superficial spreading melanomas.

All melanomas may show regression of pigment or tumor mass within their borders. Prognosis is particularly bad if the lesions are pedunculated or ulcerated. A surrounding erythema may or may not be present and the presence or absence of hair is not an accurate prognostic sign.

It appears that these tumors have three stages of growth: localized, horizontal and vertical. As long as the malignant cells lack the capacity for vertical growth the prognosis is good since metastasis is not as common. Clinically the vertical growth phase is diagnosed by a darkened color. It now appears that the deeper the lesion is allowed to penetrate the skin prior to excision, the worse will be the prognosis.

Subjective symptoms. Usually none until in the course of the disease. The patient becomes generally ill, his symptoms depend on the location of the tumor.

Etiology. Unknown. There is an apparent association with solar exposure. Blue-eyed blondes and certain families have a propensity for melanomas. Patients with xeroderma pigmentosum or large bathing trunk nevi have a greater tendency to develop melanomas than other people.

Histopathology. Nevus cells in the tumor are increased in size and amount of melanin. Mitotic figures are seen, and the cells form an alveolar arrangement as they invade the cutis. The microscopic picture is diagnostic.

In malignant lentigo the cells have unusual and different nuclei in the epidermis. The tumor does not have a dense lymphocytic band in the dermis until it begins its vertical growth phase. The malignant cells are more uniform in their appearance in superficial spreading melanoma. An inflammatory reaction around the tumor is usually regarded as a favorable sign.

Diagnostic aids. Biopsy.

Relation to systemic disease. Symptoms may be related to organs where the lesions have metastasized.

Differential diagnosis. Pigmented moles, pyogenic granulomas, angiokeratomas.

Therapy. Wide excision, possibly including removal of the regional lymph nodes. The depth of the lesions affects the type of surgery and the prognosis. The lesions are not sensitive to X-rays or radium. Immunotherapy and chemotherapy are experimental.

Miliaria

Synonym. Prickly heat.

Sites of predilection. Trunk, shoulders, neck, flexures of the extremities.

Objective signs. This disorder, associated with profuse perspiration, usually occurs in hot weather. The primary lesion is a discrete, follicular papule, papulovesicle or vesicle, which is pink to red in color. The lesions occur in patches but do not coalesce. If the lesion is very superficial a vesicle appears as a water drop on the skin surface (miliaria crystallina). If the pathology is deeper a reactive erythema surrounds the vesicle (miliaria rubra).

Subjective symptoms. Moderate to severe pruritus.

Etiology. The disease is regarded as sweat retention syndrome.

Histopathology. Dilated cystic sweat ducts, with occlusion of the duct orifice.

Diagnostic aids. Clinical appearance is characteristic.

Relation to systemic disease. None has been established.

Differential diagnosis. Folliculitis, atopic dermatitis, acne vulgaris.

Therapy. Heat and excessive perspiration should be avoided. Bathe in clear water without soap. Absorbent dusting powders may be of value. Fans and air conditioning are helpful.

Milia

Synonym. Whitehead.

Sites of predilection. Face.

Objective signs. This condition is frequently seen in association with acne vulgaris or oily skin, and consists of small, discrete, solid, whitish, cystic lesions, filled with inspissated or cheesy material. They are not inflammatory.

Subjective symptoms. None.

Etiology. Unknown.

Histopathology. A spherical, horny cyst connected to a hair follicle. The cyst contains a homogeneous lipoid substance.

Diagnostic aids. None usually necessary.

Relation to systemic disease. None has been established.

Differential diagnosis. Comedones.

Therapy. The top of the lesion may be nicked with a sharp-pointed blade or needle, and the contents expressed with a comedo expressor.

Milkers' Nodules

Synonym. None.

Sites of predilection. Fingers, wrists, forearms.

Objective signs. This condition occurs in workers in industries, as well as cattle and dairy workers. The primary lesion is a small inflammatory papule, which increases to 1-2 cm in diameter within about a week, becoming bluish-red and firm. The center of the nodule is umbilicated and may break down. Lymphangitis may occur.

Subjective symptoms. Pain.

Etiology. Virus.

Histopathology. The microscopic picture is not diagnostic.

Diagnostic aids. Biopsy.

Relation to systemic disease. Usually no constitutional symptoms accompany the lesions.

Differential diagnosis. Verrucae, pyogenic granulomas, orf, vaccinia.

Therapy. The disease is self-limited and tends to clear in 6-10 months.

Molluscum Contagiosum

Synonym. Contagious epithelioma, water wart.

Sites of predilection. Face, trunk, genitalia, extremities.

Objective signs. In this mildly contagious disease there are few to numerous, discrete, globular, umbilicated, flesh-colored to pinkish papules, which sometimes form groups. The lesions are usually waxy in appearance. The center of the lesion is occupied by a firm caseous mass called the molluscum body. The individual lesions vary from a few millimeters to 1 cm in diameter. They may become secondarily infected. The disease is autoinoculable.

Subjective symptoms. None to slight pruritus.

Etiology. Virus. Several strains of this agent have recently been detected.

Histopathology. The microscopic picture is diagnostic. Pear-shaped proliferations of prickle cells invaginate the cutis. The basal layer and lower layers of the cutis are normal, but the more superficial prickle cells show variously sized vacuoles and eosinophilic hyaline bodies, which may occupy almost the entire cell. Basophilic granules are also present at first, but these disappear with the formation of a keratin membrane about the periphery. There is no evidence of viral proliferation in the dermis.

Diagnostic aids. Smears of the expressed molluscum body, biopsy.

Relation to systemic disease. None.

Differential diagnosis. Adenoma sebaceum, verrucae, benign cystic epithelioma, pigmented nevus, acne vulgaris.

Therapy. Expression of the molluscum body.

Mycosis Fungoides

Synonym. None.

Sites of predilection. Generalized.

Objective signs. Mycosis fungoides is a systemic lymphoma which has three stages: the eczematous or premycotic stage, the infiltrated stage and the tumor stage.

    The eczematous or premycotic stage may resemble eczema, parapsoriasis en plaque, psoriasis or exfoliative dermatitis. The lesions are multiform and are not characteristic. This stage may last several years.

    During the infiltrative stage the lesions become more well-defined and elevated, with circinate or gyrate lesions which form plaques. These lesions occasionally ulcerate.

    The period of tumor formation gradually follows within several months after the infiltrative stage. Tumors occasionally arise from normal skin, but more frequently from previously involved areas. No area of the body is exempt. Tumors may involute spontaneously or may ulcerate. When the face is involved, a leonine expression, similar to that seen in lepromatous lep-

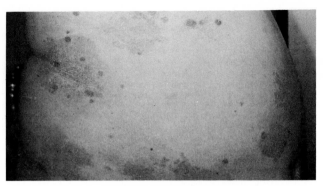

Mycosis fungoides

rosy, may be noted.

    One severe form, Sézary syndrome, is characterized by a generalized erythroderma. These patients have circulating mononuclear cells with convoluted nuclei. The prognosis is poor once the infiltrative stage is reached.

Mycosis fungoides

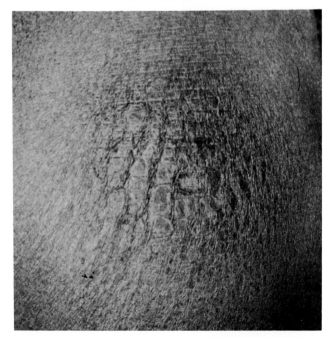

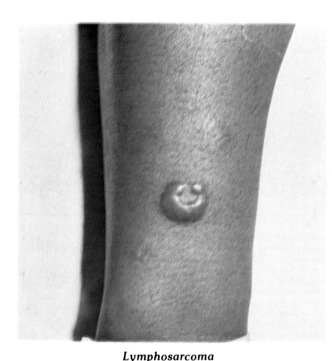

Lymphosarcoma

Mycosis fungoides, tumor stage

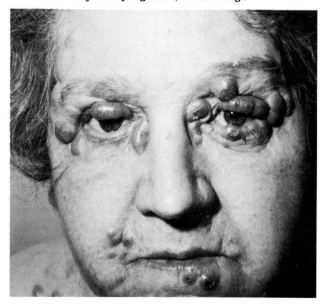

Subjective symptoms. During the early stages, pruritus is a prominent feature.

Etiology. Unknown. Some experts regard this disease as one of "antigen excess." In Sézary syndrome the malignant cell is a T cell with helper function for B cells.

Histopathology. In the eczematous phase the changes are not characteristic. In the infiltrative and tumor phases there is a polymorphous infiltrate with invasion of the epidermis. Epidermal abscesses (Pautrier) develop. An abnormal mononuclear cell with a very convoluted nucleus may be seen in the infiltrate.

Diagnostic aids. History and physical examination, biopsy, blood count, sternal marrow studies, lymphangiogram.

Relation to systemic disease. Mycosis fungoides is a systemic lymphoma which may last for many years.

Differential diagnosis. Other lymphomas, late cutaneous syphilis, leprosy.

Therapy. Supportive measures. Roentgen, grenz and cathode rays cause temporary involution of the cutaneous lesions. Antimetabolites are of value. In more superficial lesions, topical applications of nitrogen mustard are effective.

Necrobiosis Lipoidica

Synonym. Necrobiosis lipoidica diabeticorum.

Sites of predilection. Lower extremities. Lesions have been reported on the upper extremities and trunk.

Objective signs. The primary lesion is a sharply defined, reddish papule, which may be slightly scaly and varies from 1-3 cm in diameter. This lesion slowly spreads peripherally, becoming an irregularly round or oval, scleroderma-like plaque. The central portion is depressed and assumes a yellowish tinge. The lesion is shiny and translucent. Numerous telangiectatic vessels may be seen in the central portion. Ulceration rarely occurs.

Subjective symptoms. None.

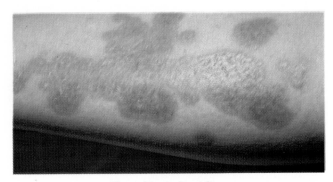

Necrobiosis lipoidica

Etiology. Unknown.

Histopathology. Necrobiotic changes in the collagen fibers, with homogenization and degeneration of the fibers. Perivascular infiltrate with obliterative vascular changes. Extracellular lipoid deposits are seen. Palisading of epithelioid cells may occur.

Diagnostic aids. History and physical examination, biopsy, urinalysis, blood sugar determinations.

Relation to systemic disease. One-third to one-half of the cases occur in diabetics.

Differential diagnosis. Localized scleroderma, localized myxedema, xanthoma, scar, erythema ab igne.

Therapy. None effective.

Neurofibromatosis

Synonym. von Recklinghausen's disease, molluscum fibrosum, fibroma.

Sites of predilection. Trunk; to a lesser extent the head, face, extremities.

Objective signs. Numerous, soft, flesh-colored tumors vary from 1 mm to several centimeters in diameter. Smaller lesions may be pressed into the skin as into a hollow. Older lesions may be dark brown. The growths are sessile or pedunculated. An occasional tumor may be large and pendulous. Widespread freckling over the entire skin is possible. There are usually one or more light brown macules, varying from 2-10 cm or more in diameter (café au lait spots). Nevus anemicus (pale avascular areas) may also be found.

Subjective symptoms. Usually none except the emotional trauma associated with the cosmetic defect.

Etiology. Unknown. The disease usually appears about the time of puberty or early in adult life, but may be present at birth.

Histopathology. Tumors of nerve sheaths that arise from connective tissue or the sheath of Schwann. They are well-circumscribed and have a light fibrous capsule. Tumors are composed of wavy fibrils of young collagen which tend to form whorls. A variable amount of older collagen is present.

Diagnostic aids. Biopsy; the clinical picture is usually characteristic.

Relation to systemic disease. There may be developmental defects in the nervous system, muscles and bone. Idiocy and epilepsy may be present. Pheochromocytoma may be associated with this disorder. Malignant degeneration of these tumors may occur.

Differential diagnosis. Multiple lipomas, skin tags, multiple sebaceous cysts, verrucae, leprosy (lepromatous type).

Therapy. None effective. Recurrence of the cutaneous lesion usually follows excision.

Nevoxanthoendothelioma

Synonym. Juvenile xanthoma, juvenile xanthogranuloma.

Sites of predilection. Face, scalp, upper part of the trunk.

Objective signs. Usually beginning in the first few weeks of life, the lesions consist of one or more groups of yellowish or yellowish-brown papules or nodules. The lesions tend to disappear spontaneously over a prolonged period. An adult form of this disease has been recently reported in which the yellowish globular lesions resemble molluscum contagiosum.

Subjective symptoms. None.

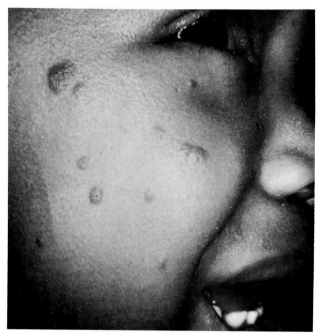

Juvenile xanthogranuloma

Etiology. Unknown.

Histopathology. Proliferation of endothelial cells and histiocytes with endothelial giant cell formation, associated with xanthoma cells and Touton cells. The microscopic picture is diagnostic.

Diagnostic aids. History and physical examination, biopsy.

Relation to systemic disease. Eye lesions which cause blindness may develop. Lesions may also develop on the genitalia, mucous membranes and in the lungs.

Differential diagnosis. Various other nevoid lesions, molluscum contagiosum, xanthomas.

Therapy. None necessary since the lesions tend to disappear spontaneously.

Nevus, Blue

Synonym. Jadassohn-Tièche nevus.
Sites of predilection. Face, forearms, hands.

Objective signs. Well-defined, firm, round or oval papules, varying from 2-15 mm in diameter. The lesion is usually dark gray or blue. The lesions begin in infancy or early childhood and do not increase in size.

Subjective symptoms. None.

Etiology. None.

Histopathology. Histopathologic picture is characteristic. Irregular masses of spindle-shaped melanocytes are seen in the lower two-thirds of the cutis.

Diagnostic aids. Biopsy.

Relation to systemic disease. None.

Differential diagnosis. Melanoma, mongolian spots, tattoo, ecchymosis.

Therapy. Wide and deep surgical excision.

Nevus Pigmentosus

Synonym. Mole, pigmented mole, benign melanoma.
Sites of predilection. Any area of the body.
Objective signs. Pigmented nevi are flesh-colored to brown or black, circumscribed tumors, which vary from a few millimeters to many centimeters in diameter. Hairs may protrude from the surface of these noninflammatory lesions. Lesions are most frequently sessile but pedunculated forms do occur. Some lesions become verrucous.

Subjective symptoms. None.

Etiology. Congenital.

Histopathology. Nevus cells tend to form alveolar ar-

Nevus pigmentosus

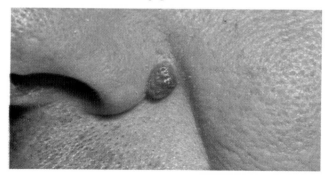

rangements or strands in the cutis. Increased cellular activity may occur at the dermal-epidermal junction.

Diagnostic aids. Biopsy.

Relation to systemic disease. None.

Differential diagnosis. The lesions are characteristic. If a lesion has grown in size or changed shape, biopsy may be indicated to rule out malignant degeneration.

Therapy. None usually necessary. Excision for cosmetic purposes may be desirable. All excised specimens should be examined histologically.

Nevus, Sebaceous

Synonym. Sebaceous nevus of Jadassohn.

Sites of predilection. Within the hairline of the scalp.

Objective signs. Yellowish-brown sessile papule with smooth or verrucous surface. Lesions vary from 5 mm-2 cm or more in diameter. Hair growth is sparse or absent in the lesions.

Subjective symptoms. None.

Etiology. Congenital.

Histopathology. The sebaceous glands are normal, but their basal layer may be atrophic or absent. The epidermis is hyperkeratotic and acanthotic.

Diagnostic aids. Biopsy.

Relation to systemic disease. None.

Differential diagnosis. Other types of nevi, xanthoma.

Therapy. Excision is mandatory. A large percentage of these lesions develop into carcinoma or may contain other hamartomas such as syringocystadenoma papilliferum.

Panniculitis, Relapsing Febrile Nonsuppurative

Synonym. Nodular nonsuppurative panniculitis, Weber-Christian disease, atrophy of the fatty layer of the skin.

Sites of predilection. Trunk, extremities.

Objective signs. In this unusual condition, round or irregular, subcutaneous nodules, varying in size up to 10 cm in diameter, gradually form atrophic sclerotic plaques. The skin over the lesions is bluish but has normal texture. Occasionally the lesions become cystic, and discharge an oily or fatty fluid.

Subjective symptoms. Fever, malaise, vomiting and muscular pain.

Etiology. Unknown.

Histopathology. Large numbers of phagocytic cells or histiocytes replace the fat cells. A marked perivascular reaction is present, and occasionally foreign body giant cells are seen.

Diagnostic aids. Biopsy.

Relation to systemic disease. None has been established.

Differential diagnosis. Erythema nodosum, low-grade cellulitis, mycobacterial infection of the skin, erythema induratum, morphea, subcutaneous fat necrosis, nodular migratory panniculitis, paraffinoma. Pancreatic disease may produce a liquefying panniculitis.

Therapy. None effective.

Papular Mucinosis

Synonym. Scleromyxedema, lichen myxedematosus, lichen fibromucinoidosus.

Sites of predilection. Lower face, ears, neck, upper chest, genitalia.

Objective signs. This disease begins in middle-aged or elderly patients with the insidious onset of flesh-colored or erythematous, asymptomatic, clustered papules or nodules. Accentuation of the skin folds appear. Deeper folds appear over the exposed areas of the skin or joints as the infiltration of these lesions becomes more pronounced. Localized urticarial or lichenoid plaques can be scattered about the upper torso. In summary, the clinical presentation may be lichenoid, scleroderma-like or a scattering of plaques.

Subjective symptoms. None to slight pruritus.

Etiology. This disease is thought to be due to an idiopathic, abnormal, intracutaneous deposition of globulins.

Histopathology. The dermal collagen fibers are separated by a slight blue staining material. Large stellate and fusiform fibroblasts are present in association with increased collagen. The blue material stains positive with colloidal iron or alcian blue for acid mucopolysaccharides.

Diagnostic aids. Biopsy, serum protein electrophoresis, bone marrow for increased plasmacytes.

Relation to other diseases. This disorder is regarded as a generalized depository disease of acid mucopolysaccharides.

Differential diagnosis. Lymphoma, myeloma, scleroderma, urticaria cysticum, sarcoid.

Therapy. Melphalan therapy should be further evaluated.

Parapsoriasis, Guttate

Synonym. Parapsoriasis en gouttes, pityriasis lichenoides chronica, parapsoriasis guttata.

Sites of predilection. Generalized except for hands, face, scalp.

Objective signs. The eruption consists of discrete, small, reddish papules, with varying amount of scale. The condition is chronic.

Subjective symptoms. None.

Etiology. Unknown.

Histopathology. The microscopic picture is not diagnostic. The histopathologic picture varies with the chronicity of the disease. The infiltrate, which is predominantly lymphocytic, surrounds the dilated capillaries in the dermis. Some parakeratotic scale may be present.

Diagnostic aids. Biopsy.

Relation to systemic disease. None has been established.

Differential diagnosis. Psoriasis, secondary syphilis, lichen planus, pityriasis rosea, drug eruption.

Therapy. None effective.

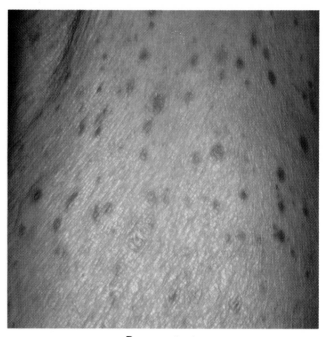

Parapsoriasis

Parapsoriasis Lichenoides

Synonym. Retiform parapsoriasis, parakeratosis variegata.

Sites of predilection. Generalized.

Objective signs. The lesions of this form of parapsoriasis are so extensive that the patient appears to have been covered with a net. The primary lesion is a scaly, flat-topped papule, which appears to be intermediate between the lesions of lichen planus and those of psoriasis. The condition is chronic and does not respond to therapy.

Subjective symptoms. None.

Etiology. Unknown.

Histopathology. See Guttate Parapsoriasis.

Diagnostic aids. Biopsy.

Relation to systemic disease. See Guttate Parapsoriasis.

Differential diagnosis. Psoriasis, lichen planus.

Therapy. See Guttate Parapsoriasis.

Parapsoriasis en Plaques

Synonym. None.
Sites of predilection. Trunk, extremities.
Objective signs. The primary lesion is a scaly macule which is not infiltrated, but forms plaques, resembling seborrheic dermatitis. The color varies from pinkish-red to brownish. The condition is chronic and recalcitrant.
Histopathology. In early lesions the microscopic picture is not diagnostic; however, biopsy studies may reveal white cells with convoluted nuclei similar to those seen in mycosis fungoides.
Diagnostic aids. Biopsy.
Relation to systemic disease. Some authorities state that parapsoriasis en plaques eventuates into mycosis fungoides; others believe that the lesions which eventuate into mycosis fungoides have the characteristic histopathologic picture from the beginning.
Differential diagnosis. Mycosis fungoides, psoriasis.
Therapy. If this is an early form of mycosis fungoides, topical nitrogen mustard is effective therapy. Ultraviolet light therapy alone or with the Goeckerman or PUVA techniques can be effective.

Pearly Penile Papules

Synonym. None.
Sites of predilection. Proximal edge of the penile corona.
Objective signs. Pearly gray, smooth-topped, small, noninflammatory papules.
Subjective symptoms. None.
Etiology. Unknown.
Histopathology. These papules are angiofibromas without any glandular structures.
Diagnostic aids. Biopsy.
Relation to systemic disease. None.
Differential diagnosis. Warts, molluscum contagiosum, seborrheic keratosis.
Therapy. None needed.

Periarteritis Nodosa

Synonym. Polyarteritis nodosa.
Sites of predilection. Trunk, extremities.
Objective signs. The cutaneous lesions of periarteritis nodosa are multiform. Nodules, purpuric lesions, urticaria, erythema nodosum or erythema multiforme-like lesions may be seen. Tender nodules may be felt along the course of a superficial artery. Ulceration may occur.
Subjective symptoms. Malaise, weakness, pain.
Etiology. Unknown.
Histopathology. Inflammatory degeneration of segments of the arterial wall, with perivascular leukocytic infiltrate. There may be intimal proliferation.
Diagnostic aids. History and physical examination, biopsy, hemograms, blood chemistries.
Relation to systemic disease. Periarteritis nodosa is a systemic disease which often has a fatal outcome. The course is marked by irregular fever, tachycardia, eosinophilia and nephritis. The condition may be marked by remissions and exacerbations or may be fulminating. Skin lesions may be entirely absent.
Differential diagnosis. Erythema nodosum, urticaria, erythema multiforme, purpura.
Therapy. Search for and eliminate any possible systemic stimulus such as drugs, foci of infection, *etc.* Systemic corticosteroid therapy may give temporary relief.

Pityriasis Rosea

This eruption is usually macular and is described in Chapter 14: Macular Eruptions. Occasionally, the early lesions are tiny, grouped papules, which eventuate into the characteristic macular lesions, or persist as a papular or follicular eruption. For more details see Pityriasis Rosea in Chapter 14.

Pityriasis Rubra Pilaris

Synonym. Lichen ruber, lichen ruber acuminatus.

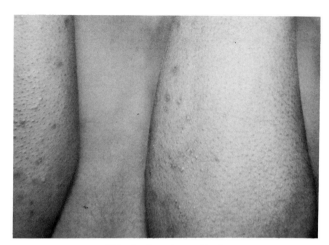

Pityriasis rubra pilaris

Sites of predilection. Dorsal surfaces of the proximal phalanges of the fingers, extensor surfaces of the wrists and forearms, anterior axillary folds, elbows, knees.

Objective signs. The characteristic lesions are hard, dry, follicular papules, surrounding a lusterless hairshaft. They are pink to bright red in color. The lesions may coalesce to form exfoliating areas.

The face, head and scalp may develop a scaly eruption which simulates seborrheic dermatitis. The condition may progress to a generalized exfoliative dermatitis.

Subjective symptoms. None to slight pruritus.

Etiology. Unknown.

Histopathology. Marked follicular hyperkeratosis, with a collarette of parakeratosis. Liquefaction of the basal layer. There is an infiltrate of polymorphonuclear leukocytes and lymphocytes. The elastic tissue is intact.

Diagnostic aids. Biopsy.

Relation to systemic disease. No specific relation, although late in the course of the disease the patient may become cachectic.

Differential diagnosis. Lichen planus, exfoliative dermatitis, keratosis pilaris, eczema.

Therapy. None effective; emollients, antipruritics and topical retinoic acid may help. Oral cis-retinoic acid is experimental.

Plantar Corn

Synonym. Clavus.

Sites of predilection. Plantar surface over the head of one of the metatarsal bones.

Objective signs. Appears as a callus. When this is trimmed away there is a solid, central avascular, translucent body. There is usually a single lesion.

Subjective symptoms. Pain on pressure.

Etiology. Local chronic irritation.

Histopathology. Avascular keratin plug.

Diagnostic aids. Clinical appearance.

Differential diagnosis. Plantar wart, foreign body.

Therapy. Avoid surgical excision. Use comfortable well-fitting shoes. Apply keratolytic plaster and keep lesions trimmed.

Porokeratosis, Actinic

Synonym. None.

Sites of predilection. Exposed areas of extremities.

Objective signs. Discrete, small, saucer-shaped lesions. The margins are hyperkeratotic and elevated; the central portion is depressed and atrophic. The skin in involved areas is dry, and freckle formation may be present.

Subjective symptoms. None.

Etiology. Chronic actinic exposure.

Histopathology. Similar to changes observed in porokeratosis of Mibelli.

Diagnostic aids. Biopsy.

Relation to systemic disease. None.

Differential diagnosis. Porokeratosis of Mibelli, actinic keratosis.

Therapy. Cryotherapy of individual lesions.

Porokeratosis of Mibelli

Synonym. Keratoderma eccentricum, hyperkeratosis figurata centrifuga atrophicans.

Sites of predilection. Any part of the body.

Objective signs. This rare disease usually begins as a small wart-like papule which enlarges peripherally, developing an atrophic center and a sharply defined, elevated border which is ridged and hyperkeratotic. The ridge is gray or brownish and the central portion is usually atrophic. A zosteriform variety has been described. These lesions are unilateral and form a linear arrangement.

Subjective symptoms. None.

Etiology. Unknown.

Histopathology. Hyperkeratosis and acanthosis. There is a deep groove filled with a large horny plug containing parakeratotic cells (coronoid lamella). Lymphocytic infiltration is present in the cutis, with vascular dilatation. The microscopic picture is diagnostic.

Diagnostic aids. Biopsy.

Relation to systemic disease. None has been established.

Differential diagnosis. The condition is characteristic. These patients rarely develop malignancies.

Therapy. Excision or destruction by electro-desiccation.

Prurigo nodularis

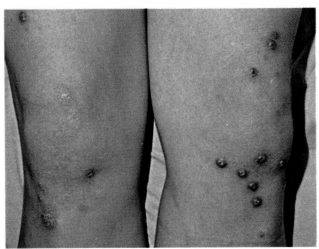

Prurigo

The term prurigo has been applied to many different forms of nodular cutaneous affections. The disease may be mild (prurigo mitis) or severe (prurigo agria). A rare condition, supposedly limited to adult women, is prurigo nodularis. All forms of prurigo itch intensely and are characterized by the formation of nodules. These lesions are probably a form of neurodermatitis, the nodules resulting from chronic irritation. Whether or not the cutaneous nerves in the lesions are altered is controversial.

Pseudofolliculitis of the Beard

Synonym. Folliculitis barbae traumatica, pseudofolliculitis barbae.

Sites of predilection. Bearded portion of the neck.

Objective signs. Numerous hyperpigmented solid, small papules and small hyperpigmented scars occur on the sides of the neck. The hair growth is sparse and the hairs grow in all different directions. The condition occurs primarily in black men.

Subjective symptoms. Moderate pruritus. The skin is traumatized when the patient shaves and causes marked discomfort.

Etiology. Probably caused by the tightly coiled hair which reenters the skin before it protrudes from the follicle. Close shaving contributes to this problem.

Histopathology. Foreign body reaction due to the ingrown hair.

Diagnostic aids. Clinical appearance.

Differential diagnosis. Sycosis vulgaris.

Therapy. Stop shaving and let the beard grow. A depilatory can be used to remove hair instead of a razor.

Pseudoxanthoma Elasticum

Although this condition frequently begins as a papule, its eventual lesion is a macule and is described fully in Chapter 14.

Psoriasis

Synonym. None.

Sites of predilection. Extensor surfaces of the extremities (elbows, knees), the scalp, trunk, penis, intertriginous folds, nails. Lesions rarely occur on the face.

Objective signs. Psoriasis is a chronic, relapsing disease. The primary lesion is a well-defined, flat-topped papule or circumscribed plaque. The lesions are pinkish to reddish-brown and are covered with a profuse, dry, silvery-white, imbricated scale. The individual lesions vary from a few millimeters to 20 cm or more in diameter. They are round, irregular, or gyrate in shape. The lesions may be linear following areas of trauma (Koebner's phenomenon). The eruption is frequently symmetrically distributed. If the scale is removed, bleeding points are exposed (Auspitz's sign). Central involution may occur, forming annular lesions. The nails may become thickened, eroded and brittle, and show pit formation. Well-defined, scaly lesions form in the scalp, and are difficult to differentiate from seborrheic dermatitis. The hair may fall out because of excoriation, entrapment within scale formation or the inflammatory reaction. The pathologic reaction does not involve the papillae.

The general health of the individual is usually not affected. Small shotty pustules may occur on the palms and soles.

Subjective symptoms. Pruritus is a variable. The cosmetic defect is distressing. Should the lesion exfoliate, the thermoregulatory contract is compromised. In severe cases hyperuricemia is present and secondary gout may occur. Patients with prior existing cardiac disease and extensive psoriasis may acquire forward heart failure due to extensive cutaneous shunting of blood. Severe exfoliation may produce loss of body protein.

Etiology. Unknown. Psoriasis is currently regarded as a generalized genetic disease. There is an in-

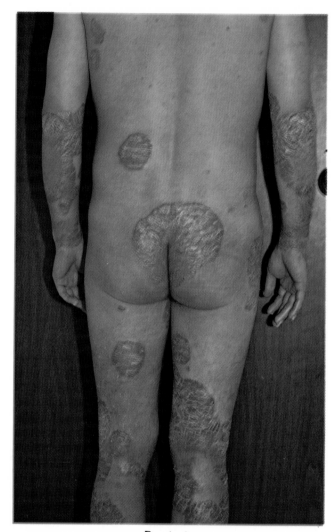

Psoriasis

creased epidermal turnover, but it has not been determined whether the primary defect is epidermal or dermal.

Histopathology. There is an increase in the keratin layer with much parakeratosis, long rete pegs with corresponding long narrow dermal pegs, and a thin layer of epidermis over the dermal

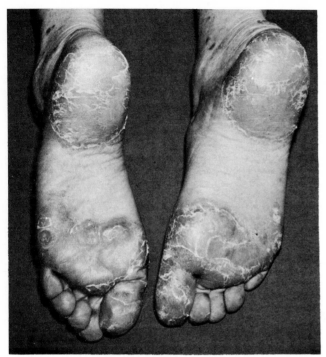

Psoriasis, plantar lesions

Koebner's phenomenon

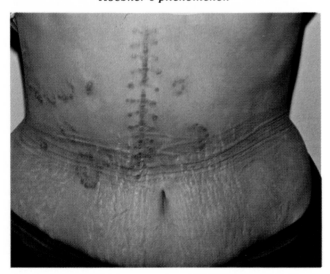

pegs. The capillaries in the dermal pegs are dilated, long and rigid. There is moderate edema and a mixed subacute infiltrate in the papillary and subpapillary layers.

Diagnostic aids. History and physical examination, biopsy.

Relation to systemic disease. Rheumatoid arthritis may be associated with the eruption. The nomenclature of this associated joint disorder is unclear.

Differential diagnosis. Seborrheic dermatitis, secondary syphillis, lichen planus, pityriasis rosea, nail lesions simulate onychomycosis or lichen planus.

Therapy. There is no specific therapy for psoriasis. Many patients will respond to systemic placebo or keratolytic therapy and others seem to improve with ultraviolet therapy or natural sunlight. Systemic administration of antimetabolites is effective. The Goeckerman technique (tar and UVL) helps many patients. Topically applied corticosteroid preparations are helpful. Coal tar and coal tar distillates are also effective. PUVA therapy (psoralen-UVA) is very effective in 70% of patients.

Sarcoidosis

Synonym. Sarcoid, multiple benign sarcoid, benign miliary lupoid (Boeck), lupus pernio (Besnier), benign lymphogranulomatosis (Schaumann), subcutaneous sarcoid (Darier-Roussy).

Sites of predilection. Any part of the body may be affected, but the inner canthi, alae nasi and sides of the neck are involved especially in black patients.

Objective signs. The cutaneous lesions of sarcoidosis are protean. Nodules, papules, macules and infiltrating plaques may be present. Atrophic or scarred lesions may occur. The lesions may be white, yellow, dull red or dark. Annular and circinate indurated plaques, especially with hypopigmented halos are distinctive. Small, discrete and

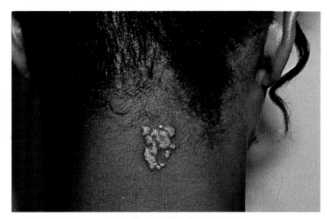

Sarcoidosis

Sarcoidosis

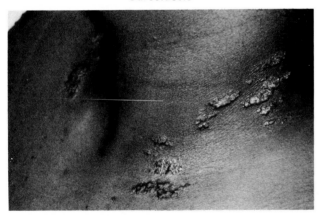

confluent, translucent, dull reddish or flesh-colored papules occurring on the alae nasi and the back of the neck are a characteristic form of the disease. There is frequently a generalized lymphadenopathy. Fusiform swelling of the phalanges and destruction of the distal portions of the digits are not uncommon. Swelling of the parotid glands and iridocyclitis (uveoparotid fever) are also symptoms of this disease. The nodules may be small and superficial or large and subcutaneous.

Subjective symptoms. Variable. Localized lesions are asymptomatic. If the uveal tract is involved, the patient may become blind. Malaise, cough, cachexia and general debility are symptoms of pulmonary involvement.

Etiology. Unknown.

Histopathology. Circumscribed nests of epithelioid cells surrounded by a fibrous network. Foreign body giant cells are present.

Diagnostic aids. Biopsy. The tuberculin test is negative unless there is underlying tuberculosis. Chest X ray may reveal infiltrations or lymphadenopathy in the hilar regions. Elevations in the blood SGOT and alkaline phosphatase, as well as hypoproteinemia with reversal of the albumin-globulin ratio may be present. Hypercalcemia or hypercalciuria may occur.

Relation to systemic disease. Sarcoidosis is always a systemic disease.

Differential diagnosis. Lupus vulgaris, lymphoblastoma, lupus erythematosus, leprosy.

Therapy. Sarcoidosis will respond to systemic corticosteroid therapy, but if used, isoniazid must be given concurrently. This type of treatment must be reserved for extensive involvement. Intralesional corticosteroids can be used for local lesions.

Sarcoma, Idiopathic Hemorrhagic

Synonym. Kaposi's sarcoma.

Objective signs. The initial lesion is a dark violaceous macule which usually first appears on the extremities. The tumors which develop retain the same color and enlarge to from 1-3 cm in diameter. The nodules may be both discrete and confluent. The affected extremity may enlarge due to edema and simulate elephantiasis. The tumors may ulcerate. The process is multifocal with lesions arising *de novo* in the mucosae and internal organs. Lymph nodes may be involved.

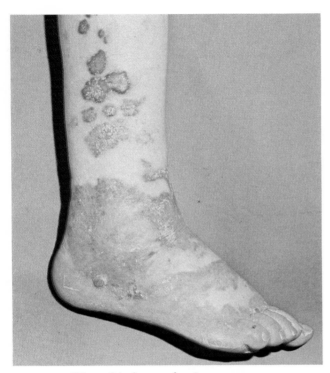

Idiopathic hemorrhagic sarcoma

Subjective symptoms. The local lesions do not produce discomfort unless they develop over pressure areas. Visceral involvement may be accompanied by fever and weight loss.

Etiology. Unknown. It occurs more commonly among European Jews, Italians, and African blacks. This disorder is becoming more frequently recognized in immunosuppressed patients.

Histopathology. In the mid-dermis there are interweaving bands of spindle cells embedded in a network of reticulin, and a network of vascular spaces. Hemosiderin-laden macrophages and an inflammatory reaction surround the cellular masses. Foci of necrosis appear in some of the masses.

Diagnostic aids. Biopsy.

Relation to systemic disease. Hepatosplenomegaly may occur. Anemia and hypergammaglobulinemia have been reported. Visceral involvement is not common.

Differential diagnosis. Lymphomas, sarcoma, granuloma.

Therapy. Radiation therapy may be used on limited areas. Perfusion with nitrogen mustard may have some value.

Sclerosis, Tuberous

Synonym. Bourneville's disease, steatadenoma, sebaceous nevus, adenoma sebaceum, epiloia.

Sites of predilection. Symmetrically distributed over cheeks and nose.

Objective signs. Yellowish to reddish, translucent papules, 1-4 mm or more in diameter. Plaques may occur on the forehead or other areas of the face. There is relative sparing of the upper lip.

Tuberous sclerosis

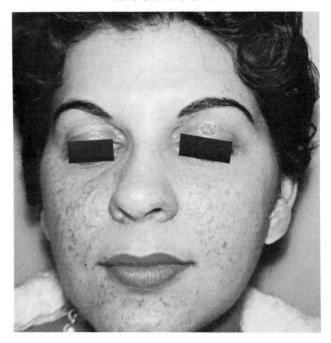

Papillomatous growths beneath the nails (Konen's tumors or subungual fibromas) are a common finding. Telangiectasia may be present. The lesions of the Pringle type are small, pink, soft and fleshy and are frequently associated with other nevi. Shagreen patches are collections of lesions which develop on the trunk. Whitish oval, "ash leaf" macules of hypopigmentation may be present on the trunk and are visualized under the Wood light. Lesions of the Balzar variety are large, pale, firm, and not symmetrically distributed (trichoepitheliomas).

Subjective symptoms. None usually, except the psychic trauma of the cosmetic defect.

Etiology. A congenital hamartomatous disease.

Histopathology. Hyperplasia of the sebaceous glands with vascular dilatation.

Diagnostic aids. History and physical examination, biopsy, Wood light to visualize "ash leaf" lesions.

Relation to systemic disease. The Pringle type of lesion is frequently associated with tuberous sclerosis, mental deficiency, and epilepsy (the triad known as epiloia), osteoporosis, cerebral calcification and bilateral renal tumors. Hamartomas may exist in any organ.

Symptoms of epiloia do not usually become apparent until the child is 6-9 years of age. This is a neurocutaneous disease. von Recklinghausen's disease and Sturge-Weber disease are also neurocutaneous, and cross-overs between these three may occur.

Differential diagnosis. Acne vulgaris, benign cystic epithelioma, nevi.

Therapy. To repair the cosmetic defect, lesions may be removed by fulguration. The major thrust of treatment should be to the underlying disease.

Skin Tags

Synonym. Cutaneous tags, acrochordon.

Sites of predilection. Neck, upper chest wall, axillae in middle-aged and elderly people.

Objective signs. Few to numerous, small (1-3 mm), flesh-colored or dark brown papules, or filiform tags. The lesions are discrete and may become secondarily infected.

Subjective symptoms. None.

Etiology. Unknown; probably associated with senescent changes in the skin.

Histopathology. Slight acanthosis, thinning of the horny layer and a spongy areolar arrangement of the fibers of the corium. There is loss of elastic tissue.

Diagnostic aids. Biopsy.

Relation to systemic disease. None has been established.

Differential diagnosis. Nevi, seborrheic keratoses, verrucae.

Therapy. Excision, desiccation or application of liquid nitrogen.

Sporotrichosis

Synonym. None.

Sites of predilection. Most common on the distal portions of the extremities; however, a disseminated form also occurs.

Objective signs. The organism is inoculated through traumatic contact, the fungus contained within infected animal excreta or vegetation. The first lesion that appears is an indurated nodule, called the sporotrichotic chancre. A localized abscess or

Sporotrichosis

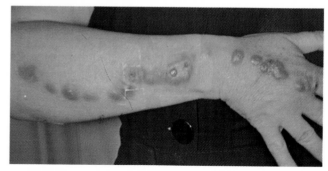

ulcer forms at this site, and the infection ascends along lymphatic channels, leaving a succession of violaceous, painless nodules (1-2 cm) which may become fluctuant. The plaque form of this disease occurs especially on the waistline. Regional lymphadenopathy is uncommon. Visceral involvement, especially pulmonary, frequently occurs. Osseous involvement and chronic draining sinuses may develop.

The disseminated form has an entirely different clinical appearance with an insidious onset of a widespread papular or papulovesicular eruption. Nodules may form and subsequently ulcerate.

Subjective symptoms. The cutaneous lesions cause few if any subjective symptoms.

Etiology. *Sporothrix schenckii.*

Histopathology. Nonspecific granuloma containing plasma cells, epithelioid cells and Langhans' cells. It is extremely rare to demonstrate the organism in biopsy specimens.

Diagnostic aids. Culture on fungus media, biopsy, chest X ray.

Relation to systemic disease. The disease may become systemic.

Differential diagnosis. Syphilis, localized pyogenic abscesses, other deep mycoses, tularemia, tuberculosis cutis.

Therapy. Potassium iodide, 2-6 gm daily by mouth, or sodium iodide daily, 1-6 gm intravenously for the localized form. For the disseminated form or when visceral involvement develops, amphotericin B is the drug of choice.

Syphilis, Late Cutaneous

Synonym. Gumma.

Sites of predilection. Lower third of the legs, thighs, trunk, face, scalp. Any area of the body may become involved.

Objective signs. The cutaneous lesion of late syphilis may appear as a solitary nodule or plaque-like lesion.

Solitary gumma. These are usually solitary, subcutaneous nodules, which appear from 5-30 years after onset of infection. These lesions grow slowly; the overlying skin gradually becomes hyperpigmented. When the lesions attain a size of 5 cm or larger, they become fluctuant, and the overlying skin sloughs to form a crateriform or cup-shaped ulcer with precipitous sides.

Nodular syphiloderm. These plaque-like lesions are a form of late syphilis which appear from 2-5 years after onset of infection. They begin as a group of nodules which coalesce to form a serpiginous plaque; subcutaneous nodules may be felt in the border. The lesions may ulcerate, forming a nodular ulcerative syphiloderm. When the nodules ulcerate, characteristic gumma-like ulcers are formed. These lesions may heal and subsequently recur in the scarred site.

Subjective symptoms. None.

See Chapter 9: Sexually Transmitted Diseases for etiology, histopathology, diagnostic aids, relation to systemic disease and therapy.

Syphilis, Papular Secondary

Synonym. The pox.

Sites of predilection. Generalized.

Objective signs. The lesions may be small monomorphic conical papules, 1-2 mm in diameter, reddish-brown (coppery or raw ham) in color, discrete or forming small groups (false corymbose grouping). The lesions occur all at one time.

The lesions may also be large and flat (lenticular papules) varying from 2 mm-1 cm in diameter. These lesions also have the characteristic color. They may form groups, with a central lesion surrounded by a ring of papules (true corymbose grouping).

Annular papules occur most commonly on the face. When these occur at the corners of the mouth or in the nasolabial folds, they form split papules. These ringed lesions have the distinctive

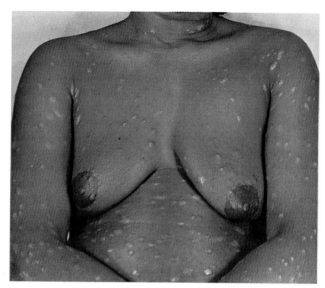

Papillary secondary syphilis

feature of radial groove formation in the margins. They are rarely observed in white patients.

In the genitocrural areas, under the breasts, between the toes and in the perianal region, papules become hypertrophic and eroded, with a grayish, moist surface. These lesions are usually discrete but may become confluent and are known as hypertrophic eroded papules or condylomata lata. They are highly contagious, usually teeming with spirochetes. Condylomata lata occur almost invariably between the buttocks or about the genitalia in patients who have annular papular syphilids on the face.

Subjective symptoms. Usually none, except occasional pruritus in blacks.

Etiology. Treponema pallidum.

Histopathology. The picture is suggestive but not pathognomonic. There is some parakeratosis and the rete shows a varying degree of acanthosis without much edema. The infiltrate, which consists of mononuclear cells (small and large) and plasma cells, tends to be dense toward the sur-

face and decreases like an inverted cone. There is endothelial swelling of the superficial and deep vessels which are surrounded by a "coat sleeve" infiltrate.

Diagnostic aids. Darkfield microscopic examination, STS, history and physical examination.

Relation to systemic disease. Syphilis is always a systemic disease. See Chapter 9.

Differential diagnosis. Psoriasis, papular pityriasis rosea, lichen planus, verruca acuminata, drug eruption.

Therapy. See Chapter 9.

Syringocystadenoma

Synonym. Syringocystoma.

Sites of predilection. Trunk, extremities.

Objective signs. This is a rare condition with numerous, small (1-3 mm) shiny, pinkish to brownish or yellowish, translucent papules.

Subjective symptoms. None.

Etiology. Congenital. These lesions are small tumors derived from misplaced embryonic sweat ducts or sweat glands.

Histopathology. Large number of round or oval masses of epithelium and epithelial lined tubules. Malformed sweat tubules in aimless coils are present in the dermis.

Diagnostic aids. Biopsy.

Relation to systemic disease. None has been established.

Differential diagnosis. Benign cystic epithelioma, papular syphiloderm, xanthomas, milia.

Therapy. None is effective. The lesions may be destroyed locally or excised if desired.

Syringoma

Synonym. None.

Sites of predilection. Eyelids, cheeks, forehead, neck, upper chest.

Objective signs. Few to numerous, small, flat, skin-colored papules.

Subjective symptoms. None.

Etiology. This is a nevoid lesion.

Histopathology. Sweat ducts are dilated and convoluted. A characteristic feature is the presence of "tadpole" or "comma" formation of the ducts.

Diagnostic aids. Biopsy.

Relation to systemic disease. None.

Differential diagnosis. Moles, trichoepithelioma.

Therapy. None is effective unless complete excision is performed.

Tuberculid, Papulonecrotic

Synonym. Folliclis, acnitis, tuberculosis papulonecrotica.

Sites of predilection. Trunk, extremities, face.

Objective signs. There are few to numerous, discrete, deep-seated, dull red to purplish, rounded, sessile papules. The center of each lesion undergoes necrosis. The crusted lesions may persist for years.

Subjective symptoms. None except the mental distress caused by the unsightly lesions.

Etiology. This entity is regarded as a tuberculid or a cutaneous reaction to a focus of tuberculosis elsewhere in the body.

Histopathology. Obliterative endovasculitis in the cutis and subcutis with caseous tubercle formation and small necrotic, crusted ulcers.

Diagnostic aids. History and physical examination, biopsy, studies for systemic tuberculosis.

Relation to systemic disease. Probably a sensitization reaction, associated with visceral tuberculosis.

Differential diagnosis. Folliculitis, papulopustular secondary syphilis.

Therapy. Treatment of the underlying condition.

Tuberculosis, Primary Cutaneous

Synonym. Primary tuberculous complex, tuberculous chancre.

Sites of predilection. Face, extremities, genitalia.

Objective signs. The lesion may vary from an inconspicuous, spontaneously healing nodule, to a large, bluish-red nodule or plaque, with a central crusted ulcer and rolled border. Regional lymph nodes may become enlarged from 3-5 cm in diameter. These are frequently productive of draining sinuses.

Subjective symptoms. None to slight local pain.

Etiology. M tuberculosis.

Histopathology. Tubercle formation with caseous necrosis. Each tubercle consists of nests of epithelioid cells and giant cells, surrounded by a zone of lymphocytes and plasma cells.

Diagnostic aids. History and physical examination, chest X ray, biopsy. Patients in whom these lesions occur should be followed with serial roentgenograms of the chest for a minimum of 18 months to rule out systemic dissemination of the disease from the primary cutaneous lesion.

Relation to systemic disease. Tuberculosis is a systemic disease.

Differential diagnosis. Initial lesions of sporotrichosis, syphilis or tularemia.

Therapy. Streptomycin, isoniazid, rifampin and para-aminosalicylic acid.

Tuberculosis Cutis

Tuberculosis of the skin occurs with less frequency in the United States than in most countries of Europe and Asia. The type of clinical manifestation depends on the site and mode of inoculation, and the degree of immunity of the individual.

Cutaneous tuberculosis may be caused by inoculation of the tubercle bacillus from an outside source, or associated with hematogenous spread or "sensitization reaction" (tuberculid).

I. Cutaneous tuberculosis caused by inoculation into the skin.

A. Primary tuberculous complex is known as a tuberculous chancre, and results from local inoculation of the M tuberculosis into the skin, in the absence of immunity.

B. Tuberculosis verrucosa cutis is a localized warty lesion which results from local inoculation of the *M tuberculosis* into the skin of individuals who have developed partial immunity.

C. Tuberculosis cutis orificialis lesions are ulcers which occur about the nose, mouth and anus in persons who have extensive, active, visceral tuberculosis.

D. Scrofuloderma (Tuberculosis cutis colliquativa). These rare granulomatous lesions result from sinus tracts which originate in lymph nodes, joints or bones. The initiating infection usually resides in the gastrointestinal tract secondary to the ingestion of infected milk.

E. Lupus vulgaris (tuberculosis cutis luposa) forms nodular lesions which usually occur on the face.

II. Cutaneous tuberculosis caused by hematogenous spread of the disease or sensitization reactions.

A. Acute miliary tuberculosis is a fulminating form of the disease in which the lesions are not limited to the skin. There is little or no immunity present; the condition is fatal.

B. Tuberculosis papulonecrotica (folliclis, papulonecrotic tuberculid).

C. Lichen scrofulosorum.

D. Lupus miliaris disseminatus faciei.

E. Tuberculosis cutis indurativa (erythema induratum).

Tuberculosis Cutis Colliquativa

Synonym. Scrofuloderma.

Sites of predilection. Areas overlying lymph nodes, joints or bones.

Objective signs. Scrofuloderma is manifested by a deep-seated nodule that gradually increases in size, becomes fluctuant and ulcerates, forming a granulomatous mass, which is the termination of a sinus tract. There may be numerous orifices which exude a thin, serous, sanguinous or sanguinopurulent material. Dense linear bands of scar tissue may form in the granulating area.

Subjective symptoms. Only slight discomfort.

Etiology. M tuberculosis.

Histopathology. Tubercles within lymph nodes undergo caseous necrosis with subsequent sinus tract formation. Tubercles may be found in the borders of the ulcers.

Diagnostic aids. History and physical examination, biopsy, chest X ray, cultures for tuberculosis.

Relation to systemic disease. The lesion is a manifestation of active tuberculosis.

Differential diagnosis. Malignancy, lymphogranuloma venereum, late cutaneous syphilis, blastomycosis, other deep fungus diseases.

Therapy. Streptomycin, isoniazid and para-aminosalicylic acid. Rifampin may also be used.

Tuberculosis Cutis Orificialis

Synonym. Tuberculous ulcers.

Sites of predilection. About the nose, mouth, anus.

Objective signs. This form of cutaneous tuberculosis is associated with the late stages of widespread tuberculosis of the lungs or other internal organs. It begins with the formation of small, yellowish nodules, which break down to form shallow, granulating ulcers. These lesions spread peripherally and show no tendency to heal.

Subjective symptoms. Some discomfort, especially when the tongue is involved.

Etiology. M tuberculosis.

Histopathology. Large numbers of circumscribed tubercles in the corium. Tubercle bacilli are easily demonstrated in the tissue.

Diagnostic aids. History and physical examination, chest X ray, sputum examination, biopsy.

Relation to systemic disease. Related to advanced visceral tuberculosis. The tuberculin test may be negative.

Differential diagnosis. Blastomycosis, pyodermas, leukemia, lymphoma, mucocutaneous leishmaniasis, midline lethal granuloma.

Therapy. Streptomycin, rifampin, isoniazid, para-aminosalicylic acid.

Tuberculosis Verrucosa Cutis

Synonym. Anatomic tubercle, prosector's wart, verruca necrogenica.

Sites of predilection. Hands, knees or other areas subject to trauma.

Objective signs. This condition begins at the site of an abrasion or wound, with a deep-seated, circumscribed, bluish-red or dull red, subcutaneous nodule, which usually has a verrucous surface. The lesion may become hypertrophic, or may involute in the center with an atrophic scar. The lesions are irregular plaques varying from 2 mm-5 cm in diameter. Pustules may develop within the lesion.

Subjective symptoms. Usually none.

Etiology. M tuberculosis.

Histopathology. Marked acanthosis and hyperkeratosis are present and there is a heavy plasma cell and round cell infiltrate in the upper cutis. Tubercle formation may be demonstrated.

Diagnostic aids. Biopsy, history and physical examination, chest X ray.

Relation to systemic disease. Tuberculosis is a systemic disease.

Differential diagnosis. Blastomycosis, verrucae, chronic pyoderma, granuloma annulare, foreign body granuloma, granuloma pyogenicum, sporotrichosis, swimming pool granuloma.

Therapy. Streptomycin, isoniazid, rifampin, and para-aminosalicylic acid.

Tularemia

Synonym. Rabbit fever, Francis' disease, deerfly fever, Pahvant Valley plague.

Sites of predilection. The initial lesion of tularemia may occur at any site.

Objective signs. Tularemia is an infectious disease of polymorphic symptomatology. The disease may be ulceroglandular, oculoglandular, pneumonic, typhoidal, meningeal or glandular. Cutaneous manifestations are important only in the ulceroglandular type.

After an incubation period of 2-9 days, a papule or nodule appears at the site of inoculation. This rapidly ulcerates, leaving a tender, firm and indolent ulcer with a necrotic base, which separates, giving a punched-out appearance. This heals with scar formation in about 6 weeks. Lymphangitis spreads from the initial lesion, and the regional lymph nodes become swollen, painful and gradually fluctuant, but rarely ulcerative.

Other skin lesions, which are probably of toxic origin, are herpetic, erythema multiforme-like eruptions and localized pustules.

Subjective symptoms. Headache, chills, generalized malaise and hyperpyrexia. The local lesions are painful and tender.

Etiology. Pasteurella tularensis. The disease occurs chiefly in the southwestern United States, although sporadic cases have been reported in almost all parts of the country. Lesions develop in people who handle infected, small animals, such as wild rabbits, squirrels and other game. The disease is also transmitted by the deerfly and some ticks.

Histopathology. The granulomatous microscopic changes in the tularemic ulcer are not diagnostic.

Diagnostic aids. Culture, history and physical examination.

Relation to systemic disease. Tularemia is always a systemic disease.

Differential diagnosis. Syphilis (primary lesion), sporotrichosis.

Therapy. Tetracycline or chloramphenicol, 250-500 mg 4 times daily for 1-2 weeks. Streptomycin, 2 gm daily for 1 week.

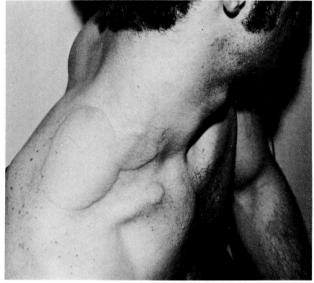

Urticaria

Urticaria

Synonym. Hives, nettle rash.

Sites of predilection. Any area may be affected.

Objective signs. The primary lesion or wheal is a whitish-pinkish or reddish, well-defined area of localized edema. The lesions assume many shapes and sizes varying from a few millimeters in diameter to involvement of an entire eyelid, lip or finger (angioneurotic edema, Quincke's edema). They may be nummular, annular or gyrate, and may be topped by a vesicle. Pseudopods may develop. There is no scale present. The lesions are usually transitory but recurrent. Slight trauma may result in wheal formation (dermatographia).

Subjective symptoms. Moderate to intense pruritus.

Etiology. Urticaria is an allergic phenomenon in which the shock organ is the small capillary in the cutis. Ingestants such as drugs, shellfish, chocolate, nuts or spoiled foods may be precipitating factors. Inhalants or injected substances such as penicillin and tetanus antitoxin are frequent offenders. Sys-temic disease and focal infections may precipitate urticaria. Psychic stimuli play a role. Isolated wheals may result from the bites of animal or plant vectors such as insects, *eg,* mosquitos, *Cimex lectularius* (bedbug), sea nettles, fleas and grain itch mites. Urticaria may also occur after exposure to cold, heat, pressure, vibrating objects or water.

In serum sickness, generalized lymphadenopathy accompanied by high fever develops. Urticarial lesions are extensive and the patient is acutely ill. Edema of the larynx and pharynx may present serious complications.

Histopathology. Edema of connective tissue and fixed tissue cells with cellular infiltration, swelling of the sweat gland cells and deposit of fibrin.

Diagnostic aids. History and physical examination.

Relation to systemic disease. Urticaria is a systemic allergic disturbance.

Differential diagnosis. The disease is characteristic.

Therapy. Detect and eliminate the cause. As an emergency measure, injections of adrenalin may give temporary relief. Systemic corticosteroid therapy is indicated in cases of extensive involvement. Antihistamine therapy is of value in mild cases. Hydroxyzine can be a useful drug. Cyproheptadine is the current drug of choice for cold urticaria.

Urticaria, Papular

Synonym. Urticaria papulosa, lichen urticatus, prurigo simplex.

Sites of predilection. Generalized.

Objective signs. This condition usually occurs in childhood as a chronic, recurrent eruption in the spring and summer. The primary lesion is a small urticarial papule or papulovesicle which subsides, leaving a small, firm, persistent papule. Numerous excoriations and blood crusts are noted. Secondary pyogenic infection is frequently present.

Subjective symptoms. Moderate to severe pruritus.

Etiology. The condition is usually attributed to insect bites. It is to be emphasized that insects may feed on other family members without producing this disease in them. Also many insects can bite without being seen or felt by the patient.

Histopathology. The microscopic picture is not diagnostic.

Diagnostic aids. Examination of the patient's environment for insect vectors, history and physical examination.

Relation to systemic disease. None.

Differential diagnosis. Scabies, varicella.

Therapy. The living quarters and bed should be thoroughly fumigated with an insecticide. An insect repellant should be placed on the body several times daily. Antihistamines should be administered. Local therapy with calamine lotion or corticosteroid creams to relieve pruritus and erythema is helpful.

VERRUCAE (WARTS)

Warts have a common virus etiology. The appearance of the lesion varies according to its location.

Verruca Acuminata

Synonym. Venereal wart, condyloma acuminatum.

Sites of predilection. Genital and perianal region.

Objective signs. Verruca acuminata is a pedunculated or sessile, round or leaf-shaped lesion which may be discrete or form confluent, cauliflower-like masses. The lesion remains intact or becomes eroded, flat and moist, and varies from flesh-colored to grayish-brown. It may be slowly growing, persisting for months, or grow to enormous size (5 cm or larger) within a few weeks.

Subjective symptoms. None to slight pruritus.

Etiology. Virus.

Histopathology. Proliferation of the prickle cell layer, with intracellular edema. Numerous mitotic figures are present, and there is a multicellular

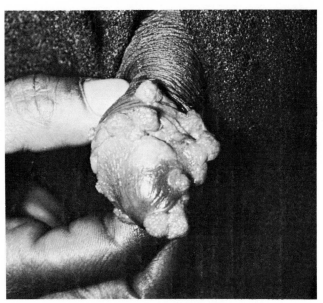

Condylomata acuminata

infiltrate. Papillary bodies are elongated. Very few viral particles are seen.

Diagnostic aids. Biopsy, darkfield microscopic examination to rule out secondary syphilis.

Relation to systemic disease. None has been established.

Differential diagnosis. Condyloma latum (secondary syphilis), ecthyma.

Therapy. Surgical excision or electrodesiccation are usually not successful. The lesions may be successfully treated with applications of a 25% solution of podophyllin in compound tincture of benzoin. The patient must be warned that the application will cause a violent local reaction.

Verruca Plana Juvenilis

Synonym. Flat warts of childhood.

Sites of predilection. Face, neck, hands, wrists, knees.

Objective signs. This condition usually occurs in children or young adults as numerous, slightly raised, flat-topped, circinate, small, skin or tan-colored

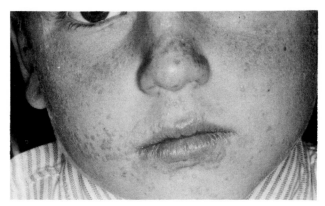

Verruca plana juvenilis

papules which may be discrete, or form irregular groups with a tendency towards linear arrangement (Koebner's phenomenon).

Subjective symptoms. None.

Etiology. Virus.

Histopathology. The histopathologic picture is similar to that seen in verruca vulgaris, but the changes are not as marked. The stratum corneum is thickened in a "basket weave" pattern.

Diagnostic aids. Biopsy.

Relation to systemic disease. May be associated with tension states.

Differential diagnosis. Lichen planus, lichen nitidus, molluscum contagiosum, perioral dermatitis, follicular acne.

Therapy. Gentle cryotherapy to avoid scar formation. Topical retinoic or salicylic acids applied topically are sometimes effective.

Verruca Plantaris

Synonym. Plantar wart.

Sites of predilection. Pressure points on the plantar surfaces.

Objective signs. The lesion may appear as a callus; removal reveals a central core in which there are usually black dots or bleeding points. These are actually hypertrophied papillae, filled with small masses of coagulated blood. This portion of the lesion is surrounded by a zone of hyperkeratosis. Plantar warts may be single, or appear in groups. A large central wart and closely aggregated smaller satellite lesions form an area known as a mosaic wart.

Subjective symptoms. None to severe pain.

Etiology. Virus. There is recent evidence that several strains of this agent exist.

Histopathology. The microscopic picture is similar to that of verruca vulgaris. Many virus particles can be seen.

Diagnostic aids. Clinical appearance.

Relation to systemic disease. None.

Differential diagnosis. Plantar corns.

Therapy. There is no specific form of therapy. Surgical removal of lesions is usually ineffective and the recurrence rate is high. Conservative therapy is indicated. The use of salicylic acid plaster (40%) followed by trimming of the lesion is frequently effective. Even with optimal therapy, recurrence (20%) is not unusual.

Plantar warts

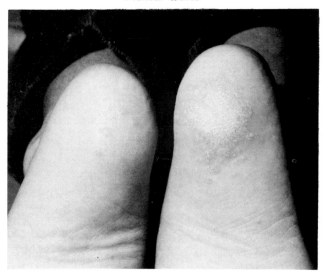

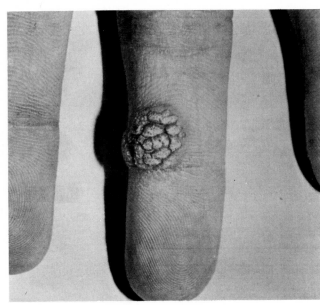

Verruca vulgaris

Verruca Vulgaris

Synonym. Common wart.

Sites of predilection. Hands; less frequently the face, lips, eyelids and other areas.

Objective signs. One or more discrete or confluent lesions may occur. The lesions are grayish, dark brown or grayish-brown, round or oval, well-defined papules, varying from 2 mm-1 cm or more in diameter. The early lesion is usually smooth and shiny, but gradually becomes rough and gray. They are occasionally seen as thread-like projections called filiform warts on the face or eyelids. Pedunculated lesions may develop.

Subjective symptoms. None.

Etiology. Virus. Evidence is present that more than one viral strain exists.

Histopathology. Marked acanthosis and hyperkeratosis, with graduating proliferation of the rete ridges, deepest at the center. Parakeratosis in the stratum corneum is evidenced by swollen, vacuolated cells which retain their nuclei. Numerous mitotic figures and viral particles are present in the epidermis.

Diagnostic aids. Biopsy.

Relation to systemic disease. These lesions frequently occur in immunosuppressed or atopic patients.

Differential diagnosis. Molluscum contagiosum.

Therapy. One of the more effective forms of therapy is the careful application of liquid nitrogen to each lesion. Electrodesiccation may be effective. Surgical excision is not advised.

Xeroderma Pigmentosum

Synonym. Atrophoderma pigmentosum, melanosis lenticularis progressiva, angioma pigmentosum et atrophicum.

Sites of predilection. Exposed surfaces.

Objective signs. This rare, progressive disease usually begins early in life, and is first characterized by a mottling of the skin in the areas exposed to sunlight, with hyperemia and some roughening of the surface. Within the next 2-3 years, pigmentation appears in the form of small, freckle-like spots, which scale and appear like flat warts. These lesions become less pronounced in the winter, but in warm weather or when exposed to sunlight, they become slightly raised. Telangiectasia develops and whitish atrophic spots appear. Angiomas and warty growths occur. The lesions frequently scar and undergo malignant degeneration and become squamous cell carcinomas, melanomas or basal cell carcinomas. Unexposed areas may become involved. The skin becomes thin and parchment-like. Corneal opacities may occur.

Subjective symptoms. Photophobia, lacrimation, increased sunburning, general debility.

Etiology. Congenital. There is an inherited defect in the repair of DNA damaged by ultraviolet light. There are several subtypes of disease corresponding to different enzymatic defects. One type

(DeSanctis-Cacchione syndrome) is associated with idiocy and a variety of neurologic disorders.

Histopathology. The changes vary with the stage of the disease and are not diagnostic. They simulate the changes seen in senescent skin and actinic dermatitis, with atrophy of the epidermis and senile elastosis.

Diagnostic aids. Biopsy, history, enzymatic determination of ultraviolet injured tissue, culture fibroblasts of the skin or amniotic cells for DNA repair enzymes.

Relation to systemic disease. These children usually die at an early age, frequently before the second or third year.

Differential diagnosis. Chloasma, freckles (early), roentgen-ray dermatitis.

Therapy. Treatment is of no benefit. Protection from sunlight is essential.

Yaws

Synonym. Frambesia.

For a description of this disease, see the description of Yaws in Chapter 22: Tropical Diseases.

XANTHOMATOSIS

Xanthomas are yellow, fatty infiltrations of the skin which occur in many forms. They may develop as nodular (tuberous), flat (planar), papular or papulonodular, yellow lesions around joints or tendons (tendinous), over bony prominences, on the eyelids (xanthelasma) or on other parts of the body. These may also appear as small streaks on the palmar and plantar surfaces or as large verrucoid structures. The lesions may be localized or widespread and may occur insidiously or rapidly (eruptive). Xanthomas may appear in persons having hyperlipidemia, apparently normal individuals, or in patients having another disorder such as diabetes or a reticuloendothelioma, which has pro-

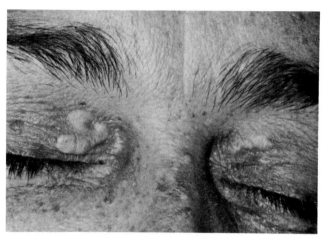

Xanthelasma

duced a fat metabolism disorder. The many forms of hyperlipidemia are included in the Table on page 193.

Xanthelasma

Synonym. Xanthoma palpebrarum.

Sites of predilection. Eyelids.

Objective signs. The primary lesion develops slowly as a flat, yellow papule which spreads in streaklike fashion across the eyelid. The lesions may be small and discrete or form large confluent areas covering much of the lid. The lesions usually develop in persons over the age of 40.

Subjective symptoms. Usually none except for the annoyance caused by the cosmetic defect.

Etiology. A defect in lipid metabolism.

Histopathology. This is a true xanthoma and is characterized by nests of foam cells and Touton giant cells.

Diagnostic aids. Biopsy, blood lipid studies, physical survey, electrocardiogram, liver function tests.

Relation to systemic disease. See Table on page 193.

Differential diagnosis. Milia.

Therapy. Treat the systemic disease responsible for producing the lesions. The cutaneous lesions may be removed by light fulguration.

Hyperlipidemia

Type	Frequency	Blood Lipids	Clinical Characteristics	Therapy	Associated Diseases	Cutaneous Manifestations
I	Rare	Creamy top layer of sera, increased chylomicrons, increased triglycerides, decreased lipoprotein, lipase	Childhood onset, abdominal pain, hepatosplenomegaly, low incidence of heart disease	Low fat diet	Pancreatitis, diabetes	Eruptive xanthomas
II	Common	Increased lipoprotein, moderate increased pre-beta-lipoproteins, increased cholesterol, increased triglycerides	Any age, advanced athero-sclerosis	Low saturated fat diet; d-thyroxine; clofibrate	Hyperthyroidism, liver disease, kidney disease, myeloma, macroglobulinemia	Arcus senilis of cornea; xanthelasma; palmar, tuberous and tendinous xanthomas
III	Infrequent	Turbid sera, increased beta and pre-beta-lipoproteins, increased cholesterol and triglycerides	Adult onset, cardiovascular disease	Low carbohydrate, low saturated fat diet; nicotinic acid; clofibrate	Diabetes, liver disease, dysproteinemia	Same as II; eruptive xanthomas
IV	Common	Turbid sera, increased pre-beta-lipoproteins, increased triglycerides	Adult onset, obesity, abdominal pain, cardiovascular disease	Low carbohydrate diet; clofibrate; nicotinic acid	Hypothyroidism, diabetes, pancreatitis, nephrosis, myeloma, glycogen storage disease	Tuberous and eruptive xanthomas; xanthelasma
V	Common	Creamy top layer and turbid sera, increased pre-beta-lipoproteins, increased chylomicrons, increased triglycerides, cholesterol may or may not be increased	Early adult onset, abdominal pain, obesity, hepatosplenomegaly	Low fat, calorie and carbohydrate diet; clofibrate	Diabetes, pancreatitis, alcoholism	Eruptive xanthomas

Xanthoma, Eruptive

Synonym. Xanthoma diabeticorum.

Sites of predilection. Palms, soles; lesions may develop on the face and other parts of the body.

Objective signs. Small discrete papules develop primarily on the palms and soles. Yellow streaks may appear in the creases of the palms. Occasionally lesions appear on the face and other parts of the body.

Subjective symptoms. The cutaneous lesions do not produce discomfort.

Etiology. A defect in lipid metabolism.

Histopathology. Nests of foam cells and Touton giant cells.

Diagnostic aids. Biopsy, blood lipid studies, electrocardiogram, urinalysis, blood sugar.

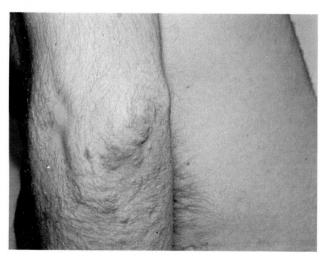

Xanthoma

Relation to systemic disease. Associated with diabetes and pancreatitis.

Differential diagnosis. Milia, carotenemia, warts.

Therapy. None for the cutaneous lesions. Treat the underlying disease.

Xanthoma, Tuberous

Synonym. Xanthoma tuberosum multiplex.

Sites of predilection. Elbows, knees and over tendon sheaths are the most common sites but lesions may occur anywhere.

Objective signs. Discrete, solid, lemon yellow papules and nodules which vary in size from single lesions 1 cm in diameter, to confluent lobulated plaques 10 cm or more in diameter. The surfaces of the lesions are smooth. Some telangiectasis is usually present.

Subjective symptoms. The cutaneous lesions rarely cause discomfort but the cosmetic defect may cause the patient some embarrassment.

Etiology. Hyperlipidemia.

Histopathology. Nests of foam cells and Touton giant cells in a fibrous tissue stroma.

Diagnostic aids. Biopsy, physical survey, blood lipid studies, electrocardiogram, liver function studies.

Relation to systemic disease. Diabetes, pancreatitis, nephrosis, glycogen storage disease, myeloma.

Differential diagnosis. Histiocytoma and other cutaneous neoplasms.

Treatment. Treat the underlying disease.

CHAPTER 16

Vesicular Eruptions

Acrodermatitis Enteropathica

Synonym. None.

Sites of predilection. Perioral, perianal and acral areas.

Objective signs. Apathetic child (3 weeks to several years old) with diarrhea develops a vesiculobullous, symmetrical eruption that later appears chapped. The lesions crust, scale and may be superinfected by *Candida* or bacteria. The tissues around the mouth, anus and on the hands, knees and feet are eventually involved. Periungual involvement precedes loss of the nail. Noncicatrical alopecia appears on the scalp, eyebrows and eyelashes. Conjunctivitis, stomatitis, photophobia, glossitis and perlèche occur. The course of the disease is marked by exacerbations and remissions.

Subjective symptoms. Pain, lassitude.

Etiology. This disorder is due to an inability of the intestine to transport adequate amounts of zinc into the body.

Histopathology. Nonspecific dermatitis.

Diagnostic aids. Clinical picture, examine stool to confirm malabsorption.

Relation to systemic disease. This disease is a generalized disease with malabsorption, diarrhea and dermatitis.

Differential diagnosis. Candidiasis, pellagra, epidermolysis bullosa, pachyonychia congenita, congenital ectodermal defect.

Therapy. Zinc sulfate is specific therapy. Supplemental vitamins should be given; appropriate antibiotics when indicated.

Dermatitis, Allergic Contact

Synonym. Contact dermatitis, dermatitis venenata.

Sites of predilection. Any exposed part of the body.

Objective signs. Erythema, edema, vesiculation, serous exudation and later secondary pyogenic infection may be present. The vesicles are characteristically arranged in linear groups in cases caused by plant sensitivity, or when a sensitizing liquid is applied to the skin and flows on to an adjacent area. When the face is involved, moderate to intense edema of the periorbital area usually occurs. After the acute stage subsides one may note scaling and slight hyperpigmentation in the involved areas.

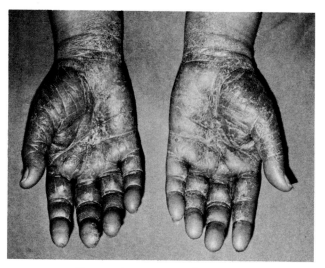

*Eczematous contact dermatitis
from rubber gloves*

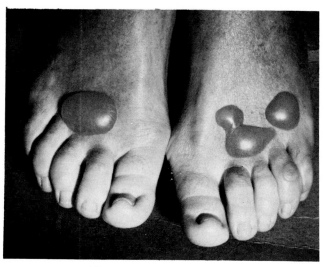

Allergic contact dermatitis

Chronic eczematous contact dermatitis

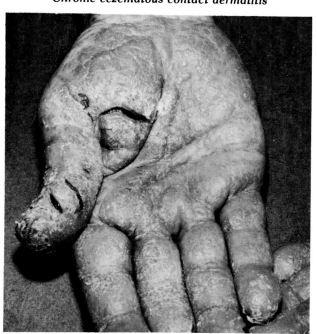

Subjective symptoms. Mild to severe pruritus and burning. Pain may accompany severe swelling.

Etiology. Acquired contact sensitivity. See the Table on page 198 for some of the offending agents. Plants, local medicaments, creams, lotions, antifungal preparations and eye drops are also causative agents. Substances or agents handled in industry are other etiologic factors. Allergic contact dermatitis differs from primary irritant dermatitis: not everyone in a population is susceptible and the patient must contact the allergen more than once to acquire the disease.

Histopathology. In the epidermis there are varying degrees of intraepidermal vesiculation. There is also intercellular edema with spongiosis. Lymphocytes and polymorphonuclear leukocytes are scattered throughout the involved epidermis with evidence of parakeratosis of the horny layer. In the cutis there is vascular dilatation and a mild perivascular infiltrate consisting of

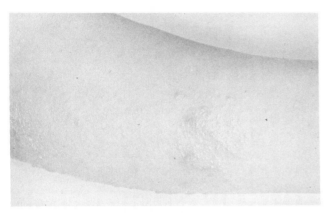

*Dermatitis venenata, showing
linear group of vesicles*

*Allergic contact dermatitis
from shoes*

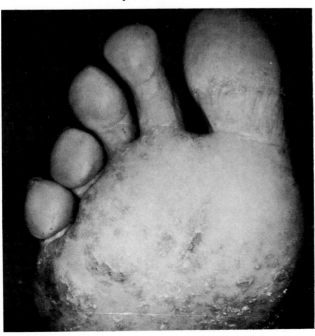

leukocytes.

Diagnostic aids. Careful history and patch testing with the suspected responsible agents.

Relation to systemic disease. None.

Differential diagnosis. Primary irritation dermatitis, neurodermatitis, atopic eczema, tinea pedis and dyshidrosis.

Therapy. Removal of the offending agent. Locally, apply compresses of cold Burow's solution (solution of aluminum acetate) diluted 1:32. If large areas of the body are involved, use lukewarm colloidal oatmeal baths. Corticosteroid creams applied locally to the affected parts give relief. Calamine lotion containing 0.5% menthol may also be effective in relieving pruritus. If the involvement is extensive, and there is no physical contraindication, systemic corticosteroid therapy for 5-7 days in adequate dosage should be administered.

Dermatitis, Primary Irritant Contact

Synonym. None.

Sites of predilection. Area of contact.

Objective signs. Clinical findings vary with the type of irritant, duration of contact with the offending agent and the area exposed. Lesions produced by chronic contact with solvents or detergents are ill-defined, dull, red and become lichenified. As time passes, these areas become dry and fissured with loss of skin tone. If caustic substances come in contact with the skin the areas may develop vesicles, blebs and subsequent erosions or ulcerations.

Subjective symptoms. Moderate to severe pruritus and pain.

Etiology. Soap, solvents, detergents, gasoline, cement, acids, alkalis, *etc.*

Histopathology. Not specific.

Diagnostic aids. History and clinical appearance. Patch tests cannot be used because the primary irritant will cause a reaction in any patient's skin, and therefore they have no diagnostic value.

Some Offending Agents in Contact Dermatitis

Involved Areas	Responsible Agents	Involved Areas	Responsible Agents
Scalp	Hair lotions, hair tonics, shampoos, pomades, hair dyes, cold wave chemicals, spray nets, hair lacquers	Neck	Scarf, cosmetics, fur collar, jewelry, plastic bib, dye from dress, religious medal, identification tag
Forehead	Hat band, rubber bathing cap, nylon or rubber elastic hairnets, scalp and hair preparations	Axillae	Deodorants, depilatories, perfume and cologne, dress shields, dye from dress or shirt
Eyes	Nail polish, nail polish remover, eye drops, eye washes, mascara, rubber eyelash curler, plants (poison ivy, sumac, *etc*)	Trunk	Elastic in brassiere, rubber girdle, underwear, cosmetics
Ears	Earrings, perfume, cosmetics used in the hair, eyeglass frames, telephone receiver, ear drops, ear phones, hearing aids	Genitalia, buttocks	Contraceptive creams and jellies, douching agents, condoms, men's shorts, bathing trunks, panties, girdles
Face	Cosmetics such as cleansing creams, hormone wrinkle removers, foundation lotions, *etc*. Shaving cream, after-shave lotions, soap, rubber powder puffs, rubber masks, pillows, plant pollen, insecticide sprays, sun protective creams and lotions, photographic materials	Arms and hands	Soaps, detergents, plastic watch band, jewelry, photographic materials, occupational agents and chemicals
Periorbital, lips and nose	Bubble gum, tooth paste and powder, mouth wash, lipstick, nose drops, pipe stem, cigarette holder, mouth piece of musical instruments, whistles, foods	Legs and feet	Shoes (thermoplastic substance, rubber cement, leather, shoe polish, *etc*) dye in socks and stockings, depilatory agents, fur-lined galoshes, external medicament applied locally to the feet for epidermophytosis

Relation to systemic disease. None.
Differential diagnosis. Allergic contact dermatitis, neurodermatitis.
Therapy. Avoid exposure to offending agent. Application of corticosteroid creams and ointments. The use of systemic corticosteroids may be indicated in severe cases.

Dermatitis Herpetiformis

Synonym. Duhring's disease.
Sites of predilection. Sacral and scapular areas, buttocks, extensor surfaces of extremities, scalp.
Objective signs. This condition may attack any age group. The vesicular type is the most common

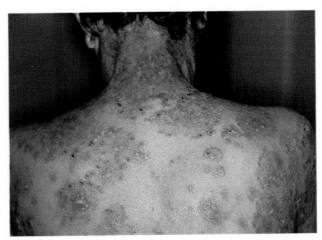

Dermatitis herpetiformis

variety seen. There are usually few to numerous groups of vesicles on an erythematous base. The vesicles are tense and have little tendency to rupture. The groups of lesions may form complete rings or segments of rings. Older lesions, which have healed, leave residual pigmentation. There are periods of remissions and relapses. The disease usually runs a chronic benign course.

Subjective symptoms. Constitutional symptoms, *eg,* elevation of temperature, generalized malaise; intense pruritus. The patient may also complain of a burning sensation of the skin.

Etiology. Unknown. Recent evidence indicates that this disease may be a genetic entity in which gluten possibly renders reticulin fibers immunogenic. Patients with this disease have an increased incidence of HLA-B8.

Histopathology. The vesicles and bullae are subepidermal. Large numbers of eosinophils are present in the early vesicle cavity. The cellular infiltrate in the cutis consists of eosinophils with intermingling mononuclear or polymorphonuclear cells. Ultramicroscopic study of the skin reveals membrane bound vesicles in the upper dermis which disappear on gluten-free diets.

Small bowel biopsies may show villous atrophy and an infiltration containing greater than 200 lymphocytes per 1000 epithelial cells.

Diagnostic aids. Biopsy; eosinophils may account for 10-30% of the total white cell count. Direct immunofluorescence studies show a deposit of IgA in normal skin surrounding the vesicles.

Relation to systemic disease. Affected areas may flare after local or systemic exposure to halogens.

Differential diagnosis. Pemphigus vulgaris, erythema multiforme, bullous pemphigoid, scabies, pediculosis corporis.

Therapy. Gluten-free diets should be considered. Dapsone in doses of 100-200 mg daily is usually effective. When the condition is controlled, the dose may be reduced. Drug administration should be monitored by periodic blood studies. Sulfapyridine in doses of 1-2 gm daily is an effective treatment but hematologic side effects occur frequently.

Dermatitis, Infectious Eczematoid

Synonym. Engman's disease.

Sites of predilection. Any part of the body.

Objective signs. Circumscribed confluent areas of erythema and edema with vesiculation, pustulation, scaling and crusting, which occur around a draining sinus, fistulous tract or an infected ear canal. These lesions become plaques which enlarge by peripheral extension. Satellite lymphadenopathy may be present.

Subjective symptoms. Moderate to severe pruritus.

Etiology. A localized allergic phenomenon associated with a draining staphylococcic infection, *eg,* otitis media, chronic ulcer, infected sinus, *etc.*

Histopathology. Acanthosis, crust formation, intraepidermal vesicle and abscess formation, edema of the prickle cell layer and presence of bacteria scattered throughout the epidermis.

Diagnostic aids. Culture of exudate from originating focus, serologic tests. See Impetigo.

Relation to systemic disease. This disease occurs in association with otitis media, cervical cancer, postoperative fistula, *etc.*

Therapy. Appropriate systemic antibiotic to treat the underlying infection. Compressing the affected areas with saline can give some symptomatic relief. Topical antibiotics may be of value in some cases.

Dyshidrosis

Synonym. Pompholyx, acrodermatitis continua, pustular bacterid.

Sites of predilection. Hands, feet.

Objective signs. The lesions are usually located on the palmar and plantar surfaces, in the interdigital spaces, and on the dorsal surfaces of the digits. They are numerous small, deep-seated, tense-walled vesicles. There is usually absence of any gross inflammatory process. Secondary pyogenic infection may develop or the condition may become eczematized. In addition to the small, deep-seated vesicles, small, tense-walled, deep-seated, sterile pustules may develop. Localized areas consisting of numerous small vesicles and pustules may be surrounded by an exfoliating margin.

Subjective symptoms. Moderate to intense pruritus. If secondary pyogenic infection develops, pain is the predominating subjective symptom.

Etiology. The condition may be associated with emotional tension, atopic dermatitis, focal infection or a combination of these factors.

Histopathology. There is a subepidermal vesicle surrounded by a chronic inflammatory infiltrate.

Diagnostic aids. Cultures on Sabouraud's medium must be performed to rule out the possibility of fungus infection. The pustules are usually sterile.

Relation to systemic disease. The condition may be associated with emotional tension, focal infections, nutritional disturbances or atopic states. This condition may eventuate into psoriasis.

Differential diagnosis. Tinea pedis, dermatophytid, contact dermatitis.

Therapy. Avoid the use of soap, detergents and other cleansing agents on the hands. Burow's solution (diluted 1:32) may be of value in relieving the edema and drying the vesicles. Topical corticosteroid preparations may aid the involution of the lesions. This is a chronic recurring condition. If the process is extensive a short course of systemic corticosteroid therapy may be indicated.

Epidermolysis Bullosa

Synonym. None.

Sites of predilection. Extremities and other areas which are frequently traumatized.

Objective signs. The table on the following page lists the various types.

Epidermolysis bullosa appears shortly after birth with variously sized bullae, 1-4 cm in diameter, following trauma. Lesions occurring over the heels, toes, feet, ankles, knees, elbows and hands are not preceded by erythema. Less frequently one sees bullae on the back, chest, abdomen, head and face. The bullae become turbid, then

Dyshidrosis

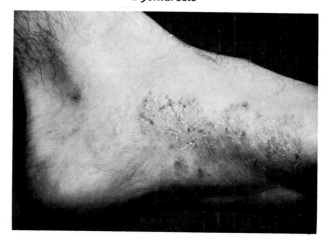

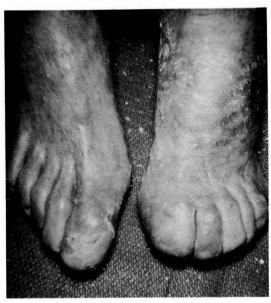

***Epidermolysis bullosa
with dystrophic lesions***

Types of Epidermolysis Bullosa

	Location	Onset	Features
Generalized Recessive Dystrophic	Below basal lamina	At birth or early life	Severe widespread blister formation, scars, milia, dystrophic nails, digital fusion, oral lesions
Localized Recessive Dystrophic	Below basal lamina	At birth or early life	Scarring, milia, nail dystrophy, mild mouth involvement
Recessive Letalis	Intermembranous spaces	At birth	Widespread involvement. Large granulating ulcers, variable nail dystrophy. Severe oral lesions, anemia
Dominant Dystrophic	Below basal lamina	Infancy or early life	Hands, feet, elbows, knees, scars, milia, nail dystrophy
Dominant Simplex	Basal epidermis	Young child	Palms, elbows, knees, hands, feet. Tendency to improve with age
Weber-Cockayne	Mid-epidermis	Adult	Blisters form only after unusual trauma

rupture, with resulting denuded areas. Epidermal cysts, resembling colloid milia, develop on the extremities. Scarring may occur depending upon the type of disease. In some cases, the toenails and fingernails may become atrophic, and dystrophic changes occur, resulting in destruction of the bones of the fingers and toes (see Table). In the recessive lethal type, patients usually die in childhood.

Subjective symptoms. In the dystrophic type, walking may be painful because of marked bony changes in the toes, *etc.*

Etiology. Unknown. The condition is congenital and may be familial. At times it occurs in *several gen-erations of one family (see Table).

Histopathology. Vesicles and bullae are usually sub-epidermal. A mild to moderate, chronic, inflammatory infiltrate is seen in the upper cutis. In the dystrophic form one may note epidermal cysts (milia) in the upper cutis.

Diagnostic aids. Biopsy.

Relation to systemic disease. None.

Differential diagnosis. Pemphigus neonatorum, pemphigus vulgaris, dermatitis herpetiformis, bullous syphilis in infants, factitious dermatitis, erythema multiforme.

Therapy. Protect patient from trauma. In the advanced recessive types, systemic corticosteroid therapy may be lifesaving.

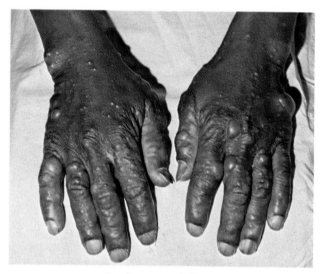

Erythema multiforme

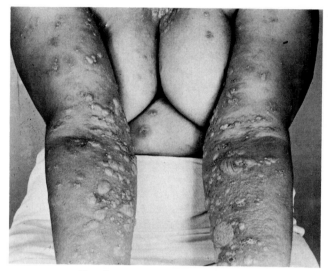

Erythema multiforme bullosum

Erythema Multiforme Bullosum

Synonym. Stevens-Johnson syndrome, ectodermosis erosiva pluriorificialis.

Sites of predilection. Lips, tongue, mouth, genitalia, hands, feet, forearms, legs.

Objective signs. Variously sized tense vesicles measuring 2 mm-3 cm arising on an erythematous base. Rings within rings, or circles within circles (iris or target lesions) may develop. These iris lesions are commonly seen on the palms and soles. Erosions with shreds of epithelium occur in the mouth and, when the lips are involved, crust formation may be marked. Bullous lesions, 1 cm or more in diameter, may develop and leave residual pigmentation after involution. This invariably occurs in fixed drug eruptions. The condition is characterized by frequent relapses.

Subjective symptoms. Slight to moderate pruritus and burning may be present. When the oral cavity is involved there is usually marked discomfort in chewing and swallowing.

Etiology. May be caused by a focus of infection, herpes simplex, bacterial infection or drug sensitivity. One type (Hebra's disease) has a seasonal preference for fall or spring.

Histopathology. Subepidermal vesicle formation with a perivascular inflammatory infiltrate in the cutis.

Diagnostic aids. Biopsy; direct or indirect cutaneous immunofluorescence to exclude a band at the dermal-epidermal junction.

Relation to systemic disease. May be evidence of an allergic reaction to penicillin, vaccines or other drugs. The condition occurs in association with rheumatic fever and other infectious diseases. Without adequate treatment this condition may be fatal.

Differential diagnosis. Pemphigus vulgaris, dermatitis herpetiformis, pyoderma, bullous pemphigoid.

Therapy. Elimination of the cause. Systemic corticosteroid therapy in adequate dosage is necessary when extensive involvement occurs.

Grain Itch

Synonym. Straw itch.

Sites of predilection. Trunk, neck. Rarely occurs on face, hands or feet.

Objective signs. The primary lesion is an erythematous wheal with a small central vesicle (1-3 mm) which may become a pustule. Secondary pyogenic infection may develop.

Subjective symptoms. Moderate to severe pruritus which is intensified at night. Malaise and slight temperature elevation may be present.

Etiology. Pyemotes ventricosus (grain itch mite). This condition develops in persons who handle straw.

Histopathology. Intraepidermal vesicle. Edema of the cutis with an infiltrate of leukocytes and eosinophils. Vascular dilatation is also present. Parasites are not found.

Diagnostic aids. History and physical examination, biopsy.

Relation to systemic disease. None.

Therapy. Antipruritic lotions, liniments or creams. Eliminate contact with contaminated material.

Herpes Gestationis

Synonym. Dermatitis herpetiformis associated with pregnancy.

Sites of predilection. Trunk, extremities.

Objective signs. The lesions are grouped papules, vesicles or bullae occurring on erythematous bases. The bullae are tense and residual hyperpigmentation may appear. The condition usually begins in the second trimester of pregnancy although it may start very shortly after conception. The eruption is persistent through the early postpartum period. The dermatosis may or may not recur with succeeding pregnancies. It may however recur at the time of menses.

Subjective symptoms. Intractable pruritus.

Etiology. Unknown. Speculation that the eruption is a hypersensitivity reaction to fetal or placental products or the increased hormones during pregnancy is common.

Diagnostic aids. Direct immunofluorescence shows a deposition of immunoglobulin throughout the dermal side of the lucid lamina and around the dermal anchoring fibrils.

Relation to systemic disease. Occurs in association with pregnancy.

Differential diagnosis. See Dermatitis Herpetiformis.

Therapy. This condition is benefited by systemic corticosteroid therapy. Therapeutic abortion may be indicated.

Herpes Simplex

Synonym. Herpes labialis, fever blisters, cold sores, herpes febrilis. On the genitalia, these lesions are called herpes progenitalis.

Sites of predilection. Lips, nose, chin, mucous membranes and other areas. May occur on the glans penis, under surface of the prepuce and the labia minora.

Primary herpes simplex

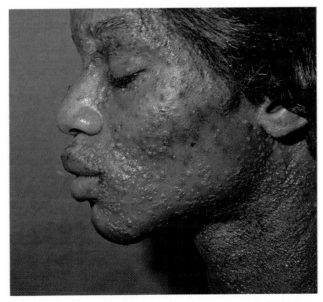

Objective signs. The clinical appearance of this disease differs depending upon whether the patient has had no prior infection with this virus (primary) or whether it is a disease due to secondary or recurrent exposure.

Primary herpes simplex may be a subclinical disease a keratoconjunctivitis, a gingivostomatitis, a vulvovaginitis, localized vesicles, or generalized lesions. It may also be a serious systemic infection with encephalitis, hepatosplenomegaly, high fever and serious sequelae. The vesicles in this form of disease are mostly discrete but may be confluent.

Secondary or recurrent herpes simplex are usually more localized infections exhibiting grouped, small vesicles on an erythematous base. One or more groups may develop at the same time. The individual vesicles range from 1-3 mm in diameter. The vesicle fluid is at first serous, but after a day or two becomes purulent. In a few days the lesions form a serous crust and usually heal without scar formation. Submental adenopathy may occur when the lesions occur on the lower lip or regional adenopathy may accompany the lesions at other sites. Lesions tend to recur in the same site. If the lesion is localized on a digit it is called a herpetic whitlow. In immunosuppressed or debilitated patients large ulcerations on the skin may occur.

Subjective symptoms. In primary herpes simplex the patient may be asymptomatic or seriously ill with a variety of symptoms. In secondary or recurrent herpes, tingling, burning and pruritus may precede the eruption. Slight fever and headache may be present during the height of the process.

Etiology. It is caused by a virus. Recent evidence has demonstrated that there are at least two types of this virus. In general, type I virus infects above the waist whereas type II infects the body below the waist. There are, however, many exceptions to this generality. There is some cross reactivity between the two types. It is not clear where the virus

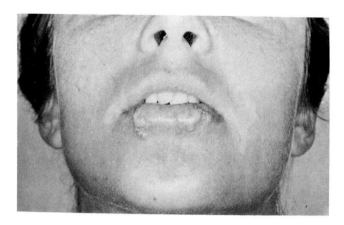

Herpes simplex

resides in the latency period between attacks. It may reside in the nerves, the skin or in the mouth and become activated or ''triggered'' by actinic rays, cold, febrile illnesses, gastrointestinal disturbances, sensitivity to certain foods (*eg*, hot mustard) and menstruation. Secondary attacks of the disease by an entirely new strain have been recorded.

Histopathology. Multilocular intraepidermal vesicles with degeneration of epidermal cells, giving rise to reticular degeneration. In the cutis there is an infiltrate of leukocytes. Special stains will reveal intranuclear inclusion bodies.

Diagnostic aids. Tissue culture of vesicular fluid or crusts, Giemsa-stained smear of vesicular fluid (Tzanck smear), complement fixation or viral neutralization tests.

Relation to systemic disease. At times herpes simplex occurs in acute febrile illnesses or toxic states when the temperature remains elevated for several days or weeks. It may occur more often in immunosuppressed patients. Generalized cutaneous herpes simplex infection occurs in patients with active or inactive atopic dermatitis.

Differential diagnosis. Impetigo contagiosa, chancre of lips or genitalia, chancroid, contact dermatitis, herpes zoster, thrush, varicella, variola.

Therapy. Systemic adenine arabinoside is used for the primary disease. There is no specific therapy for the secondary or recurrent diseases. Analgesics and emollients are recommended.

Hidrocystoma, Apocrine

Synonym. None.
Sites of predilection. Face.
Objective signs. A solitary, firm dome-shaped, blue or flesh-colored papule which may contain colored fluid.
Subjective symptoms. None.
Etiology. Unknown.
Histopathology. A cyst lined with columnar cells surrounded by myoepithelial cells is located in the dermis. Papillary projections may extend into the lesion.
Diagnostic aids. Biopsy.
Relation to systemic disease. None.
Differential diagnosis. See Eccrine Hidrocystoma.
Therapy. Simple puncture or destruction.

Hidrocystoma, Eccrine

Synonym. None.
Sites of predilection. Face: especially prominent on the forehead, infraorbital and cheek areas.
Objective signs. Single or multiple, discrete, non-inflammatory, whitish or bluish, deep-seated vesicles. These tense vesicles do not readily rupture.
Subjective symptoms. None.
Etiology. Occurs in middle-aged women who work in hot environments and perspire freely.
Histopathology. There are large, dilated, cystic cavities lined by two or more layers of epithelial cells in the cutis. Papillary projections may extend into the cyst. The cysts develop as a result of sweat retention in the ducts of the eccrine sweat glands.
Diagnostic aids. Biopsy.
Relation to systemic disease. None.
Differential diagnosis. Miliaria crystallina (sudamina), syringoma, apocrine hidrocystoma.
Therapy. Puncture each lesion with a sharp needle to release the fluid.

Impetigo Contagiosa

Synonym. Impetigo vulgaris, pyoderma.
Sites of predilection. Mouth, central face, buttocks.
Objective signs. Impetigo is a term applied to a superficial infection of the skin which begins as a flaccid or tense, well-defined vesicle, originating on normal skin or on an erythematous base. The vesicle is filled with clear, yellowish fluid which becomes pustular. After a few days the lesion is covered with a thick, yellow ("honey") crust. The lesions may become confluent and spread, with the development of more lesions because of the contagious nature and autoinoculability of the disease. Annular lesions may occur. Constitutional symptoms rarely occur. Regional lymphadenopathy may be seen in streptococcal disease. Leukocytosis is present in a minority of patients. The more superficial the lesion is, the more contagious the disease.

Impetigo

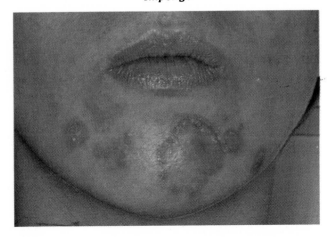

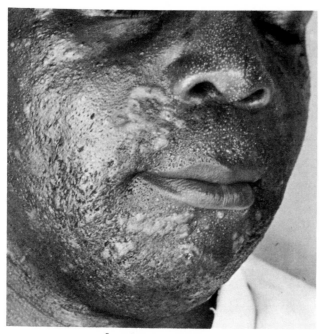

Impetigo contagiosa

Etiology. *Staphyloccocus aureus* and *Streptococcus pyogenes*. Staphylococci cause bullous lesions. Most of the crusted impetigo lesions contain both the streptococcus and staphylococcus. The former is regarded as the primary pathogen and the latter as a secondary invader. Impetigo may be spread in schools and camps by direct contact or may occur secondary to some other underlying dermatosis such as pediculosis capitis, pediculosis pubis, scabies and other pruritic conditions.

Histopathology. A subcorneal vesicle containing polymorphonuclear leukocytes, lymphocytes, fibrin and bacteria. The upper third of the cutis contains an inflammatory infiltrate consisting primarily of polymorphonuclear leukocytes and lymphocytes.

Diagnostic aids. Culture, sensitivity tests. Serologic tests for streptococci such as anti DNase-B or antihyaluronidase.

Relation to systemic disease. Acute nephritis may be seen as a complication of impetigo contagiosa. Impetigo in the newborn may cause fatal bacteremia.

Differential diagnosis. Herpes simplex, contact dermatitis, pemphigus vulgaris, varicella, tinea sycosis.

Therapy. Isolation precautions should be practiced. Systemic antibiotic therapy is preferable. Penicillin in adequate dosage is the drug of choice, with erythromycin as the first alternate. In some cases the use of topical antibiotic ointments may be of value.

Impetigo, Bockhart's

Synonym. Superficial pustular perifolliculitis.
Sites of predilection. Scalp, thigh, forearms.
Objective signs. This is follicular impetigo which is usually pustular from its onset. The superficial small pustules occur at the orifices of the pilosebaceous apparatus.
Etiology. Staphylococcus.
Histopathology. See Impetigo Contagiosa.
Diagnostic aids. See Impetigo Contagiosa.
Relation to systemic disease. It is secondary to some preexisting dermatosis.
Differential diagnosis. See Impetigo Contagiosa.
Therapy. See Impetigo Contagiosa.

Impetigo, Bullous

Synonym. Pemphigus neonatorum.
Objective signs. It occurs in infants, with formation of staphylococcal induced bullae on the neck, trunk and buttocks. Large areas of the body may be involved and systemic toxic complications such as septicemia may develop.
Subjective symptoms. Pruritus and burning. Pain is rarely present.
Etiology. S aureus.
Histopathology. See Impetigo Contagiosa.

Diagnostic aids. Culture.
Differential diagnosis. See Impetigo Contagiosa.
Therapy. See Impetigo Contagiosa.

Lymphangioma Circumscriptum

Synonym. None.
Sites of predilection. Any part of the body.
Objective signs. Groups of deep-seated, thick-walled vesicles develop in infancy or early childhood. The tense vesicles are thick-walled and contain a colorless or pinkish fluid (lymph). The lesions become crusted or hyperkeratotic, eventually resembling verrucae. Involvement of the tongue produces macroglossia.
Subjective symptoms. None.
Etiology. Congenital.
Histopathology. In the papillary and subpapillary layers of the cutis there are large numbers of dilated lymphatics or cysts lined by a single layer of endothelial cells. The cysts contain coagulated lymphocytes.
Diagnostic aids. Biopsy.
Relation to systemic disease. None.
Differential diagnosis. Herpes simplex, herpes zoster, dermatitis venenata.
Therapy. Surgical excision, desiccation and cryotherapy are of value in the destruction of small lesions.

Miliaria Crystallina

Synonym. Sudamina.
Sites of predilection. Neck, trunk, extremities.
Objective signs. Discrete, pinpoint to pinhead size, translucent, thin-walled vesicles, containing a droplet of clear sweat. They develop and involute in a short period of time leaving a slight superficial scale.
Subjective symptoms. Mild pruritus.
Etiology. Result from excessive sweating associated with fever, steam baths, exercise or occlusive plastic mattress covers.

Histopathology. The superficial vesicles are situated in the stratum corneum in direct communication with the sweat ducts. The orifices of the ducts are plugged.
Diagnostic aids. Biopsy.
Relation to systemic disease. May be associated with any disease which caused fever.
Differential diagnosis. Varicella, miliaria rubra, drug eruption.
Therapy. Oatmeal baths, calamine lotion, dusting powders. Place patient in a cool, well-ventilated or air conditioned room.

Miliaria Rubra

Synonym. Prickly heat, heat rash, summer rash.
Sites of predilection. Neck, trunk, extremities.
Objective signs. Numerous erythematous, pinpoint to pinhead size, discrete, closely aggregated vesicles, vesicopapules and papules.
Subjective symptoms. Stinging, prickling, pruritus or burning in the affected areas.
Etiology. High temperature and humidity associated with increased or profuse perspiration.
Histopathology. Keratin plugs in the sweat duct orifices, and distention of the sweat ducts in the epidermis and upper cutis. A lymphocytic infiltrate surrounds the sweat ducts in the upper cutis.
Diagnostic aids. Biopsy.
Relation to systemic disease. None.
Differential diagnosis. Urticaria, varicella, eczema, dermatitis venenata, drug rash.
Therapy. Remove to cool environment. Apply talc, calamine lotion or initiate cooling baths.

Necrolysis, Toxic Epidermal

Synonym. Scalded skin syndrome, Lyell's disease.
Sites of predilection. Generalized.
Objective signs. This condition occurs in males and females of all ages. The bullous phase is preceded by erythema and skin tenderness. The eruption usually begins in the groin and axillae and

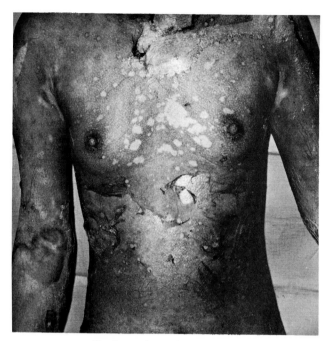

Toxic epidermal necrolysis

spreads rapidly. Within 24 hours flaccid bullae develop, Nikolsky's sign becomes positive, and the epidermis peels off leaving extensive, moist, denuded areas which resemble scalded tissue. At the onset the eruption may simulate bullous erythema multiforme but the lesions rapidly coalesce to produce generalized involvement. The eyelids, vagina and other orifices may be sealed together due to fibrin and necessitate surgical lysis. Hyperpyrexia and varying constitutional signs may be present.

Subjective symptoms. Severe pain, malaise.

Etiology. In infants the condition is most frequently due to a toxin (exfoliatoxin) liberated by a group 2 staphylococcus, whereas in adults it is most commonly due to an adverse drug reaction. Penicillin, sulfonamide phenylbutazone and phenolphthalein are among the more frequent causes of this syndrome in adults.

Histopathology. Superficial bullous formation and necrosis. The basal layer and the skin appendages are not involved. Mild inflammatory changes are observed in the dermis. The bullae are at the dermal-epidermal junction in the drug-induced type and intraepidermal at the malpighian or granular layer in the infection-induced form of the disease.

Diagnostic aids. Biopsy, history, culture for bacteria.

Differential diagnosis. Erythema multiforme, pemphigus vulgaris, bullous pemphigoid.

Therapy. Early diagnosis and institution of the proper treatment is essential. In young babies the outcome may be fatal. If the condition is due to infection, selection and administration of the proper antibiotic will stop further toxin production. If the condition is due to a drug reaction, prednisone or another corticosteroid should be prescribed in adequate dosage. Good nursing care is essential.

Pemphigoid, Benign Mucous Membrane

Synonym. Pemphigus of the mucous membranes, ocular pemphigus, pemphigus conjunctivae.

Mucous membrane pemphigus

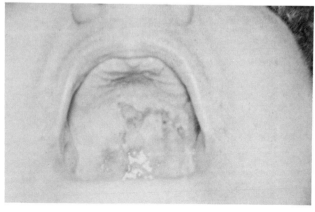

Sites of predilection. Conjunctivae, buccal mucosa, pharynx, larynx, esophagus, nasal mucosa, penis, vulva, anus. In 50% of the patients the skin is also involved.

Objective signs. Lesions begin on the buccal mucosa as vesicles and result in denuded areas. The lips are rarely involved. Scars form in the mouth and involvement of the larynx results in hoarseness. When adhesions occur in the esophagus, strictures and stenosis develop with impairment in eating and swallowing. Adhesions may also complicate genital involvement. There may be scarring and shrinking of the conjunctivae, resulting in adhesions (symblepharon), corneal damage with ulceration and opacities. Due to scarring the lower lids turn in (entropion) and the lashes cause further irritation.

Subjective symptoms. Scarring of the conjunctivae and corneal opacities may lead to partial blindness. Burning, smarting and photophobia may be an early complaint when the eyes are involved. Hoarseness and difficulty in swallowing are experienced when the mouth, throat, larynx and esophagus are involved.

Etiology. Unknown.

Histopathology. Subepidermal bulla. There is ab-sence of acantholysis in the epidermis. Marked inflammatory infiltration is present with subsequent fibrosis of the outer dermis.

Diagnostic aids. Biopsy. Direct immunofluorescence reveals the deposit of IgG on the dermal-epidermal membrane. Some patients also have a positive indirect immunofluorescence test.

Relation to systemic disease. None.

Differential diagnosis. Pemphigus vulgaris, erythema multiforme.

Therapy. None specific. Systemic corticosteroid therapy is effective. It is frequently necessary to remove the lower lashes by electrolysis. Topical corticosteroids are ineffective.

Pemphigoid, Bullous

Synonym. None.

Sites of predilection. Trunk, extremities.

Objective signs. Tense bullae of considerable size which do not break as easily as the blebs of pemphigus vulgaris. The denuded areas resulting from the rupture of some of the bullae heal rapid-

Bullous pemphigoid

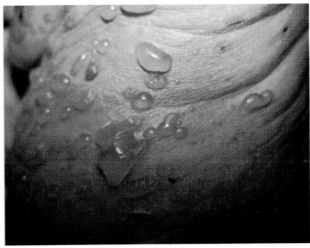

Ocular pemphigus

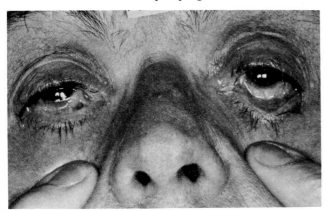

ly and do not spread. There may be erythematous patches where the bullae become confluent, forming a serpiginous configuration, or the blebs may be grouped as in dermatitis herpetiformis. Mucous membrane involvement may occur but the blisters heal rapidly. The condition occurs most frequently in adults but may also develop in young children. The disease may persist for months to many years with remissions and exacerbations.

Subjective symptoms. Pruritus is usually moderate to severe but may be entirely absent. In older patients the general health may be impaired.

Etiology. Unknown. Complement activation appears to be important in this disease.

Histopathology. The picture is similar to that of dermatitis herpetiformis, except more eosinophils are present in the bullae along with neutrophils.

Diagnostic aids. Biopsy. Direct and indirect immunofluorescence reveal deposition of IgG and C3 on the dermal epidermal membrane. Properdin, factor B, C1, C3 and C4 have been deposited within the lesion.

Relation to systemic disease. None.

Differential diagnosis. Pemphigus vulgaris, dermatitis herpetiformis, erythema multiforme.

Therapy. Systemic corticosteroids alone or in combination with immunosuppressive drugs is the only effective therapy.

Pemphigus, Chronic Benign Familial

Synonym. Hailey-Hailey disease.

Sites of predilection. Neck, axillae, crural areas.

Objective signs. Vesicles and bullae with crusted erosions are seen over the affected areas. The lesions may spread peripherally, producing a circinate or serpiginous border. There are relapses and remissions. The condition runs a chronic course.

Subjective symptoms. Mild to moderate pruritus. Symptoms may be more severe in warm, humid weather.

Etiology. This is an incomplete autosomal dominant

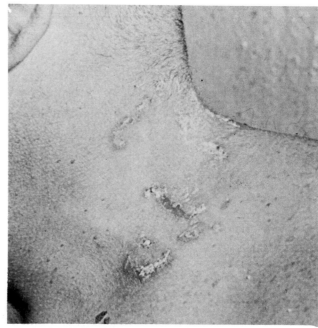

Chronic benign familial pemphigus

genodermatosis.

Histopathology. Large bullae develop, separating the basal layer from the rest of the epidermis. Acantholytic cells, some of which show keratinization, are present. Dyskeratosis occurs occasionally. Corps ronds are not a constant feature.

Diagnostic aids. Biopsy.

Relation to systemic disease. None.

Differential diagnosis. Contact dermatitis, intertrigo, dermatitis herpetiformis, pemphigus vulgaris.

Therapy. During exacerbations administer systemic antibiotics such as erythromycin. Topical corticosteroids may be effective. Systemic corticosteroids should be reserved for severely ill patients. Genetic counseling is advised.

Pemphigus Vulgaris

Synonym. Pemphigus malignus.

Sites of predilection. Mucous membranes, scalp, face, neck, extremities, trunk.

Objective signs. The bullae are tense at first but become flaccid as they increase in size. Bullae may arise from normal appearing skin, or on an erythematous base. The fluid content is serous at first but may become purulent or hemorrhagic. The flaccid blisters rupture easily to form denuded lesions which involve large areas. The lips, buccal mucosa, tongue, palate, pharynx and larynx are involved. The mucous membranes of the conjunctivae, nostrils, vulva and anal region may also be affected. Nikolsky's sign is elicited by making pressure with the finger over so-called normal skin, and rubbing off the epidermis.

Subjective symptoms. The eruption is preceded or accompanied by malaise, chills and fever, slight to moderate pruritus and burning, and soreness of the involved areas. When lesions are present in the oral cavity, swallowing and talking may become difficult. The condition occurs most commonly in the middle-aged group and is somewhat more prevalent in Jewish people. Untreated, the disease runs a fatal course.

Etiology. This is an autoimmune disease in which afflicted patients have a circulatory antibody to their mucosal and epidermal intercellular cement. Immune globulins, complement and possibly circulatory immune complexes are important pathogenic factors.

Histopathology. Tzanck (acantholytic) cells are present in a unilocular, intraepidermal vesicle. There is little or no inflammatory reaction in the cutis.

Diagnostic aids. Biopsy. Direct and indirect immunofluorescence studies show IgG bound to the intercellular cement of the mucosa and epidermis. C3 deposition can be demonstrated more frequently than properdin or factor B.

Relation to systemic disease. Pemphigus vulgaris is a serious systemic illness.

Differential diagnosis. Erythema multiforme, dermatitis herpetiformis (Duhring's disease), impetigo contagiosa.

Therapy. Systemic corticosteroid therapy is a life-saving measure in this disease; without its use, the prognosis is grave. The drug must be given in adequate dosage and with utmost care and supervision. Immunosuppressant drugs such as azathioprine or methotrexate may also be important.

Other Types of Pemphigus

Pemphigus erythematosus (Senear-Usher syndrome). This variant of pemphigus may start with a butterfly lesion on the face and resemble lupus erythematosus. The disease is regarded as a variant of pemphigus foliaceus because the bullae are superficial in the epidermis. The bullae are flaccid and, when they become crusted and impetiginized, resemble seborrheic dermatitis. The condition usually runs a chronic but relatively benign course.

Pemphigus foliaceus. The lesions are superficial bullae which leave shallow erosions. There are also areas of erythema, scaling, oozing and crusting. The denuded areas are more superficial than those of pemphigus vulgaris. At first the eruption may be limited to the scalp, face and portions of the back and chest, but as the condition progresses, most of the body surface is involved. In this type of pemphigus the patients are usually free of oral lesions. The disease runs a chronic course for a period of many years. The same immunofluorescence findings are present in this disease as in all other forms of pemphigus.

Pemphigus vegetans. This is a variant of pemphigus vulgaris which at first cannot be differentiated. As the disease progresses, the denuded areas develop vegetations or papillomatous, hypertrophic surfaces covered with pustules. The mucous membranes are also involved in this type. The course of the disease is the same as that of pemphigus vulgaris.

Porphyria Cutanea Tarda

Synonym. Acquired porphyria.

Sites of predilection. Hands, face and other areas exposed to sunlight.

Objective signs. The typical cutaneous lesions are more severe during the summer months but may occur at any time during the year. Following exposure to sunlight or minor trauma, bullae, sometimes with hemorrhagic contents, develop. There are crusted lesions, superficial scars and subsequent milia. The skin becomes hyperpigmented and somewhat hirsute. Porphyria cutanea tarda can be accompanied by sclerodermatous changes. The urine becomes dark in color or has a reddish tint which fluoresces coral red under the Wood light.

Subjective symptoms. Discomfort produced by the presence of bullae and embarrassment due to cosmetic defect. Secondary pyogenic infection may develop.

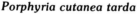

Porphyria cutanea tarda

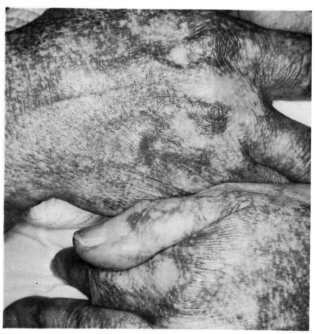

Etiology. Some cases appear to be congenital, whereas others are acquired presumably from liver disease such as alcoholism, hepatitis or tumor. In some instances it has been attributed to occupational exposure to chlorinated hydrocarbons.

Histopathology. Subepidermal bullae appear. Superficial arterioles reveal PAS-positive material. The liver has intracellular porphyrin deposition, varying degrees of cellular damage and subsequent fibrosis.

Diagnostic aids. Biopsy of the skin for light microscopy, biopsy of the liver for fluorescent microscopy, examination of the urine under the Wood light. Quantitative determination of liver function tests, uroporphyrins and coproporphyrins in the feces and urine.

Relation to systemic disease. These patients have chronic alcoholism and liver damage. Some patients with lipoid proteinosis also have this form of porphyria.

Differential diagnosis. Epidermolysis bullosum, erythema multiforme bullosum, bullous pemphigoid.

Therapy. Discontinue ingestion of alcoholic beverages, avoid sunlight. Venesection and systemic chloroquine under controlled conditions.

Scabies

Synonym. "The itch."

Sites of predilection. Interdigital spaces of the fingers, flexor surfaces of the wrists and forearms, the elbows, anterior folds of the axillae, the breasts, buttocks, male genitalia, the abdomen. Rarely occurs on the face or scalp. May occur on the feet of infants.

Objective signs. Scabies is a prevalent contagious disease. The initial lesion is an irregular vesicle, 1-5 mm in diameter. Traversing the center of some of these lesions is a black dotted line, or "burrow," composed of the eggs and fecal matter of the parasite. Intact vesicles are found only on the

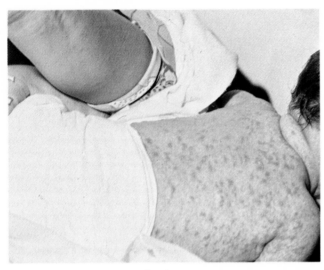

Scabies

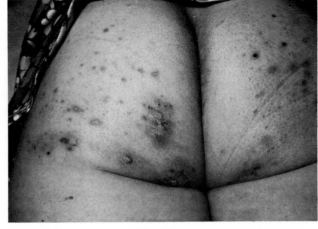

Scabies

palms and between the fingers. Papules, pustules, crusts, nodules and excoriations occur elsewhere on the body. Secondary pyogenic infection frequently occurs. Rarely the lesions may become hyperkeratotic (Norwegian scabies).

Subjective symptoms. Severe pruritus, especially at night when the patient is in bed.

Etiology. *Sarcoptes scabiei.* The female burrows into the skin, especially at night, where she deposits eggs and feces.

Histopathology. The burrow is located in the horny layer and the head of the mite is buried in the prickle cell layer. The vesicles occur because of edema of the prickle cell layer.

Diagnostic aids. Confirmation of diagnosis by biopsy with serial sections or microscopic examination of vesicle contents for presence of the parasite.

Relation to systemic disease. None.

Differential diagnosis. Papular urticaria, contact dermatitis, "id" reactions, atopic dermatitis, neurotic excoriations.

Therapy. Isolate the patient and treat all infested contacts. Specific therapy for adults and older chil-

dren is the single application of gamma benzene hexachloride lotion to the entire body. Crotamiton cream applied for 2 consecutive days is the drug of choice for the treatment of infants.

Tinea Pedis

Synonym. Athlete's foot, dermatophytosis, epidermophytosis.

Sites of predilection. Feet, hands.

Objective signs. The eruption begins with the development of variously sized (1-5 mm), thick-walled, discrete and confluent, deep-seated vesicles on the feet. The first lesions appear in the interdigital spaces, plantar surfaces of the toes, or the medial aspects of the feet. Later, because of the wearing of shoes, trauma or overzealous therapy, the areas become macerated. The tissues in the interdigital spaces appear whitish and boggy. Fissures develop with exfoliating margins, and secondary pyogenic infection may occur. Eroded areas appear on the medial and lateral surfaces of the feet, and the lesions assume an eczematous appearance. Chronic lesions de-

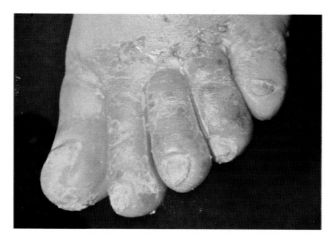

Tinea pedis

velop in the interdigital spaces as the vesicle fluid is absorbed, resulting in the appearance of hyperkeratotic lesions, or "soft corns." Vesicles appear on and between the fingers and on the palms (epidermophytid). This manifestation is thought to be an allergic response to the fungus infection on the feet. It may develop as a response to onychomycosis. Secondary pyogenic infection may complicate the infection on the hands and feet. Cellulitis, lymphangitis and inguinal adenopathy may occur.

Subjective symptoms. Pruritus. Pain predominates if secondary infection develops.

Etiology. The initial eruption is caused by one of the superficial dermatophytes. The secondary pyogenic infection is caused by staphylococci or streptococci. Superimposed allergic contact dermatitis may develop because of overzealous therapy. Latent fungus infections may be precipitated into activity by systemic antibiotic therapy.

Histopathology. Intracellular edema, spongiosis and intraepidermal vesicle formation. Infiltration of leukocytes in the upper cutis. The PAS stain reveals hyphae in the stratum corneum.

Diagnostic aids. Direct examination of vesicle top or scales with 20% potassium hydroxide or the ink-potassium hydroxide stain to demonstrate fungi in tissue. Culture on fungus medium to determine the offending organism.

Relation to systemic disease. None.

Differential diagnosis. Contact dermatitis, dyshidrosis, pustular psoriasis, pustular bacterid, pyodermas.

Therapy. In the absence of secondary infection, establish good hygiene. Following the bath, rinse the feet in alcohol and thoroughly dry. Apply 5% salicylic acid ointment, 5% salicylic acid in 95% alcohol, or half-strength Whitfield's ointment. Clotrimazole cream or lotion and tolnaftate preparations are specific antifungal agents. Do not attempt to sterilize the shoes. In warm weather wear perforated leather shoes, sandals or amounts of talcum in the shoes sufficient to absorb all moisture. If possible avoid rubber shoes or synthetic soles. If secondary infection, cellulitis or lymphangitis is present, systemic antibiotic therapy will be necessary. Conventional X-ray or grenz-ray therapy is of no value in superficial fungus infections.

Griseofulvin, administered systemically, is effective but usually not necessary.

Varicella

Synonym. Chicken pox.

Sites of predilection. Face, trunk, scalp.

Objective signs. The condition, which has an acute onset, is initiated with a macular eruption, but rapidly becomes papular, and then vesicular, in a 24-hour period. Discrete, scattered vesicles, measuring 2-4 mm in diameter first appear on the face. The vesicles are thin-walled, translucent, and later become turbid. They have the so-called "dewdrop" appearance, with an erythematous areola. The lesions appear in successive crops and show polymorphism with varying stages of development from a fresh vesicle to a drying, crusted lesion. Central umbilication develops in the lesions prior to involution. Healing is followed

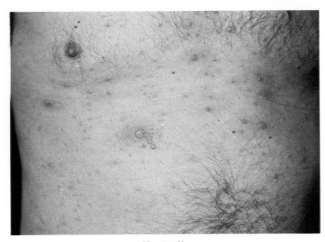

Varicella

by pitted scars (pock marks). Scattered vesicles occur on the buccal mucosa or the hard or soft palate. Involution of the individual vesicles usually begins after 48 hours.

Subjective symptoms. There may be prodromal symptoms of coryza, slight elevation of temperature and malaise. The eruption is accompanied by pruritus.

Etiology. A virus identical to the virus that causes zoster.

Histopathology. Unilocular vesicles with large multinucleated balloon cells are seen within the epidermis. There is a sparse leukocytic infiltration occupying the upper portion of the cutis.

Diagnostic aids. Biopsy, tissue culture, complement fixation or virus neutralization tests.

Relation to systemic disease. Cerebral complications such as encephalitis have been reported. Pneumonia, middle ear infections, cellulitis and septicemia are also complications of varicella.

Differential diagnosis. Variola, impetigo contagiosa, folliculitis, drug eruptions, eczema herpeticum, eczema vaccinatum, papular urticaria, scabies, rickettsialpox.

Therapy. Isolation, bed rest, antipyretics and fluids.

Antipruritic lotions locally for relief of pruritus. Zoster immune globulin may be given to seriously ill patients or to debilitated, susceptible contacts.

Varicelliform Eruption, Kaposi's

Synonym. This name applies to a clinical syndrome which can be produced by two different viruses. Generalized cutaneous herpes simplex infection (eczema herpeticum), generalized cutaneous vaccinia (eczema vaccinatum).

Sites of predilection. Face, neck, shoulders, upper chest, upper arms.

Objective signs. Occurs on eczematous areas and also normal skin. It is usually seen in patients with atopic dermatitis or a history of other atopic disease. Groups of vesicles and pustules, some showing umbilication, occur on the sites of predilection. The lesions are uniform in size. As a

Kaposi's varicelliform eruption complicating atopic dermatitis

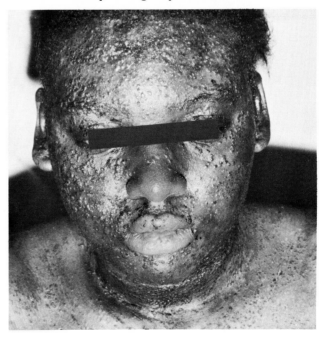

general rule, unlike varicella, successive crops do not occur. Crusting occurs about 24 hours before the eruption makes its appearance, and continues for a week or more. The face is usually the area most extensively affected and may be edematous, especially in the periorbital region. The eruption may involve a limited area or it may become generalized. The cornea may also be involved, with ulcer formation. Encephalitis may ensue if overwhelming toxicity occurs.

Subjective symptoms. Elevated temperature, headache, toxicity.

Etiology. Herpes simplex or vaccinia viruses can cause this disease.

Histopathology. Vesiculation and pustulation with reticular and balloon cell degeneration. Contained within the degenerated epidermal cells one may see inclusion bodies. A moderate to severe inflammatory reaction is present in the cutis. Herpes simplex virus will produce intranuclear inclusion bodies whereas vaccinia will produce intracytoplasmic inclusions.

Diagnostic aids. Recovery of the causative virus, tissue culture, biopsy, serologic tests such as viral neutralization, Tzanck smear.

Relation to systemic disease. The disease may be fatal. Involvement of the eye with corneal ulceration leads to impairment of vision.

Differential diagnosis. Varicella, variola.

Therapy. Nonspecific. Bed rest, cool, normal saline compresses to the affected areas, fluids, and sedation are indicated. If involvement is extensive adenine arabinoside given intravenously is indicated for herpes simplex infections and vaccinia hyperimmune globulin can be administered for eczema vaccinatum.

Zoster

Synonym. Shingles, zona, herpes zoster.

Sites of predilection. The eruption follows a unilateral course along a nerve trunk such as an intercostal

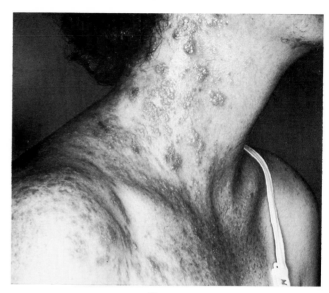

Zoster

nerve, ophthalmic branch of the trigeminal nerve, sciatic nerve, *etc.*

Objective signs. Grouped vesicles on an erythematous and edematous base follow the course of the involved nerve. Careful examination of the patient may reveal a few discrete lesions at distant sites from the main infection. The tense, deep-seated vesicles measure 2-6 mm in diameter. The eruption is unilateral. After 10-14 days from the onset, the vesicles dry and become crusted. In some instances the lesions may become necrotic or gangrenous. Regional adenopathy may develop. When the ophthalmic division of the trigeminal nerve is involved the lesions may develop over the forehead, eyelids and cornea. Blindness may ensue. A generalized form of herpes zoster (varicelliform) may occur at times with certain systemic diseases such as the lymphomas. In this instance most of the lesions are discrete except over the initially involved dermatome.

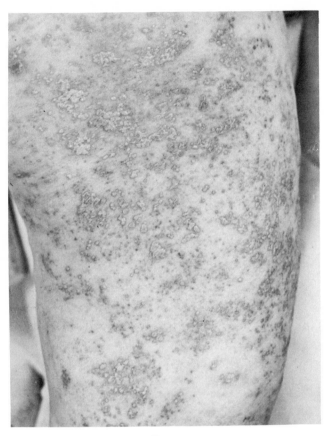

Zoster

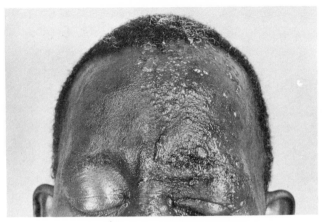

Zoster, trigeminal distribution

Subjective symptoms. Neuritis may be present over the area for several days before the vesicles appear. The pain may be severe and if the area involved is over the abdomen an erroneous diagnosis of acute appendicitis, cholecystitis or renal colic may be made. Postherpetic pain over the involved region may remain for many months after the eruption has completely cleared. This is especially true in elderly patients.

Etiology. A virus identical with the virus causative of varicella. Zoster is a reactivation of latent varicella or a reinfection of a partially immune person by a different viral strain.

Histopathology. Intraepidermal unilocular vesicles which contain leukocytes and altered epithelial cells showing balloon cell degeneration. Within these balloon cells one sees eosinophilic inclusion bodies, known as Lipschütz bodies. Dilated blood vessels are present in the cutis with an inflammatory infiltrate consisting of lymphocytes and scattered polymorphonuclear leukocytes.

Diagnostic aids. Tzanck smear, biopsy, tissue culture, virus complement fixation or neutralization tests.

Relation to systemic disease. The rare generalized form may occur in association with lymphoblastomas such as leukemia, Hodgkin's disease, *etc.* Herpes zoster may be associated with chronic infectious diseases such as malaria, neurosyphilis, multiple sclerosis, leprosy or tuberculosis.

Differential diagnosis. Herpes simplex, eczema, dermatitis herpetiformis, vaccinia.

Therapy. No generally accepted specific therapy is available. Adenine arabinoside, given intravenously, early in the course of the disease will dry the vesicles and shorten the convalescent period. It may also abort the herpetic neuralgia. Chlorprothixene in small doses will relieve pain in some patients. Sublesional corticosteroid injections are being investigated as a therapeutic measure.

CHAPTER 17

Pustular Eruptions

Acne Vulgaris

Synonym. Acne, pimples.

Sites of predilection. Face, neck, shoulders, chest, buttocks.

Objective signs. This is a chronic inflammatory disease of the pilosebaceous apparatus, characterized by papules, pustules and nodules, and associated with seborrhea oleosa and comedones. In the superficial type there are few to numerous, conical or round, pink to reddish papules and pustules, varying in size from 2-5 mm in diameter. Numerous comedones are present, and the skin is usually very oily. In the deep, indurated type, acne conglobata, there are large dull red or bluish, cystic lesions, indolent abscesses and discharging sinuses, which heal slowly, leaving dense scars.

Subjective symptoms. Pain on pressure. Slight pruritus or burning.

Etiology. Unknown. Acne occurs most commonly between the ages of 12 and 30 years. The production of acne may be a result of the interaction of sex hormones and surface bacteria at the sebaceous gland in an unknown manner. Androgenic drugs and other agents such as lithium or hyperalimentary feedings may produce acne-like eruptions.

Histopathology. Perifollicular inflammation. Abscesses surrounded by a dense inflammatory infiltrate of lymphocytes and polymorphonuclear leukocytes. There is hyperkeratosis of the lining of the hair follicle outlet above the infundibulum.

Diagnostic aids. Biopsy, history and physical examination.

Relation to systemic disease. None. The cosmetic defect may produce serious mental illness. Cystic acne patients may develop normochromic, normocytic anemia; low-grade fever; arthritis; arthralgia or osteomyelitis in rare instances. Some patients with cystic acne may also have deficiencies in cell mediated immunity.

Differential diagnosis. Actinomycosis, bromide and iodide intoxication, scrofuloderma, acneform eruptions produced by petroleum products.

Therapy. *Systemic treatment.* The tetracyclines are of value. Dietary restrictions include the elimination of oily foods, nuts, chocolate, carbonated beverages and fried foods, if history indicates their

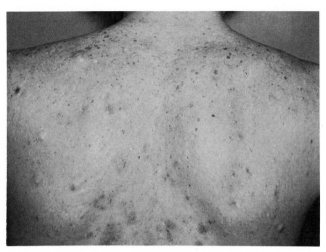

Acne vulgaris

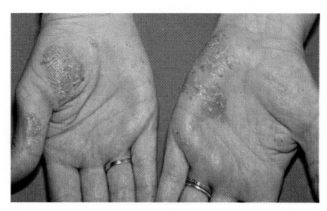

Acrodermatitis continua

role in the eruption.

Topical treatment. Retinoic acid in solution or gel. Benzoyl peroxide in cream or gel. Colloidal sulfur lotions may be of value. Topical antibiotics such as clindamycin are commonly used.

Acrodermatitis Continua

Synonym. Hallopeau's acrodermatitis, acrodermatitis perstans, dermatitis repens.

Sites of predilection. Hands, feet.

Objective signs. The condition begins as a group of vesicles or vesicopustules which extend peripherally on an erythematous base. Exfoliation occurs, leaving an eroded or crusted area, surrounded by an exfoliating margin in which there are deep-seated vesicles and vesicopustules. New lesions continue to appear. The condition is chronic and progressive. Crust formation may be present.

Subjective symptoms. Burning, pruritus and pain.

Etiology. Staphylococcic or streptococcic infection complicating previously existing eczematous eruptions.

Histopathology. Epidermal vesicles and abscesses are

present. These lesions usually do not extend into the corium, but the inflammatory reaction does.

Diagnostic aids. Culture of the exudate, history and physical examination.

Relation to systemic disease. Usually none.

Differential diagnosis. Pustular psoriasis, pustular bacterid, dyshidrosis.

Therapy. Local debridement of the exfoliating infected material. Systemic antibiotic drugs are indicated if the infection is severe.

Actinomycosis

Synonym. Lumpy jaw.

Sites of predilection. Face, neck, thorax, tongue.

Objective signs. The infection usually begins in the mouth and the skin lesions are secondary. Deep, subcutaneous, slowly developing, dusky red nodules rupture, forming sinuses in the skin from which exudes a purulent discharge containing tiny, whitish or yellowish granules (sulfur granules).

Subjective symptoms. Pain, especially on mastication.

Etiology. Actinomyces bovis.

Histopathology. Deep nodular infiltrations with granulation tissue, epithelioid cells, plasma cells and giant cells. The ray fungus is present in the infiltrate.

Diagnostic aids. Demonstration of ray fungus by direct examination, culture on Sabouraud's medium, biopsy, history and physical examination.

Relation to systemic disease. The fungus may invade internal organs, producing generalized involvement.

Differential diagnosis. Furuncle, carbuncle, blastomycosis, tuberculosis cutis, late syphilis (gumma).

Therapy. Penicillin in adequate dosage may be curative. Chloramphenicol is of value. Sulfonamides may also be useful.

Anthrax

Synonym. Malignant pustule, woolsorter's disease.

Sites of predilection. Face, extremities.

Objective signs. The primary lesion develops as a reddish papule at the site of inoculation. A bleb forms over this lesion and the involved area becomes edematous and indurated. The lesion assumes the characteristics of a discharging carbuncle, with suppurative satellite adenopathy. Metastatic abscesses frequently develop. Vesicles and pustules occur about the periphery of the crusted, necrotic area.

Subjective symptoms. This is a serious, generalized, constitutional illness. Systemic symptoms include chills, fever and malaise. Pruritus, burning and pain occur at the site of the lesions.

Etiology. *Bacillus anthracis.* Infection usually develops in persons who handle hides or infected animals. Infection may result from careless handling of infected dressings.

Histopathology. Numerous bacilli are present in the subpapillary vascular net. In the corium and subcutaneous tissue there is vascular dilatation and interstitial edema. Collagen bundles are swollen and split. Marked generalized leukocytic infiltration is present.

Diagnostic aids. Biopsy, history and physical examination, culture.

Relation to systemic disease. The primary lesion is evidence of a generalized systemic illness. Fatal termination may result from overwhelming infection.

Differential diagnosis. Furunculosis, carbunculosis.

Therapy. Chloramphenicol, the tetracyclines and penicillin are of value given in adequate dosage early in the course of the illness.

Atopic Dermatitis

Synonym. Dermatitis, eczema.

Sites of predilection. Face, scalp, upper extremities.

Objective signs. These pustular lesions always represent secondary pyogenic infection of a previously existing eruption. Pustule formation may complicate vesicular eczema or develop as small pustules on an eczematous dermatitis. The areas are ill-defined, confluent lesions which are covered with small, yellowish or greenish-yellow pustules and pus crusts.

Subjective symptoms. Moderate to severe pruritus.

Etiology. This is a staphylococcic or streptococcic infection superimposed on a previously existing allergic dermatitis.

Histopathology. Nonspecific. Superficial abscesses are present in the epidermis.

Diagnostic aids. History and physical examination, culture.

Relation to systemic disease. See Atopic Dermatitis in Chapter 14: Macular Eruptions.

Bacterid, Pustular

Synonym. Pustular psoriasis, dyshidrosis.

Sites of predilection. Hands, feet.

Objective signs. The condition begins on the palmar and plantar surfaces as deep-seated, small vesicles (1-2 mm in diameter). Eventually, practically all the lesions become pustular. Tiny, hemorrhagic puncta commonly develop among the pustules. In extensive cases the pustules coalesce to form large, honeycombed lesions in the epidermis. When the pustules rupture or dry, scaling, crusting and fissuring occur. New pustules usually appear in crops and are accompanied by marked pruritus. When the condition becomes quiescent, adherent scaling is the predominant feature.

Subjective symptoms. Pruritus, burning and pain.

Etiology. Unknown. It appears that this is the same entity as dyshidrosis.

Histopathology. There are pustules in the epidermis with a slight inflammatory reaction in the cutis. The pustules contain numerous leukocytes and epithelial cells.

Diagnostic aids. Biopsy, culture, history and physical examination.

Relation to systemic disease. No specific relationship.

Differential diagnosis. Pustular psoriasis, dermatitis repens, epidermophytosis.

Therapy. See Dyshidrosis.

Blastomycosis

Synonym. Dermatitis blastomycetica, North American blastomycosis, Gilchrist's disease.

Sites of predilection. Face, hands, wrists, forearms. May occur at any site.

Objective signs. The fully developed lesion is a chronic, slowly progressive granuloma, characterized by the formation of thick crusts, verrucous vegetations and draining sinuses. The lesion usually begins as a papule or papulopustule, which spreads peripherally and is covered with a crust. The pustules coalesce to form a verrucous granuloma. Thick mucoid pus is present under the crusts or exudes through the sinuses. The central portion of the lesion involutes and forms a thick scar. Small pustules are present in the granulomatous margin. The lesions spread by autoinoculation. Papillomatous projections are pronounced in lesions on the hands and feet. The

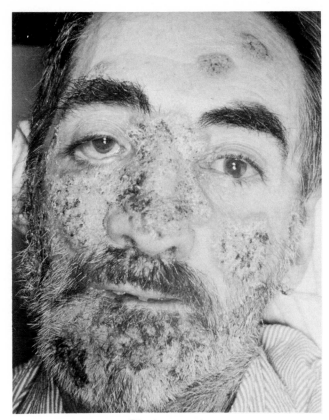

Blastomycosis

lesions are vascular and bleed after slight trauma. Lesions may spread by lymphatic extension.

Subjective symptoms. Little or no pain.

Etiology. *Blastomyces dermatitidis.*

Histopathology. Debris consisting of pus, blood and epithelial cells is present on the surface. The horny layer may be destroyed or may extend in thickened masses between distorted papillae. Miliary abscesses containing the *Blastomyces* are found throughout the epidermis and cutis. Pseudoepitheliomatous hyperplasia is present.

Diagnostic aids. History and physical examination, biopsy, culture, intradermal blastomycin test.

Relation to systemic disease. This is a progressive disease in which all organs may be involved.

Differential diagnosis. Tuberculosis verrucosa cutis, granuloma inguinale, drug eruptions, gumma, chronic pyodermas.

Therapy. Amphotericin B is the drug of choice.

Bromoderma

Synonym. Drug eruption, dermatitis medicamentosa.

Sites of predilection. Face, trunk, lower extremities.

Objective signs. The most common lesions are follicular pustules which vary from 2-6 mm in diameter. The eruption resembles acne vulgaris without comedones. Granulomatous lesions occur most frequently on the lower extremities, although they may develop on the face in infants. The granulomatous lesions may coalesce to form large areas, which become suppurative, crusted or vegetative. There is a striking resemblance to the lesions of blastomycosis.

Subjective symptoms. Pruritus and burning.

Etiology. Hypersensitivity to bromide. Bromides are contained in some commercially available headache remedies.

Histopathology. Follicular lesions are nonspecific pustules. The granulomatous lesions have a nonspecific picture.

Diagnostic aids. Biopsy, blood bromide level, history and physical examination.

Relation to systemic disease. The condition that necessitated continuous consumption of bromides. Mental illness.

Differential diagnosis. Acne, syphilis, furuncles, blastomycosis.

Therapy. The ingestion of bromides must be discontinued. Sodium chloride given by mouth and intravenously will replace the bromide in the blood. Care must be exercised in giving hypertonic intravenous saline to prevent shock.

Carbuncle

Synonym. None.

Sites of predilection. Back of the neck, trunk, extremities.

Objective signs. The lesion is usually a single, raised, indurated, acutely inflamed, red or reddish-blue, fluctuant pustule which varies in size from 1-5 cm. It has two or more openings which discharge thick yellow pus. The central part of the lesion is composed of one or more large necrotic pustular masses (core).

Subjective symptoms. Pain. Systemic symptoms include chills and fever.

Etiology. Staphylococci.

Histopathology. There is a deep, circumscribed, pyogenic infection extending well into the corium.

Diagnostic aids. History and physical examination, culture of exudate, urinalysis, blood sugar, assay of immune globulin.

Relation to systemic disease. Diabetes mellitus may predispose to the development of carbuncles. These lesions may occur in leukemias or other debilitating diseases.

Differential diagnosis. Sebaceous cysts, gumma, deep mycotic granulomas.

Therapy. Incision and drainage of fluctuant lesions. Systemic antibiotic therapy is indicated in extensive lesions. Use the drug indicated by sensitivity tests.

Coccidioidomycosis

Synonym. Coccidioidal granuloma, valley fever, San Joaquin fever.

Sites of predilection. Face, upper extremities.

Objective signs. Primary cutaneous coccidioidomycosis is rare. Pulmonary lesions are common in this serious, generalized illness. The earliest cutaneous lesion is a chancre or granuloma which may remain localized for several years. Satellite lymphadenopathy eventually suppurates and forms sinuses. The lesions spread slowly. Nodular or circumscribed granulomas may develop. Cellulitis caused by this microorganism is not unusual.

Erythema nodosum is a common allergic manifestation of pulmonary involvement. The cutaneous lesions which complicate pulmonary involvement are not distinctive. Large nodular lesions or granulomas develop on the legs, hips and buttocks. These lesions become confluent, suppurate and ulcerate. Vegetative lesions may develop. Pulmonary lesions are associated with malaise, chills, fever, night sweats and severe headaches. The disease has a poor prognosis.

Etiology. Coccidioides immitis.

Histopathology. A granuloma deep in the cutis. Plasma cells, leukocytes, giant cells and epithelioid cells form the dense infiltrate. The organisms are present in the giant cells.

Diagnostic aids. History and physical examination, culture, biopsy, intradermal skin tests.

Relation to systemic disease. This is a serious systemic disease.

Differential diagnosis. Blastomycosis, chromoblastomycosis, gumma.

Therapy. Amphotericin B is the therapy of choice.

Ecthyma

Synonym. Deep-seated impetigo contagiosa.

Sites of predilection. Legs, buttocks, hands, trunk, vulva.

Objective signs. The primary lesion is a vesicle or vesicopustule (1-3 cm in diameter) which enlarges peripherally. The surface becomes covered with a thick adherent, black or brown (hemorrhagic) crust. Removal of the crust reveals a shallow ulcer, the base of which is bathed in pus. Healing may take place with scar formation.

Subjective symptoms. Slight to severe pain.

Etiology. Staphylococcus aureus or group A beta hemolytic streptococcus. Ecthyma may develop as a complication of dermatitis venenata, scabies or atopic dermatitis.

Histopathology. Numerous abscesses involving the entire thickness of the epidermis and the upper portion of the cutis.

Diagnostic aids. Culture of the exudate, antihyaluronidase.

Relation to systemic disease. None.

Differential diagnosis. Sporotrichosis, gumma, condyloma latum on the vulva, chancroid.

Therapy. Systemic antibiotic therapy is indicated. Local hygiene is important.

Folliculitis

Synonym. None.

Sites of predilection. Buttocks, extensor surfaces of thighs, trunk, face.

Objective signs. This condition is characterized by the development of numerous superficial pustules which originate in hair follicles. These lesions vary in size from 1-4 mm in diameter. A hair shaft may pierce the pustule. Follicular papules may be intermingled with the pustules.

Subjective symptoms. Pain, mild pruritus.

Etiology. Staphylococcus aureus; contact sensitivity or local irritation. Some systemic drugs also produce folliculitis.

Histopathology. Abscess formation in and about the hair follicle.

Diagnostic aids. Culture, history and physical examination.

Relation to systemic disease. A drug sensitivity reaction may precipitate the eruption.

Differential diagnosis. Impetigo contagiosa, varicella, acne vulgaris, papulonecrotic tuberculid.

Therapy. Simple drainage is all that is necessary for a single lesion. In patients with multiple lesions, systemic antibiotic therapy or removal of the offending allergen or irritant may be necessary.

Furuncle

Synonym. Boil.

Sites of predilection. Any site.

Objective signs. The initial lesion is an acute, tender, circumscribed, deep-seated, follicular pustule which varies from 2 mm-1 cm in diameter. Perifollicular erythema and induration develop. The central area becomes soft and develops a yellowish top. When the furuncle ruptures, a thick, yellow, greenish or bloody pus is discharged, followed by the "core." Furuncles may heal with scar formation. A "blind boil" is a furuncle which does not fully develop and rupture.

Subjective symptoms. Pain.

Etiology. *Staphylococcus aureus.*

Histopathology. A deep abscess formed by necrotic material, leukocytes, and colonies of staphylococci. The lesions begin in and around the pilosebaceous apparatus, eventually forming abscesses. The inflammatory cells are densely packed. In chronic lesions, lymphocytes, plasma cells and giant cells may be present.

Relation to systemic disease. Diabetes, alcoholism, immunodeficiencies, anemias and other debilitating diseases.

Differential diagnosis. Carbuncle, sebaceous cysts.

Therapy. Systemic antibiotic selection should be based on disc or tube dilution sensitivity tests. Fluctuant lesions must be drained surgically.

Hidradenitis Suppurativa

Synonym. Abscess of the apocrine sweat gland, axillary abscesses.

Sites of predilection. Axillae; lesions occasionally occur about the external genitalia, the areolae of the breasts or the buttocks.

Objective signs. The lesions begin as small subcutaneous nodules, which may involute spontaneously or develop into abscesses. Adjoining lesions may coalesce to form band-like indurations. Sinus tracts may develop and drain for many months. The condition occurs more frequently in women.

Subjective symptoms. Varying degrees of pain.

Etiology. Unknown. May be associated with cystic acne.

Histopathology. Variable leukocytic infiltration surrounding the lumen of the apocrine gland. When

the infection is of long standing, there is a perivascular infiltration of plasma cells and lymphocytes.

Diagnostic aids. Culture, history and physical examination.

Relation to systemic disease. None has been established.

Differential diagnosis. Furuncle, cellulitis, erysipelas, lymphadenitis.

Therapy. Systemic antibiotic therapy is of limited value. Surgical excision of the entire involved area is frequently necessary, especially if scarred bridges occur between the lesions. Incision and drainage of localized lesions is not an effective form of treatment.

Kerion

Synonym. Kerion celsi, tinea kerion.

Sites of predilection. Scalp.

Objective signs. There are usually one or more raised, boggy, inflammatory, crusted lesions present. Pus exudes from the follicles and the hairs fall out. The lesions begin as a group of follicular pustules in an area of tinea capitis. Healing may be followed by scar formation and alopecia. The pyogenic infection usually destroys the fungus infection.

Subjective symptoms. Pain.

Etiology. Pyogenic infection, complicating a fungus infection of the scalp.

Histopathology. An inflammatory process in the upper part of the corium and about the follicles. The causative organism may be present in abundance within and outside of the hair follicle.

Diagnostic aids. Culture for both bacteria and fungi.

Relation to systemic disease. None.

Differential diagnosis. Impetigo contagiosa, furuncles.

Therapy. Systemic antibiotic therapy is indicated. The scalp must be cleansed frequently. Fluctuant lesions must be incised and drained.

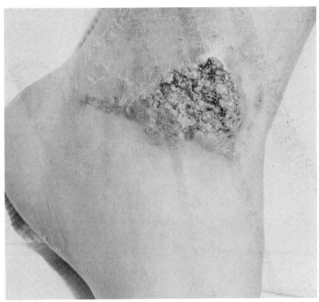

Sporotrichosis,
initial lesion on ankle

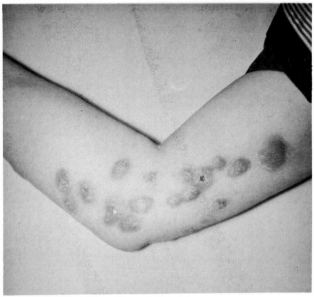

Sporotrichosis,
ascending nodules on arm

Sporotrichosis

Synonym. None.

Sites of predilection. Extremities.

Objective signs. The causative organism is inoculated by trauma in gardeners, florists and laborers. The initial lesion is usually a small nodule which breaks down to form the sporotrichal "chancre" at the site of inoculation. Numerous indolent, painless nodular granulomas develop along the course of the ascending lymph vessels. These granulomas eventually become fluctuant and form abscesses and ulcers. Lesions may develop in bone or viscera.

A papular or plaque form of the disease exists in mild cases. Also, a systemic form may develop in which the cutaneous lesions are small vesicles and papules. In this disseminated type visceral involvement occurs early in the course of the disease.

Subjective symptoms. Vary with the extent and severity of the lesions.

Etiology. *Sporothrix schenckii.*

Histopathology. An infectious granuloma with the formation of deep abscesses, sinuses and ulcers. The chronic inflammatory infiltrate is composed of epithelioid cells, giant cells, plasma cells and lymphocytes.

Diagnostic aids. Culture on Sabouraud's medium, history and physical examination. It is rare to be able to visualize the microorganism in tissue sections of the lesion.

Relation to systemic disease. Involvement of the skeletal system, lungs and other organs may occur.

Differential diagnosis. Tuberculosis cutis, blastomycosis, syphilis, bacterial infections, tularemia.

Therapy. Potassium iodide, 4-6 gm daily, continued for one month after all lesions have healed. Amphotericin B should be instituted in the disseminated form.

Sycosis Barbae

Synonym. Sycosis vulgaris, barber's itch.

Sites of predilection. Bearded portion of the face and neck.

Objective signs. This is a chronic eruption of the bearded area. It begins as scattered follicular pustules from which hairs protrude. The lesions spread and, in a brief time, cover large areas. The skin between the pustules becomes red and scaly. These pustules are ruptured by washing or shaving and the entire area may become covered with serous and pus crusts. The hairs become loosened in the follicles. Healing takes place with scar formation which may produce a large area, devoid of hair and surrounded by papules and pustules.

Subjective symptoms. Pruritus.

Etiology. *Staphylococcus aureus.* The condition may develop as a result of bacterial infection superimposed on contact dermatitis.

Diagnostic aids. Culture.

Differential diagnosis. Impetigo contagiosa, actinomycosis, furuncles.

Therapy. There is a tendency to spontaneous involution of lesions. Systemic antibiotic therapy is indicated. Improve shaving hygiene and discontinue after-shave lotions.

Vaccinia

Synonym. Cowpox, eczema vaccinatum.

Sites of predilection. Generalized.

Objective signs. This condition develops 4-10 days after vaccination in persons with atopic dermatitis or other eczematous eruptions. It may also develop following contact with a vaccination "take" in another person. Vaccinia only develops in individuals who have not been successfully vaccinated against smallpox. The eruption may occur on any part of the body.

The lesions begin as large (1-1.5 cm in diameter) vesicles which umbilicate, become globular pustules, then form crusts. Healing takes place with scar formation. Satellite lesions may occur.

Subjective symptoms. Patients become seriously ill, with chills, fever and general malaise.

Etiology. Vaccinia virus.

Histopathology. Subepidermal vesicles and marked intracellular edema in the epidermis. Intracytoplasmic inclusion bodies are present in the cells of the vesicle.

Diagnostic aids. Biopsy, tissue culture, hemagglutinin test, viral neutralization test, Tzanck smear of the vesicular cells.

Relation to systemic disease. This is a generalized disease which may be complicated by ocular paralysis, postvaccinial retinitis and encephalitis. Death may ensue.

Differential diagnosis. Variola, varicella.

Therapy. Supportive. Prophylaxis demands that vaccination is contraindicated in atopic dermatitis. Patients who have active disease may be treated with hyperimmune globulin. Isatin beta thiosemicarbazone is an agent which prevents pox virus release from cells and as such may decrease the transmission of the disease to susceptibles.

Variola

Synonym. Smallpox.

Sites of predilection. Generalized.

Objective signs. An acute, infectious and contagious disease characterized by the successive development of macules, papules, vesicles and pustules on the skin and mucous membranes. The first lesions to appear are numerous macules which become vesicles within 24 hours. These lesions umbilicate, then become pustules. Unlike varicella, variola is characterized by a single crop of lesions which progresses through the successive stages of development at the same time. When fully developed, the eruption consists of numerous, discrete, shotty, globular pustules 2-6 mm in diameter. There is facial swelling and generalized erythema. These lesions later become crusted and eventually heal with pitted scars.

Subjective symptoms. Prodromal symptoms of malaise, headache and fever (38.8-40.5°C), before the development of the exanthem. The patient is very ill and may lapse into a coma.

Etiology. Variola virus.

Histopathology. The primary lesion is an intraepidermal, multilocular vesicle which contains balloon cells and inclusion bodies (Guarnieri's bodies).

Diagnostic aids. History and physical examination, tissue culture, hemagglutinin test, virus neutralization test, Tzanck smear of cells within the vesicle fluid.

Relation to systemic disease. This is a generalized systemic disease which may be fatal. Renal failure and pulmonary complications occur.

Differential diagnosis. Pustular syphilis, varicella, generalized vaccinia, Kaposi's varicelliform eruption.

Therapy. Strict isolation of the patient is necessary. Vaccination is a preventive measure. The use of hyperimmune serum of isatin beta thiosemicarbazone should be considered.

CHAPTER 18

Eruptions Involving the Scalp and Other Hairy Areas

Alopecia Areata

Synonym. Baldness. If all scalp hair is lost the condition is called alopecia totalis. Alopecia universalis is the term when total body hair is lost.

Sites of predilection. Scalp, beard or generalized (alopecia totalis).

Objective signs. One or more circumscribed, round or irregular, noninflammatory bald areas appear suddenly without prodromal symptoms. The involved areas may be completely bald or a few scattered, discrete, isolated hairs may be present. Often the patient does not notice the hairs falling out even if hair loss is acute. The lesions extend peripherally, and occasionally all of the hair may be lost. When the hair begins to regrow it is usually fine and white. This growth is lost and is replaced by normal hair. There is a tendency to relapse. Nail changes may develop with pit formation and longitudinal ridging. Cataracts may occur as a rare complication of alopecia totalis.

Subjective symptoms. None except the emotional imbalance produced by the cosmetic defect.

Etiology. Unknown. The condition may be associated with psychogenic stimuli. Genetic predisposition but the mode of inheritance is unknown. Physical trauma may be a cause.

Histopathology. Atrophy of the hair follicles and sebaceous glands. There is a mononuclear cell infiltration around the hair follicle bulb. Attenuated follicles are seen. Telogen follicles are present in older lesions and anagen activity in the early inflammatory stages. The hairs have cuticular damage with longitudinal ultramicroscopic open fractures which look like the shaft exploded. In early lesions telogen follicles are in the center. In later stages the follicles appear to be in anagen.

Diagnostic aids. Clinical appearance, serologic test for syphilis, history and physical examination, biopsy, CBC, ANA. Serum calcium, phosphorus and T_4; autoantibodies for thyroid follicular cells, parietal cells and adrenal cortical cells.

Relation to systemic disease. Emotional imbalance, atopic diseases, vitiligo and autoimmune diseases (pernicious anemia, Hashimoto's thyroiditis, Addison's disease).

Differential diagnosis. Ringworm of the scalp, syphilitic alopecia, alopecia caused by febrile illnesses, seborrheic dermatitis.

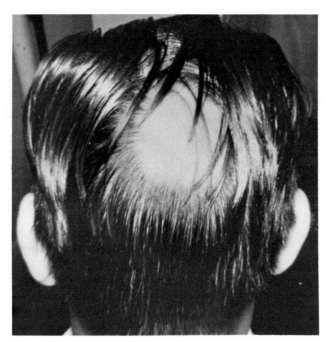

Alopecia areata

Therapy. There is no specific treatment. Rest and relief from anxiety is essential. Topical or systemic corticosteroid therapy is of temporary benefit only and is therefore avoided.

Alopecia, Congenital

Synonym. Congenital ectodermal defect.
Sites of predilection. Scalp and other areas.
Objective signs. There may be complete or partial absence of hair on all parts of the body (congenital ectodermal defect). If hair is present, it is usually fine, whitish, lusterless and occurs in scattered tufts. Associated with this deformity is partial or complete absence of sweating and sebum production, and defective nail formation. Some patients are edentulous from birth. The condition is usually incomplete and appears in the absence of any gross inflammatory process. In a variant of this disease called anhidrotic ectodermal dysplasia (Clouston's syndrome), nail dystrophy, dyskeratosis of the palms and soles, eccrine pore prominence and hyperpigmentation around the knuckles were seen in this dominant disorder. Squint, deafness, CNS and dental abnormalities were also found.

Subjective symptoms. Due to lack of sweat glands these patients are unable to tolerate heat.
Etiology. A congenital defect.
Histopathology. Absence of hair follicles and a decreased number or absence of sweat glands.
Diagnostic aids. History and physical examination, biopsy.
Relation to systemic disease. Associated with other congenital abnormalities. Many of these patients are subnormal mentally.
Differential diagnosis. The condition is characteristic.
Therapy. None effective.

Alopecia, Male Pattern

Synonym. Alopecia prematura, alopecia senilis.
Sites of predilection. Scalp.
Objective signs. Male pattern baldness may begin prior to the twentieth year (alopecia prematura), or may not have its onset until after the third decade. The hair recedes on either side in the parietal area and also on the crown. The condition may be manifested by slight thinning of the hair distribution in these areas, or it may be progressive, becoming an extensively bald area with only a fringe of hair remaining. The skin of the bald area appears normal, although varying degrees of seborrheic dermatitis may be present. The scalp may be dry or oily. In older individuals seborrheic keratoses and actinic keratoses may be found on the bald area. If male pattern baldness occurs in the adult female before age 60, it is due to hormone imbalance and may be indicative of an ovarian neoplasm.
Subjective symptoms. Usually none. If seborrheic dermatitis is present there is mild pruritus.

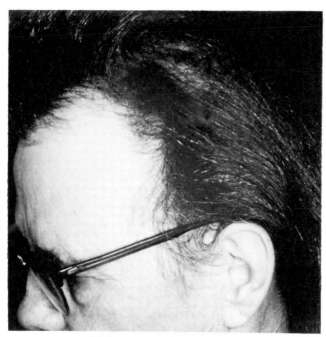

*Male pattern alopecia in a
70-year-old woman with an ovarian tumor*

Etiology. Unknown. There may be a familial tendency toward baldness.

Histopathology. Atrophy of hair follicles in the involved area.

Diagnostic aids. History, clinical appearance.

Relation to systemic disease. None. The degree of alopecia has no relationship to the state of the patient's health or virility.

Differential diagnosis. Clinical appearance is characteristic.

Therapy. None effective.

Alopecia, Symptomatic

Synonym. Essential alopecia of women, telogen effluvium.

Sites of predilection. Scalp.

Objective signs. Loss or diffuse thinning of scalp hair in the absence of any gross inflammatory process.

There are no circumscribed areas of alopecia. The hair is of normal texture. There is no excessive scale or oiliness.

Subjective symptoms. Emotional imbalance caused by hair loss.

Etiology. May be associated with factors such as emotional tension, excessive brushing, post pregnancy, hormone imbalance, estrogen administration (birth control pills).

Histopathology. The microscopic picture is not diagnostic.

Diagnostic aids. History and physical examination; use scrapings and cultures to rule out fungus infections. Most of the hairs lost are in the telogen phase.

Relation to systemic disease. Hormone imbalance, emotional tension, post pregnancy, drug administration.

Differential diagnosis. Other types of alopecia.

Therapy. Avoid excessive brushing, washing, use of mechanical devices and hair preparations. Treat the underlying disease. The condition is self-limited.

Alopecia, Syphilitic

Synonym. None.

Sites of predilection. Scalp. This type of hair loss occurs concurrently with other lesions of secondary syphilis.

Objective signs. There are numerous discrete areas of incomplete alopecia over the entire body. The individual areas vary in size from 1-2 cm in diameter. The incomplete hair loss, in these closely grouped lesions, presents a characteristic "moth-eaten" appearance. Following administration of antisyphilitic treatment the hair regrows.

Subjective symptoms. None produced by the cutaneous lesions.

Etiology. Treponema pallidum (see Chapter 9: Sexually Transmitted Diseases).

Histopathology. See Chapter 9.

Diagnostic aids. See Chapter 9.

Relation to systemic disease. Syphilis is a systemic disease.

Differential diagnosis. Alopecia areata, tinea capitis, febrile alopecia.

Therapy. Treatment of syphilis.

Alopecia, Toxic

Synonym. Febrile alopecia, telogen effluvium.

Sites of predilection. Scalp.

Objective signs. There is diffuse, general hair loss, occasionally approaching complete baldness. The underlying skin or scalp appears normal.

Subjective symptoms. None produced by the cutaneous lesions.

Etiology. This type of alopecia is associated with constitutional infections such as typhoid fever, influenza, pneumonia, scarlatina and side effects or adverse reactions to drugs. Hyperpyrexia is usually associated. Although the hair loss is produced by some constitutional disease, the mechanism of action is unknown.

Histopathology. Nonspecific.

Diagnostic aids. History and physical examination. When the hair loss is due to antitumor drugs or radiation therapy most of the damaged hairs are in the anagen phase of growth. Those hairs lost in the idiopathic form of the disorder are predominately telogen.

Relation to systemic disease. The condition is associated with some generalized systemic illness, usually accompanied by fever, drug intoxication (thallium acetate), antitumor drugs or X-ray therapy.

Differential diagnosis. Alopecia areata, alopecia prematura, syphilitic alopecia.

Therapy. Treatment of the underlying condition. The hair loss is usually temporary.

Toxic alopecia, caused by thallium acetate

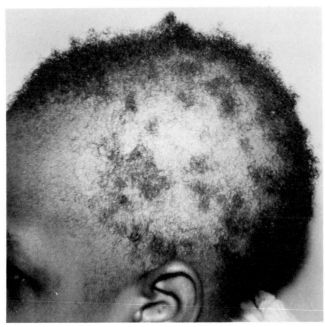

Canities

Synonym. Gray hair, poliosis.

Sites of predilection. Scalp.

Objective signs. Graying of the hair may develop prematurely in childhood, at puberty or after the third decade. There is depigmentation of the hair to gray or white in circumscribed areas, or there is generalized involvement. The texture of the hair is unchanged. Occasionally a circumscribed area of gray hair accompanies the development of vitiligo or leukoderma. A single, circumscribed lock of white hair may develop in early childhood or at puberty (poliosis circumscripta or localized canities).

Subjective symptoms. None.

Etiology. The condition may be congenital because it appears to occur in certain families.

Histopathology. Absence of pigment in the follicle and hair shaft. Air spaces are present in the medulla of the hair shaft.

Diagnostic aids. Clinical appearance is characteristic.

Relation to systemic disease. Premature graying of the hair may follow a prolonged systemic illness, emotional tension, alopecia areata or pernicious anemia.

Differential diagnosis. Clinical appearance is characteristic.

Therapy. None specific. Dyeing can be done for cosmetic improvement.

Cutis Verticis Gyrata

Synonym. None.

Sites of predilection. Scalp.

Objective signs. The skin of the scalp is overabundant and thrown into folds resembling the convolutions of the brain. The condition may be localized into one small area or it may involve the entire scalp. There is usually thinning of the hair over the convolutions, which are arranged in an irregular, sagittal manner.

Subjective symptoms. None produced by the cutaneous lesion.

Etiology. Probably due to a genetic developmental defect.

Histopathology. Nonspecific.

Diagnostic aids. Clinical appearance, history.

Relation to systemic disease. The condition has been known to develop in association with acromegaly and myxedema. Other conditions including some inflammatory diseases have been associated in anecdotal reports.

Differential diagnosis. The clinical condition is characteristic.

Therapy. None is effective.

Dandruff

Synonym. Seborrhea sicca, pityriasis capitis, mild seborrheic dermatitis.

Sites of predilection. Scalp, eyebrows, face.

Objective signs. The condition does not usually develop until puberty. After this it may appear at any age. There are ill-defined, discrete and confluent, small or large, scattered areas in which there is moderate to marked scaliness. The scale is white or gray, dry or oily. The condition is usually limited within the hair line. There is absence of inflammatory changes. More extensive lesions, in which inflammation develops, are characteristic of seborrheic dermatitis.

Subjective symptoms. None to mild pruritus.

Etiology. Some scale formation is physiologic.

Histopathology. Hyperkeratosis and parakeratosis with slight acanthosis.

Diagnostic aids. Use the Wood light and cultures to rule out fungus infections.

Relation to systemic disease. None usually.

Differential diagnosis. Ringworm of the scalp, psoriasis, pediculosis.

Therapy. Use one of the available antidandruff shampoos on a regular basis. Topically applied corticosteroid lotions will relieve pruritus and reduce inflammation. Alcoholic solution of salicylic acid (3%) will reduce the extent of scale.

Favus

Synonym. Tinea favosa.

Sites of predilection. Scalp, trunk, nails.

Objective signs. In the scalp, the lesion begins as a pinkish macule which becomes scaly. Scale formation increases until there are numerous areas of raised, cup-shaped (scutula), yellowish or grayish, scaly lesions at the bases of tufts of hair. Eventually, diffuse or circumscribed areas of thick scale formation occur. The scalp has a musty odor. Removal of the scutula exposes an atrophic scarred area which is permanently bald.

The nail plates become distorted, thickened and friable. Underlying the plates there is grayish or brownish, hyperkeratotic and caseous material. Permanent distortion of the involved nail bed occurs.

Subjective symptoms. Mild to moderate pruritus.

Etiology. *Trichophyton schoenleini.* The condition is found among immigrants from Slavic countries.

In the United States the condition is endemic in some areas of West Virginia and Kentucky.

Histopathology. Histopathologic changes depend on the clinical manifestation.

Diagnostic aids. Culture on Sabouraud's medium. Examination of a direct preparation using 20% potassium hydroxide solution. The hair shaft has a greenish fluorescence when examined under the Wood light.

Relation to systemic disease. None.

Differential diagnosis. Seborrheic dermatitis, psoriasis, tinea tonsurans, impetigo contagiosa.

Therapy. Griseofulvin may be of value on systemic administration. X-ray epilation may be necessary to stop the progress of the disease in the scalp. Nail lesions are resistant to treatment.

Folliculitis Decalvans

Synonym. Quinquaud's disease, pseudopelade.

Sites of predilection. Scalp.

Objective signs. The condition begins with the development of small, reddish, follicular papulopustules. A hair usually protrudes through each of the follicular lesions. As the pustules dry, the crust and hair fall out, leaving a thin atrophic scar. In advanced cases there are few to numerous, round or irregular, bald areas in which the surface is a shiny, pinkish or whitish scar, without follicular orifices. Active follicular pustules are usually present in the margins of the bald areas. The alopecia produced by this process is permanent.

Subjective symptoms. Moderate to intense pruritus.

Etiology. *Staphylococcus aureus.*

Histopathology. Not diagnostic.

Diagnostic aids. Cultures must be made to rule out scarring fungus infections of the scalp. Cultures on blood agar and sensitivity tests should be done.

Relation to systemic disease. No specific relationship.

Differential diagnosis. Favus, lupus erythematosus, alopecia areata, *Trichophyton tonsurans* or *Trichophyton violaceum* infection.

Therapy. Systemic antibiotic therapy is of questionable value because of the recurrent nature of the disease. Avoid trauma. Daily shampoo with hexachlorophene may be of some use.

Hypertrichosis

Synonym. Excessive hair, superfluous hair.

Sites of predilection. Face, trunk and extremities of women.

Objective signs. There is an excessive growth of hair, usually occurring on the face. This may consist of a profuse growth of fine down. Occasionally the condition is limited to the moustache area. Coarse, dark hair may be intermingled with the fine, downy growth. In some women there is a scattered growth of coarse, black hairs over the chin and upper lip. If the condition is extensive it may involve the areolae of the nipples and the extremities. If an endocrine disturbance is responsible, the hair growth on the abdomen may assume the male pattern.

The condition may be present at birth, but most commonly develops after puberty and becomes extensive with the passage of time. In many women the condition begins at the time of the menopause.

Subjective symptoms. Cutaneous lesions produce no subjective symptoms. The cosmetic defect may be causative of severe mental distress.

Etiology. The condition may be familial, idiopathic or caused by some endocrine imbalance.

Histopathology. Nonspecific.

Diagnostic aids. History and physical examination, urinary determination of 17-ketosteroids, plasma testosterone, morning and evening cortisol determinations.

Relation to systemic disease. Ovarian abnormalities, acromegaly. Cushing's syndrome, juvenile myxedema, adrenocortical hypoplasia caused by the administration of corticosteroids, intake of progestational drug.

Therapy. The use of depilatories may be of value. Mechanical removal of the hair by electrolysis may be preferred by some patients but is tedious, painful, inefficient and expensive. Correction of any underlying disorder.

Ingrown Hair

Synonym. Pili incarnati.

Sites of predilection. Bearded portion of the face, particularly the neck.

Objective signs. The hair in the affected portion grows obliquely and does not penetrate the stratum corneum, but extends beneath it, causing papules and pustules to develop. On close inspection, using a hand lens, the examiner will see the hair growing transversely just beneath the stratum corneum. When the skin surface is broken the hair may be lifted out. Following extraction of the buried hair, the papules heal with scar formation.

Subjective symptoms. Pruritus.

Etiology. An inherent defect in hair follicle direction, becoming apparent in adolescence or early adult life when shaving becomes a necessity. For unknown reasons this condition is more frequently observed in black patients.

Histopathology. The follicles in the involved areas are distorted, and in some instances form an acute angle with the skin surface.

Diagnostic aids. Biopsy.

Relation to systemic disease. None.

Differential diagnosis. Folliculitis, sycosis vulgaris.

Therapy. Correction of shaving technique is essential. Manual epilation of the hairs in the involved areas. Permanent removal of the hair by the use of electrolysis or high frequency current is frequently of value.

Keratosis, Seborrheic

Synonym. Senile warts.

Sites of predilection. Scalp, face, back.

Objective signs. This benign, superficial, epidermal tumor usually effects persons beyond the age of 35. The lesions develop as well-defined, flat-topped, grayish, brownish, or blackish papules or tumors, which vary in size from 5 mm to 2-3 cm in diameter. The lesions are round or oval in shape, usually sessile, but occasionally pedunculated, and are covered with an oily film. They are few to numerous and may persist indefinitely without change. A gray or white scale can be observed after scratching the lesions.

Subjective symptoms. None or slight pruritus.

Etiology. Unknown.

Histopathology. The acanthotic epidermis is papillomatous. The papillae of the cutis are elongated.

Diagnostic aids. Biopsy.

Relation to systemic disease. The sudden onset of multiple keratosis may be associated with internal malignancy.

Differential diagnosis. Melanoma, senile keratoses, epitheliomas, nevi.

Therapy. Removal of the lesion by light desiccation, cryosurgery or curettage under procaine anesthesia.

Lepothrix

Synonym. Trichomycosis axillaris.

Sites of predilection. Axillae.

Objective signs. There are yellow, red or black concretions on the hair shafts. The individual lesions resemble the ova of pediculosis.

Subjective symptoms. None.

Etiology. A mixture of nonpathogenic fungi and bacteria which form the waxy concretions.

Histopathology. The concretions on the hair shafts are formed of masses of microorganisms in a homogeneous waxy substance resembling chitin.

Diagnostic aids. Microscopic examination of the involved hair.

Relation to systemic disease. None.

Differential diagnosis. Pediculosis, fungus infections.

Therapy. Shave the axillae and cleanse the skin with mild antiseptics.

Lupus Erythematosus

Synonym. None.

Sites of predilection. Scalp, face and other areas. See Lupus Erythematosus in Chapter 14: Macular Eruptions.

Objective signs. The scalp lesions consist of one or more, round or irregular, discrete or confluent, depressed, atrophic scarred areas which are devoid of hair. Follicular plugging may be observed at the margin of the lesion. The edges of the scarred area are usually pink and the central portion white. The baldness is permanent. While there are usually other lesions present, the eruption in the scalp may be the only clinical evidence of the disorder.

Subjective symptoms. Pruritus or burning.

Etiology. Unknown.

Histopathology. See Chapter 14.

Relation to systemic disease. Lupus erythematosus is a systemic disease.

Differential diagnosis. Favus, folliculitis decalvans, alopecia areata, pseudopelade, scleroderma.

Therapy. See Chapter 14.

Pediculosis Capitis

Synonym. Head lice, bugs.

Sites of predilection. Scalp.

Objective signs. There are few to numerous ova appearing as minute, pearly, ovoid bodies, which adhere to the hair shafts by a layer of chitin. Live pediculi may be present. Excoriations or pyogenic infection in the scalp, on the forehead and the back of the neck are physical signs which may be indicative of pediculosis. The ova (nits) glow with grayish fluorescence when exposed to the Wood light.

Subjective symptoms. Intense pruritus.

Etiology. *Pediculus capitis.*

Histopathology. Microscopic examination of a hair shaft containing an ovum reveals the parasite within the ovum. The Wood light is an excellent method for finding ova.

Relation to systemic disease. None usually.

Differential diagnosis. Seborrhea sicca, psoriasis.

Therapy. Shampoo with gamma benzene hexachloride and thoroughly rinse. Apply the same chemical in a lotion after the hair is dry. One application will suffice. To remove the ova (nits), the next day, soak the hair in 5% acetic acid or white vinegar. Wrap the head in a towel dampened with this solution for several hours. This will soften the chitin (cement substance) which binds the nit to the hair. Comb the hair with a fine-tooth comb and follow this with a thorough shampoo. A 25% emulsion of benzyl benzoate also kills nits.

Perifolliculitis Capitis
Abscedens et Suffodiens

Synonym. Perifolliculitis of the scalp with scarring alopecia. Dissecting folliculitis of the scalp.

Sites of predilection. Scalp.

Objective signs. The condition begins as follicular pustules, which develop into multiple abscesses in the scalp. The lesions become deep-seated and confluent by burrowing into each other. As the older lesions heal, new lesions develop. The healing lesions leave irregular, permanently bald scars.

Subjective symptoms. Pain in the involved areas.

Etiology. Unknown. Probably an acneform process. Pyogenic bacteria are contributing factors.

Histopathology. Scar formation in the areas of alopecia, with obliteration of hair follicles. The histopathologic picture in the active nodules is a granulomatous process suggestive of tuberculosis.

Diagnostic aids. Culture of the exudate, disc and tube dilution sensitivity tests for antibiotic selection, general physical examination.

Relation to systemic disease. May be seen in patients with cystic acne or hidradenitis suppurativa.

Differential diagnosis. Furuncles, folliculitis decalvans.

Therapy. Systemic administration of the selected antibiotic is only of temporary value. Radiation therapy may be necessary to epilate the scalp in order to cure the infection.

Pili Annulati

Synonym. Ringed hair.

Objective signs. This syndrome may be present at birth or may develop during the first two years of life. The hairs may break off after they have obtained a length of 10-15 cm. Bright and dark bands are seen within the hair.

Subjective symptoms. None.

Etiology. Unknown.

Histopathology. Microscopic examination of the hairs to see cortical cavities.

Diagnostic aids. Microscopic examination of the hair.

Relation to systemic disease. May also be seen with hereditary wooly hair disease.

Differential diagnosis. Pseudo-pili annulati, a disorder in which the shaft axis is rotated reflecting light in bands.

Therapy. None required.

Pili annulati

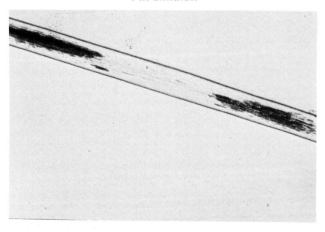

Primary Irritation Dermatitis

Synonym. Allergic contact dermatitis.

Sites of predilection. Scalp and other areas.

Objective signs. In the scalp the lesions may be macular, papular or vesicular. Secondary pyogenic infection may complicate the previously existing eruption. The lesions may be localized to the scalp or extend on to the forehead, face and neck. Small or large areas may be involved. In extensive cases the edema may spread to the forehead and the tissues about the eyes.

Subjective symptoms. Moderate to intense pruritus.

Etiology. Irritation from hair tonics, spray net, hair straighteners, hair-wave solutions, shampoos, perfume and many other agents applied to the hair or scalp.

Histopathology. Edema of the epidermis and upper cutis. Perivascular round cell infiltration in the upper cutis.

Diagnostic aids. History and physical examination; patch tests to the suspected sensitizing substance.

Relation to systemic disease. None usually.

Differential diagnosis. Seborrheic dermatitis, psoriasis, fungus infection.

Therapy. Determination and removal of the causative factor. If secondary pyogenic infection is present, administer systemic antibiotics. If there is no evidence of pyoderma, apply a corticosteroid lotion several times daily.

Psoriasis

Synonym. None.

Sites of predilection. Scalp, elbows, knees, trunk.

Objective signs. In the scalp it is frequently difficult to differentiate seborrheic dermatitis from psoriasis, unless there are characteristic lesions on the trunk and extremities.

There are few to numerous, discrete and confluent, sharply defined macular lesions, which are covered with profuse silvery or grayish scales. It is difficult to demonstrate bleeding points on the scalp. Alopecia may develop from trauma, the inflammatory process or the extirpation of hair shafts trapped in the scales. Annular lesions may be present. (See Psoriasis in Chapter 15: Papular Eruptions.)

Subjective symptoms. Mild to moderate pruritus.

Etiology. Unknown.

Histopathology. There is parakeratosis with extension of the rete pegs and dilatation of vessels in the tips of the papillae. Munro abscesses occur in the stratum corneum and a mononuclear cell infiltrate may be seen in the dermis.

Diagnostic aids. Biopsy.

Relation to systemic disease. None.

Differential diagnosis. Seborrheic dermatitis, favus, fungus infections of the scalp.

Therapy. See Chapter 15.

Pyoderma

Synonym. Impetigo contagiosa, Bockhart's impetigo.

Sites of predilection. Scalp.

Objective signs. The condition begins as a primary pyogenic infection. The initial lesion is a small vesicle or pustule which may surround a hair or occur on the scalp between hair follicles. These vesicles or pustules break down and form grayish or yellowish, thick, superficial crusts which are held in place by the hair. When the crusts are removed, pus exudes. The eruption may be localized to one or more small areas or it may become quite extensive. Healing is not followed by scar formation or alopecia.

Pyogenic infection may complicate seborrheic dermatitis of the scalp, psoriasis, pediculosis and contact dermatitis. If the pyoderma is secondary to some other eruption, evidence of the primary disease is usually found.

Subjective symptoms. Moderate to intense pruritus.

Etiology. See Impetigo in Chapter 16: Vesicular Diseases.

Histopathology. See Chapter 16.

Diagnostic aids. See Chapter 16.

Therapy. Use shampoo containing hexachlorophene on a daily basis. Administer the appropriate systemic antibiotics.

Seborrhea Oleosa

Synonym. Oily skin.

Sites of predilection. Face, scalp.

Objective signs. The skin and hair are exceptionally oily, causing the surface to have a shiny appearance. The sebum production in the scalp may be profuse as to necessitate washing the hair 2-3 times weekly.

Subjective symptoms. Usually none.

Etiology. Excessive endocrine activity (androgenic) is a hypothesis for the cause.

Histopathology. Dilated sebaceous glands.

Diagnostic aids. Clinical appearance is characteristic.

Relation to systemic disease. Parkinson's disease may be accompanied by oily skin.

Differential diagnosis. The condition is characteristic.

Therapy. Frequent cleansing of the face with a bland soap and frequent washing of the scalp with a bland shampoo.

Seborrheic Dermatitis

Synonym. Cradle cap.

Sites of predilection. Scalp, face, presternal region, interscapular area, pubic area. (See Seborrheic Dermatitis in Chapter 14: Macular Eruptions.)

Objective signs. The condition usually begins in the scalp with variously sized, discrete and confluent, round or irregular macules which are well-defined, and covered with a moderate or profuse, whitish or yellowish, oily scale. Alopecia may develop from trauma, inflammation or removal of hairs encased within scales. There is festoon formation by extension of the lesion beyond the hairline onto the forehead. Annular lesions are present.

Subjective symptoms. Moderate to intense pruritus.

Etiology. Unknown.

Histopathology. Slight hyperkeratosis and parakeratosis; moderate acanthosis. There is some cellular and perivascular round cell infiltration in the upper cutis. The picture is not diagnostic.

Diagnostic aids. Use of the Wood light, culture on Sabouraud's medium to exclude fungus infections.

Relation to systemic disease. None.

Differential diagnosis. It is frequently difficult to differentiate seborrheic dermatitis from psoriasis when the lesions occur only in the scalp. The confusion which exists between these two conditions has resulted in the development of the term "seborrhiasis."

Therapy. Use one of the available medicated shampoos on a regular basis. Apply 3% sulfur-salicylic acid ointment to remove the heavy scale. Corticosteroid lotions are also of value.

Sycosis Vulgaris

Synonym. Barber's itch, folliculitis of the beard.

Sites of predilection. Bearded portion of the face.

Objective signs. The primary lesion is a deep-seated follicular papule or pustule, pierced by a hair. In the older pustular lesions the hairs become loosened in the follicle and may be easily extracted. The condition is chronic and recurrent. Some papules and pustules undergo involution, but new lesions constantly develop. Scar formation may develop and become extensive. The onset of the condition may be preceded by a contact dermatitis. In chronic cases there is frequently associated blepharitis and folliculitis.

Subjective symptoms. Pruritus.

Etiology. *Staphylococcus aureus.* The infection may be initiated by poor shaving hygiene or an underlying allergic contact dermatitis.

Histopathology. There is a primary follicular infection and perifollicular involvement as well. The inflammatory infiltrate consists of round cells and polymorphonuclear leukocytes.

Diagnostic aids. Biopsy, culture on blood agar with sensitivity tests, culture on Sabouraud's medium to rule out fungus infections.

Relation to systemic disease. None usually.

Differential diagnosis. Tinea sycosis.

Therapy. Correct shaving hygiene. Avoid the use of perfumed after-shave lotions and shaving creams containing sensitizing antiseptics. Wash the face thoroughly, before and after shaving. Wash, disinfect and dry the razor before storing. Use a fresh blade with each shave. Shave healthy beard first then cut hairs over the lesions only once. Use 50% alcohol as an after-shave lotion. Administer systemic antibiotics.

Tinea Barbae

Synonym. Tinea sycosis, barber's itch.

Sites of predilection. Bearded portion of the face.

Objective signs. A superficial lesion, similar to ringworm infections on other parts of the body, develops as a discrete, round, pinkish, occasionally annular, scaly macule. The lesions may develop as concentric rings. The hair follicles are involved and the infected hairs, which become dry and brittle, are easily extracted.

The deep type of tinea barbae develops on the skin beneath the lower lip, on the upper lip, on the jaw or on the neck just below the jaw. The condition may begin as the superficial type and eventually develops deep-seated papules and pustules. The lesions are round or oval, bright red and covered with broken-off hairs. The nodules may ulcerate. Pus and seropurulent material are discharged through dilated follicular orifices in the lesions. A single, large, boggy, granulomatous, crusted lesion, resembling kerion may develop (Majocchi's granuloma).

Subjective symptoms. Intense pruritus.

Etiology. *Microsporum canis, Microsporum fulvum, Trichophyton gypseum* and *Trichophyton crateriforme.* An occasional case is caused by *Trichophyton rubrum.*

Histopathology. There is invasion of the hair shaft within the follicle by the offending fungus. There is also folliculitis and perifolliculitis and an in-

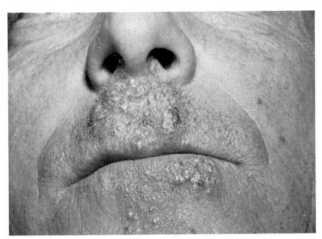

Majocchi's granuloma

filtrate of polymorphonuclear leukocytes.

Diagnostic aids. History and physical examination, use of smears with the 20% potassium hydroxide solution, culture on Sabouraud's medium to identify the offending organism, biopsy.

Relation to systemic disease. None.

Differential diagnosis. Sycosis vulgaris, folliculitis.

Therapy. There is a tendency toward spontaneous involution of lesions. Use hot normal saline compresses several times daily to keep lesions draining and remove surface detritus. Administer systemic antibiotics. Systemic griseofulvin may be necessary in some cases.

Tinea Capitis

Synonym. Ringworm of the scalp, tinea tonsurans.

Sites of predilection. Scalp, neck, face.

Objective signs. The lesions begin in the scalp as one or more small, pinkish, scaly macules which spread peripherally. Because of invasion of the hair cortex by the fungus, the hairs become weak and break off close to the scalp, leaving well-defined areas of partial alopecia. The mature lesion is well-defined, round, discrete or confluent, and covered with an adherent grayish scale. Bro-

ken-off hairs in the involved area are lusterless.

Secondary pyogenic infection may develop, producing raised, boggy, tender lesions, which are covered with pustules and pus crusts. This complication, known as kerion, may vary in size from 2-10 cm in diameter.

Lesions composed of concentric rings and annular lesions may appear on the scalp, face or neck.

Subjective symptoms. The dry scaly lesions may cause mild pruritus. The lesions of kerion cause severe pain.

Etiology. This contagious disease is most commonly caused by *Microsporum audouini* (human type) or *Microsporum canis* (animal type). *M canis* infects cats, dogs and monkeys and is transmitted to humans. *Trichophyton tonsurans* and *Trichophyton violaceum* also cause ringworm of the scalp.

Histopathology. The ectothrix organisms (*M audouini* and *M canis*), as well as the other organisms, begin invasion of the hair root within the follicle. The cortex of the hair is weakened by the hyphae and spores which may be found throughout the hair shaft.

Diagnostic aids. The Wood light is valuable in the diagnosis of tinea capitis caused by *M audouini* and *M canis*. The hair in the affected area glows with a bluish-green fluorescence, when exposed to this light. The Wood light is of no value in tinea capitis caused by other organisms.

Direct examination of hair, using 20% potassium hydroxide solution will reveal hyphae and spores, thus establishing the fungus origin of the disease in a few minutes.

Culture on Sabouraud's medium is essential to identify the specific offending organism.

Relation to systemic disease. None.

Differential diagnosis. Seborrheic dermatitis, psoriasis.

Therapy. Griseofulvin, an antifungal antibiotic, administered systemically, cures tinea capitis. In order to comply with health department regulations, the child's hair should be shaved or closely clipped and a washable cap should be worn at all times.

There is no satisfactory, commercially available topical fungicide for the treatment of these patients.

Traction Alopecia

Synonym. Alopecia liminaris frontalis.

Sites of predilection. The hair margin, on the forehead and anterior to the ears.

Objective signs. The condition may begin on the forehead or anterior to the ears as a scant, scaling, macular eruption which does not produce subjective symptoms. The eventual picture is a symmetric band-like area of baldness which extends from one preauricular area across the forehead at the hair margin to the other preauricular area. The baldness produced is usually permanent, unless the traction is discontinued. Other variants of this condition may be produced inadvertently by light hair braiding or tight hair curlers.

Subjective symptoms. None.

Etiology. The condition is more common in blacks and is caused by excessive traction on the hair in forming braids. Excessive brushing with a very stiff brush may also cause this condition.

Histopathology. There is follicular atrophy.

Diagnostic aids. Clinical appearance and history.

Relation to systemic disease. None.

Differential diagnosis. Seborrheic dermatitis, scarring alopecias of other types.

Therapy. Discontinue the practice of strenuous brushing and the formation of tight braids. Local therapy is of no value.

Trichorrhexis Nodosa

Synonym. None.

Sites of predilection. Scalp.

Objective signs. There is diminution of hair in the involved area. The lesion may be circumscribed or

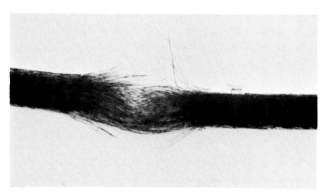

Trichorrhexis nodosa

universal. The condition most commonly occurs in the scalp but may involve the ears, the axillae or the pubic area. There is longitudinal splitting of the hair shaft at intervals producing the minute grayish nodes observed on gross examination. Several nodes may develop on a single hair. Hairs fracture easily on slight trauma.

Subjective symptoms. None.

Etiology. In many cases this defect is an acquired condition due to trauma of varying sorts to the hair shaft. In other instances this may be a genetic defect which may or may not be associated with an aminoaciduria.

Histopathology. Examination of the nodes reveals longitudinal splitting of the hair shaft producing a formation which resembles two small paint brushes pushed together end to end.

Diagnostic aids. Microscopic examination of the hair.

Relation to systemic disease. Liver disease and Addison's disease may accompany this condition and also other hair diseases such as trichoschisis, hereditary wooly hair disease and Menkes' kinky hair syndrome.

Differential diagnosis. Other idiopathic atrophies of the hair.

Therapy. None.

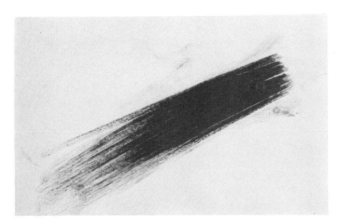

Trichostasis spinulosa

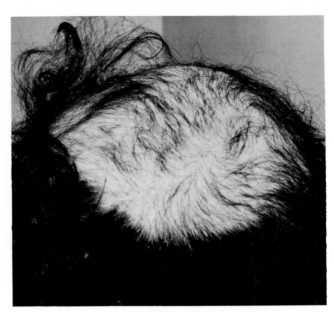

Trichotillomania

Trichostasis Spinulosa

Synonym. None.

Sites of predilection. Scalp and other hair-bearing areas.

Objective signs. This is a relatively common condition in young men and occurs in both sexes after middle age. Numerous small black spots resembling comedones develop on the scalp, forehead, temples and upper trunk. When examined with a lens, small projecting tufts of hair are found within these spots.

Subjective symptoms. None.

Etiology. Unknown.

Histopathology. The plugs removed from the follicles contain a bundle of short hairs.

Diagnostic aids. Microscopic examination.

Relation to systemic disease. None.

Differential diagnosis. Comedones.

Therapy. Manual removal of the short tufts of hair.

Trichotillomania

Synonym. None.

Sites of predilection. Scalp.

Objective signs. This type of baldness is self-inflicted. The patient forcibly extracts or twists the hair either inadvertently or purposefully. There are one or more, small or large, irregular areas of baldness without evidence of any active inflammatory process. The remaining hair in these areas of incomplete baldness varies in length from 1 mm-1 cm.

Subjective symptoms. Those produced by the mental aberrations of the patient.

Etiology. Emotional instability or accidental hair pulling.

Histopathology. Not specific.

Diagnostic aids. History, physical examination, psychoanalysis.

Relation to systemic disease. Mental illness, emotional instability.

Differential diagnosis. Alopecia areata, alopecia prematura, tinea capitis, alopecia of secondary syphilis.

Therapy. Explanation of cause, sedation or tranquilizers, psychotherapy.

CHAPTER 19

Lesions Involving the Mucous Membranes

Behçet's Syndrome

Synonym. Aphthosis. In the Middle East and Orient this entity appears to be a separate severe disorder. In the United States most physicians regard it as the serious end of a spectrum of diseases extending down to aphthosis.

Sites of predilection. Mouth, genitalia, eyes.

Objective signs. The initial lesions are small, superficial yellow ulcers on the buccal mucosa and/or the genitalia. A few weeks or months later ocular lesions initially develop as conjunctivitis but later extend into iritis and uveitis. Other complicating features which may develop are arthritis, thrombophlebitis, cardiac disorders, furunculosis, encephalitis, pulmonary lesions and other central nervous system disturbances.

Subjective symptoms. Fever and malaise may develop. Pain from ulcers. Blindness may follow uveitis. Other subjective symptoms are those attributed to organic involvement.

Etiology. The cause has not been determined.

Histopathology. The oral and genital lesions show nonspecific inflammatory changes. In central nervous system involvement there are multiple small foci of necrosis. The venules appear to be involved.

Diagnostic aids. Immune globulin studies, white count to rule out cyclic neutropenia. T and B lymphocytes may be decreased and null lymphocytes may be increased. Cellular and hormonal immunity is intact. Asian patients have pathergy, which is the ability to develop a local pustule 48 hours after a pinprick. The serum fibrinogens and alpha 2 macroglobulins may be elevated in severe cases.

Relation to systemic disease. Patients may develop systemic involvement as described above.

Differential diagnosis. Reiter's syndrome, aphthous stomatitis, cyclic neutropenia, leukemia.

Therapy. Supportive. No systemic therapy has proved beneficial.

Candidiasis

Synonym. Thrush, moniliasis.

Sites of predilection. Mouth, genitocrural region and other areas. (See Candidiasis in Chapter 14: Macular Eruptions.)

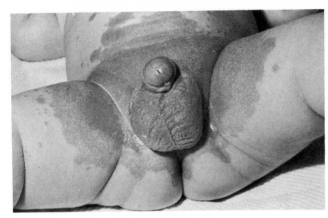

Candidal infection

Objective signs. On the tongue or buccal mucosa there are discrete or confluent whitish spots, which form a membrane resembling curdled milk. Forcible removal of this membrane produces bleeding. Similar lesions may be found in the vagina and under the prepuce. Between the thighs the lesions appear as a whitish film. For a more complete description of these and other lesions see Candidiasis in chapter 14.

Subjective symptoms. Depend on the extent of involvement. Symptoms may be absent or the patient may have pain.

Etiology. *Candida albicans.*

Histopathology. See Chapter 14.

Diagnostic aids. See Chapter 14.

Relation to systemic disease. See Chapter 14.

Differential diagnosis. Leukoplakia, lichen planus, syphilis.

Therapy. See Chapter 14.

Cheilitis, Actinic

Synonym. Cheilitis caused by sun exposure.

Sites of predilection. Vermilion surfaces of the lips.

Objective signs. There is edema of the lips and the vermilion border presents a dry, crusted and scaly appearance with radial fissures. In sailors, farmers and other individuals who are constantly exposed to sunlight, the vermilion surface becomes pale, excessively dry and covered with an adherent scale. Premalignant actinic keratoses are a frequent development.

Subjective symptoms. Discomfort because of the excessive dryness.

Etiology. Constant exposure to sunlight without adequate protection.

Histopathology. Hyperkeratosis with atrophy of the epidermis and senile elastosis in the cutis.

Diagnostic aids. Biopsy, history and physical examination.

Relation to systemic disease. None usually.

Differential diagnosis. Cheilitis exfoliativa, chronic contact dermatitis.

Therapy. Adequate protection from constant exposure to sunlight. Use of sunscreen cream. Removal of keratoses when they develop.

Cheilitis, Exfoliative

Synonym. Exfoliative dermatitis of the lips, cheilitis exfoliativa.

Sites of predilection. Lips.

Objective signs. The vermilion border of the lips is exceptionally dry and covered with a loosely adherent scale. Forcible removal of this scale may cause bleeding. Radial tissues may develop. The patient constantly moistens the lips with the tongue.

Subjective symptoms. Pain; discomfort is especially present when eating.

Etiology. The condition may be associated with atopic dermatitis or may be evidence of chronic contact reaction to dentifrices or toothpaste.

Histopathology. Hyperkeratosis and acanthosis. There is vascular dilatation of the papillary portion of the cutis and perivascular mononuclear and plasma cell infiltrate.

Diagnostic aids. History and physical examination, patch tests, search for foci of infection.

Relation to systemic disease. The condition may be

associated with atopic dermatitis.

Differential diagnosis. Erythema multiforme bullosum.

Therapy. Search for and remove the causative factor. Topical corticosteroid therapy is frequently of value. Discontinue use of toothpaste and mouth washes. Application of 2-3% salicylic acid in petrolatum to soften and remove excess scale.

Cheilitis Glandularis

Synonym. None.

Sites of predilection. Lips.

Objective signs. There is swelling of the lips caused by enlargement of the mucous glands. Over the mucous surfaces of the lips there are widely dilated openings of the mucous glands and constant exudation of mucus. Mucous glands are readily palpable and feel like small pebbles. When pressure is applied, mucous exudes through the openings. There may be associated enlargement of the mucous glands of the buccal and pharyngeal mucosae.

Subjective symptoms. Patients complain of a "sticky" feeling about the lips.

Etiology. Unknown.

Histopathology. Enlargement of the mucous glands and widely dilated mucous gland ducts.

Diagnostic aids. History and physical examination, biopsy.

Relation to systemic disease. None usually.

Differential diagnosis. Clinical appearance is characteristic.

Therapy. Discontinue smoking; use lozenges, astringent mouth washes and toothpaste. Use sodium bicarbonate as a dentifrice.

Cheilosis, Angular

Synonym. Perlèche.

Sites of predilection. Commissures of the lips.

Objective signs. These lesions, which are usually bilateral, are superficial or deep fissures at the commissures. The lesions extend a short distance onto the skin and the mucous membrane. The

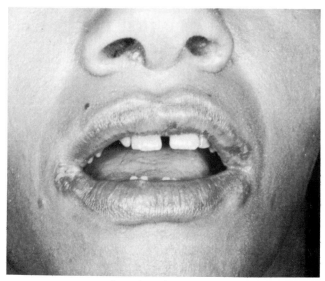

Angular cheilosis

mucous membrane in the involved area is usually thickened, macerated and covered with a whitish, boggy membrane. There may be an eczematous area on the skin surrounding the fissure, which is usually covered with a serous crust or whitish membrane. In extensive cases there may be marked discomfort when the mouth is opened.

Subjective symptoms. Vary from pruritus to severe pain.

Etiology. The condition may be associated with candidiasis, bacterial infections or nutritional deficiencies. Lip licking is the mechanical factor in the production of the lesions. Malocclusion or "sagging cheeks" are a major cause of this problem.

Histopathology. Nonspecific.

Diagnostic aids. Culture for *Candida albicans* on Sabouraud's medium, culture for other organisms on blood agar, history and physical examination.

Relation to systemic disease. The condition may be associated with candidiasis.

Differential diagnosis. The split papule of secondary syphilis.

Therapy. Clotrimazole cream or nystatin cream. Correct malocclusion.

Cysts (Retention) of the Mucous Membrane

Synonym. Mucous retention cyst.
Sites of predilection. Lips, tongue, buccal mucosa.
Objective signs. The lesions are usually single, non-tender, raised, noninflamed, fluctuant cysts. They are shiny, and covered with normal mucous membrane. They vary in size from 3-5 mm in diameter and contain a clear, thick fluid.
Subjective symptoms. None.
Etiology. Caused by closure of the mucous gland duct by trauma. Lip biting may be a causative factor.
Histopathology. A dilated mucous cyst.
Diagnostic aids. Biopsy.
Relation to systemic disease. None.
Differential diagnosis. Tumor of any type which may

Mucous retention cyst

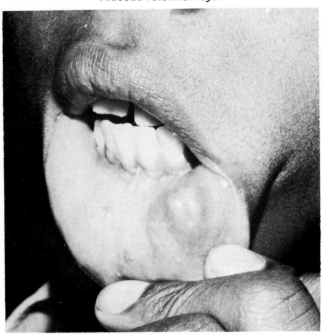

occur on the lips.
Therapy. Destruction of the cyst by electrodesiccation.

Fordyce's Disease

Synonym. None.
Sites of predilection. Lips and buccal mucosa, labia minora, penis, areolae of the nipples.
Objective signs. Few to numerous discrete, grouped or confluent, whitish or yellowish, noninflammatory, flat lesions. The condition may be extensive.
Subjective symptoms. None.
Etiology. Unknown.
Histopathology. The lesions are anomalous sebaceous glands.
Diagnostic aids. Biopsy.
Relation to systemic disease. None.
Differential diagnosis. Leukoplakia, lichen planus.
Therapy. No treatment is necessary for this benign condition. Patients should be reassured.

Leukoplakia

Synonym. None.
Sites of predilection. Tongue, buccal mucosa, genital area.
Objective signs. The lesions are sharply defined, round, oval or irregular, slightly raised, white or grayish, slow-growing, hyperkeratotic areas. The surface may not be removed by scraping. The lesions are irregular, hyperkeratotic and noninflammatory. Fissures may develop. These lesions are frequently precancerous.
Subjective symptoms. Some discomfort because of the presence of the hyperkeratotic lesion. Other symptoms may develop depending on the extent of the lesion.
Etiology. The oral lesions may be postinflammatory, due to poor dental hygiene, or associated with excessive smoking. Genital lesions of leukoplakia may develop in association with lichen sclerosus et atrophicus (kraurosis vulvae).

Histopathology. Hyperkeratosis and acanthosis, with the formation of dyskeratotic cells.

Diagnostic aids. Biopsy.

Relation to systemic disease. None.

Differential diagnosis. Lichen planus, lupus erythematosus, syphilis.

Therapy. Remove the irritating cause. Discontinue smoking. The lesion may be removed by excision or desiccation and curettage.

Lichen Planus

Synonym. None.

Sites of predilection. Buccal mucosa, flexor surfaces of the forearm, male genitalia, and lower extremities. The lesions may occur only in the mouth.

Objective signs. Well-defined, reticulated white lines, plaques or slightly elevated, smooth, whitish papules. Single white lines may appear on the

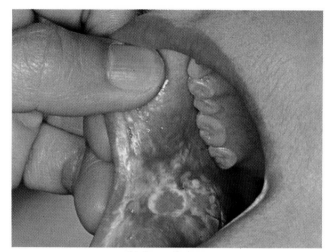

Lichen planus

buccal mucous membrane. These lesions may be the only objective sign of lichen planus or there may be associated lesions elsewhere. (See Lichen Planus in Chapter 15: Papular Eruptions.)

Diagnosis. Biopsy.

Differential diagnosis. Leukoplakia, lupus erythematosus, syphilis.

Therapy. See Chapter 15.

Lupus Erythematosus

Synonym. None.

Sites of predilection. Buccal mucosa and other parts of the body. (See Lupus Erythematosus in Chapter 14: Macular Eruptions.)

Objective signs. The lesions on the buccal mucosa are well-defined, whitish plaques, which are slightly thickened and have an irregular surface. The lesion is not a membrane and is not easily removed. Ulcers may develop.

Subjective symptoms. None.

Etiology. See Chapter 14.

Histopathology. See Chapter 14.

Diagnostic aids. See Chapter 14.

Lichen planus

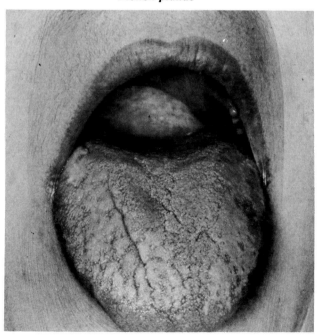

Relation to systemic disease. See Chapter 14.
Differential diagnosis. Leukoplakia, candidiasis, lichen planus, syphilis.
Therapy. See Chapter 14.

Macroglossia

Synonym. None.
Sites of predilection. None.
Objective signs. The entire tongue is enlarged.
Subjective symptoms. Obstruction of the airway may produce stridor and anxiety.
Etiology. The disease may be congenital or associated with hypothyroidism, mongolism or primary amyloidosis.
Histopathology. In hypothyroidism mucinous tissue is present in the dermis. In amyloidosis the abnormal protein allows deposition in the dermis.
Diagnostic aids. Biopsy with PAS and Congo red stains.
Relation to systemic disease. The relationship with hypothyroidism and amyloidosis has been mentioned.
Differential diagnosis. Angioneurotic edema and various benign or malignant tumors may mimic macroglossia. Usually the neoplasias do not involve the entire tongue so its structure is nodular.
Therapy. None effective.

Noma

Synonym. Cancrum oris.
Sites of predilection. Mouth.
Objective signs. This condition which is really a symptom complex and usually unilateral, may begin as ulcerative stomatitis, or it may begin with the appearance of a small bulla. The lesions become gangrenous, progress rapidly, and form large, excavated, necrotic ulcers with irregular, undermined margins. The base of the ulcer is usually covered with a thick, grayish, membranous exudate, which when removed, leaves a granulomatous surface. The condition may be quite extensive, eventually causing a portion of the face to slough.
Subjective symptoms. Those associated with the underlying systemic disease. Intense pain in the involved area.
Etiology. Chronic infections, recurrent acute infections, tumors and vasculitis may produce this condition.
Histopathology. Nonspecific.
Diagnostic aids. History and physical examination, biopsy.
Relation to systemic disease. Agranulocytosis, leishmaniasis, measles, avitaminosis, lethal midline granuloma. Lymphoma may cause this symptom complex.
Differential diagnosis. Syphilis carcinoma, tuberculosis.
Therapy. Treat the underlying condition. A high protein diet with vitamin supplements, and good nursing care are indicated.

Pemphigus Vulgaris

Synonym. None.
Sites of predilection. Mucous membranes and other parts of the body. (See Pemphigus Vulgaris in Chapter 16: Vesicular Eruptions.)
Objective symptoms. On the buccal mucosa the bullae rupture shortly after formation, leaving large denuded areas. The condition may be extensive and involve the entire buccal mucosa, the hard and soft palates and the pharynx. The lips are thickened, covered with blood crusts and bullae, and are fissured. The female genitalia may show extensive involvement, similar in character. The lesions in pemphigus vulgaris may be limited to the mucous membranes or may involve the entire body.
Subjective symptoms. Pain. Inability to swallow if the mucous membranes are extensively involved. Generalized malaise.
Etiology. Unknown.
Histopathology. See Chapter 16.

Diagnostic aids. See Chapter 16.
Relation to systemic disease. Pemphigus vulgaris is a systemic disease.
Differential diagnosis. Erythema multiforme bullosum, dermatitis herpetiformis, lesions of syphilis, benign mucous membrane pemphigus.
Therapy. See Chapter 16.

Peutz-Jeghers Syndrome

Synonym. Periorificial lentiginosis.
Sites of predilection. Oral mucosa, hands, feet.
Objective signs. Round, oval or irregularly shaped, pigmented macules, 1-5 mm in diameter are distributed over the gums, buccal mucosa, hard palate and the lips. Pigment spots may develop on the face, hands and feet.
Subjective symptoms. The cutaneous lesions are asymptomatic.
Etiology. This is an inherited condition and is due to an antosomal dominant gene.
Histopathology. Increase in melanin in the basal layer.
Diagnostic aids. Biopsy, radiologic examination of the gastrointestinal tract, gastroscopy.
Relation to systemic disease. These patients have concomitant gastrointestinal polyposis which may undergo malignant transformation.
Differential diagnosis. Addison's disease, freckles, incontinentia pigmenti.
Therapy. None for the cutaneous lesions. The underlying gastrointestinal disease should be treated.

Stomatitis, Aphthous

Synonym. Canker sores.
Sites of predilection. Buccal mucosa, tongue, genitalia.
Objective signs. The lesions are variously sized, discrete and confluent, sharply defined, shallow ulcers, which vary in size from 2 mm-2 cm in diameter. Individual ulcers have a central, yellowish-white basement membrane, and are surrounded by a bright red areola. The lesions may

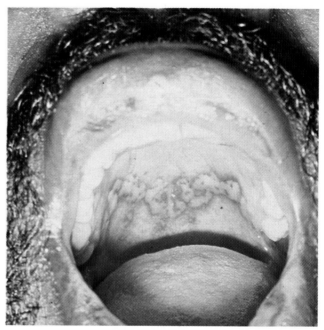

Aphthous stomatitis

be few or numerous and, if extensive, cause marked destruction of the mucous membrane. Occasionally these ulcers become gangrenous.
Subjective symptoms. The lesions are painful. If the condition is extensive the patient may have difficulty in swallowing. Lesions in the genital area cause difficulty in walking and dyspareunia.
Etiology. Unknown. This condition may represent the mild part of a spectrum varying up to Behçet's syndrome.
Histopathology. Nonspecific.
Diagnostic aids. Clinical appearance, history and physical examination.
Differential diagnosis. Syphilis, tuberculosis, cancrum oris.
Therapy. Tetracycline mouth wash every 2-3 hours promptly relieves pain and heals the lesions. The condition is marked by recurrences. Systemic prednisone may be necessary for relief.

Stomatitis, Bismuth or Mercury

Synonym. None.

Sites of predilection. Mouth.

Objective signs. There is a thin, blue or dark gray, stippled line which occurs on the gums at the insertion of the teeth, forming a peculiar festooned appearance. The condition is seen on both the buccal and lingual sides of the gums. Occasionally there is redness and swelling of the gums. The tongue may be coated and the breath is usually fetid.

Subjective symptoms. Pain may or may not be a symptom.

Etiology. Caused by deposits of metallic bismuth or mercury in the gums. They may be associated with poor dental hygiene. Heavy metal deposit is probably caused by the patient's idiosyncrasy to the drug.

Histopathology. Nonspecific.

Diagnostic aids. History and physical examination, clinical appearance.

Relation to systemic disease. The condition which necessitated the administration of the heavy metal. Kidney damage may be associated with the bismuth or mercury line.

Differential diagnosis. The normal bluish pigmentation of gums and mucous membranes common to black people.

Therapy. Discontinue the drug. Institute proper dental hygiene.

Syphilis, Early Mucous Membrane Lesions

Synonym. Mucous patches, condylomata lata, split papules, chancre.

Objective signs. Chancre. Over 95% of all initial lesions occur on the genitalia. In the remaining 5% the lesions may be found on the tongue, buccal mucosa, lips, nipples, fingers and elsewhere. The initial lesion is usually a single, well-defined, markedly infiltrated ulcer with an eroded crusted surface. Multiple chancres are unusual. The clinical appearance of the lesion is altered because of the location. There is satellite adenopathy.

Mucous erosive lesions (mucous patches). These simple erosions are oval or round, varying in size from 1-2 cm in diameter. They are well-defined, superficial, reddish or grayish, and do not have any inflammatory areola. The lesions may be elevated, infiltrated and covered with grayish or whitish membrane.

Hypertrophic eroded papules (condylomata lata). These multiple lesions are found between apposing surfaces. They are well-defined, flat-topped papules varying from 5 mm-2 cm in diameter. The surface is covered with a grayish or whitish, moist membrane.

Split papules. These lesions, which occur at the commissures of the lips, are reddish papules in which there is a central split or fissure. This fissure is covered with a grayish or whitish membrane.

Subjective symptoms. Vary from none to moderate pain.

Etiology. Treponema pallidum. All of these are moist lesions of early syphilis and the *T pallidum* may be demonstrated from any of them by darkfield examination.

Histopathology. See Chapter 9: Sexually Transmitted Diseases.

Diagnostic aids. See Chapter 9.

Differential diagnosis. Aphthous stomatitis, fusospirillosis, diphtheria, leukoplakia.

Therapy. See Chapter 9.

Syphilis, Late Mucous Membrane Lesions

Synonym. See Syphilis in Chapter 9: Sexually Transmitted Diseases.

Sites of predilection. Mucous membranes of oropharynx and the tongue.

Objective signs. The lesions are single or multiple, excavated or punched-out ulcers. The base of the ulcer may be covered with a grayish-green membrane, but there is little or no discharge. These lesions are destructive and may distort the entire pharynx. Such lesions occurring on the nasal mucosa produce perforation of the nasal septum.

When the tongue is involved by late syphilis, a solitary gumma may develop, or because of the dense inflammatory infiltration and subsequent healing, the tongue may become hard, smooth, thickened and scarred.

Subjective symptoms. Little or no pain.

Etiology. This is a late manifestation of syphilis (gumma).

Histopathology. See Chapter 9.

Diagnostic aids. See Syphilis in Chapter 9.

Relation to systemic disease. This is a systemic disease. See Chapter 9.

Differential diagnosis. Aphthous stomatitis, geographic tongue.

Therapy. See Chapter 9.

Tongue, Black Hairy

Synonym. Lingua nigra.

Sites of predilection. Tongue.

Objective signs. The lesion, which usually appears in the midline of the tongue, and may involve the entire central portion, is dark brown, black or dark gray. It is composed of hair-like projections which are actually prolongations of the papillae. The condition may develop quickly or slowly, and is of variable duration.

Subjective symptoms. Usually none, although the patient may complain of a bad taste in the mouth.

Etiology. Unknown. Local or systemic tetracyclines or penicillin have been responsible for the production of these lesions in many patients. Excessive use of tobacco is another cause.

Histopathology. The papillae are hyperkeratotic and hypertrophied.

Diagnostic aids. History and physical examination, culture on Sabouraud's medium, biopsy.

Relation to systemic disease. None.

Differential diagnosis. Condition is characteristic in appearance.

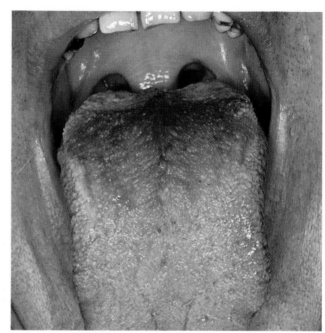

Black hairy tongue

Therapy. Reassure the patient that it is not a serious systemic disease. Eliminate causative drugs.

Tongue, Burning

Synonym. Glossodynia.

Sites of predilection. Tongue.

Objective signs. This condition, which commonly occurs in men and women beyond middle age, produces severe burning pain. The subjective symptoms may be limited to the front half of the tongue and are occasionally unilateral.

Etiology. Emotional tension or some underlying systemic disease.

Histopathology. No change noted.

Diagnostic aids. History and physical examination, adequate laboratory studies to rule out systemic disease.

Relation to systemic disease. Pernicious anemia, hypochromic anemia and avitaminoses can be causative factors.

Differential diagnosis. There is no visible abnormality.

Therapy. There is no specific treatment. Palliative therapy with topical anesthetic lozenges or solutions may be helpful. Search for and remove the underlying cause. Treat any systemic disease present.

Tongue, Geographic

Synonym. Transitory benign migrating plaques.

Sites of predilection. Tongue.

Objective signs. The condition begins as one or more small, sharply defined, grayish or yellowish, arcuate areas which spread peripherally, producing asymptomatic, superficial, bizarre, geographical figures which are reddish in color and may or may not have slightly raised, grayish or yellowish borders. The papillae are flattened. Concentric rings may be formed, or two or more patches may become confluent, producing polycyclic figures. The condition has an acute course. The lesions ultimately disappear and leave no trace. The condition is recurrent.

Subjective symptoms. None or slight discomfort.

Etiology. Unknown.

Histopathology. Acanthosis and parakeratosis with edema of the rete. There is perivascular mononuclear cell infiltration and a slight chronic in-

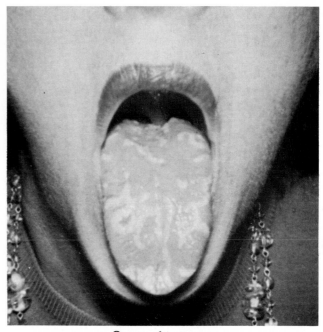

Geographic tongue

flammatory infiltrate in the upper dermis.

Diagnostic aids. The clinical appearance is diagnostic.

Relation to systemic disease. None.

Differential diagnosis. Leukoplakia, secondary syphilis, erythema multiforme.

Therapy. No specific therapy. Topical anesthetic lozenges or solutions may give relief from subjective symptoms.

CHAPTER 20

Sweat Gland Lesions

Anhidrosis

Synonym. Absence of sweating.

Sites of predilection. Generalized.

Objective signs. The skin is exceptionally dry because of the absence of sweating.

Subjective symptoms. Excessive dryness. These patients cannot tolerate heat.

Etiology. Unknown.

Histopathology. Sweat glands are absent or atrophied.

Diagnostic aids. Biopsy.

Relation to systemic disease. This condition is common in ichthyosis, exfoliative dermatitis, congenital ectodermal defect, scleroderma, extensive psoriasis and roentgen dermatitis. Localized anhidrosis may occur due to lesions in the central nervous system.

Differential diagnosis. Related to the conditions productive of the anhidrosis.

Therapy. There is no curative therapy. Use of lubricants may be of value in relieving subjective symptoms.

Bromhidrosis

Synonym. Stinking sweat, "BO."

Sites of predilection Feet, axillae, genital area.

Objective signs. This condition is not usually present until after puberty. The patient who has bromhidrosis does not necessarily have excessive perspiration. The odor varies in the same individual from time to time. It may be mildly unpleasant or a strong, penetrating stench.

Subjective symptoms. The patient is not usually aware of the body stench.

Etiology. The odor may be caused by bacterial contamination or fermentation of apocrine sweat.

Histopathology. Nonspecific.

Diagnostic aids. Clinical symptoms are diagnostic.

Relation to systemic disease. Many systemic diseases such as uremia, carcinoma and other debilitating illnesses are productive of an unpleasant body odor.

Differential diagnosis. The odor may be caused by the clothing the patient is wearing, his occupation, *etc.*

Therapy. Simple hygiene. The use of deodorants or perfumes.

Chromhidrosis

Synonym. Colored sweat.

Sites of predilection. Face, axillae, genital area.

Objective signs. This is a rare condition characterized by the appearance of colored sweat. In the majority of these cases some affection of the apocrine sweat glands is responsible for the production of this unusual symptom. The discoloration may be brown, red, green or black.

Subjective symptoms. None.

Etiology. The condition may be caused by the presence of bacteria on the skin surface, colored substances on the skin or drug ingestion.

Histopathology. Nonspecific.

Diagnostic aids. Clinical appearance is characteristic. Cultures for bacteria and fungi should be performed.

Relation to systemic disease. None usually.

Differential diagnosis. Clinical appearance is characteristic.

Therapy. Restoration of normal hygiene. The use of soap and water will remove the pigment.

Hidradenitis Suppurativa

Synonym. Sweat gland abscesses.

Sites of predilection. Axillae, genitocrural area, perianal region, areolae of the breasts.

Objective signs. Few to numerous, deep-seated abscesses occur in the axillae. These lesions, which involve the apocrine sweat glands, are discrete or confluent, variously sized, fluctuant nodules containing pus. Deep subcutaneous sinuses develop. These sinus tracts which are surrounded by dense scar formations drain constantly. Spontaneous healing seldom occurs. Involvement of the perineum may cause a clinical picture suggestive of lymphogranuloma venereum.

Subjective symptoms. Pain.

Etiology. The precipitating factor may be an allergic contact dermatitis caused by deodorants, with subsequent secondary pyogenic infection. Axillary shaving may also initiate the infection. Varieties of staphylococci or gram-negative organisms are commonly recovered on culture.

Histopathology. This is cystic dilatation of the deep part of the glands with destruction of the epithelial lining. There is evidence of an acute inflammatory reaction and subcutaneous abscess formation.

Diagnostic aids. Cultures of the pus on blood agar with sensitivity tests for antibiotic selection.

Relation to systemic disease. Patients with this disease often have perifolliculitis of the scalp and cystic acne.

Differential diagnosis. Clinical picture is characteristic.

Therapy. Drainage of the large fluctuant lesions will temporarily relieve discomfort, but may also help form chronic draining sinuses. Systemic administration of the antibiotic of choice as determined by sensitivity tests should be used, but is only partially effective. If the response to antibiotic therapy is not satisfactory, surgical excision of the involved areas is necessary.

Hyperhidrosis

Synonym. Excessive sweating.

Sites of predilection. May be generalized or localized. The lesions may occur on the palms, soles, the axillae, over the entire body, or may be unilateral.

Objective signs. There is an excessive production of sweat, particularly in times of stress. The or slightly to one side. As the nail grows, fine On the palms and soles the skin becomes soggy, pale pink in color, and appears water-logged. The feet may become tender.

Localized, unilateral hyperhidrosis may involve half the face, a small area over one scapula, one arm or any discrete or isolated area of the body. This condition exists as a result of some organic neurologic lesion.

Subjective symptoms. Discomfort caused by excessive sweating.

Etiology. In generalized cases, or in those involving only the palms and soles, the condition may be caused by emotional tension, drugs, excessive heat, or debilitating diseases such as tuberculosis, pneumonia and leukemia.

Histopathology. Dilatation of the sweat glands in the involved area.

Diagnostic aids. The clinical appearance is characteristic. The patient should have a thorough physical examination and history. Study for systemic disease.

Relation to systemic disease. Tuberculosis, leukemia, nutritional disturbances, hyperthyroidism, mental illness.

Differential diagnosis. None necessary. The clinical appearance is characteristic.

Therapy. Treatment of the underlying cause. Topical aluminum chloride solutions may provide temporary relief.

Miliaria Rubra

Synonym. Prickly heat.

Sites of predilection. May be generalized. Frequently limited to the folds of the neck, the axillae and the crural regions of infants.

Objective signs. There is an acute onset of a profuse eruption of numerous pinpoint or slightly larger papules, vesicles or papulovesicles. Occasionally, numerous small pustules are scattered throughout the eruption. One or more of these pustules may develop into furuncles. The eruption is common in infants during hot weather. It may be precipitated in the winter by the wearing of too much clothing. It may appear in the winter months if the child is kept in an overheated room with poor ventilation. If the condition is neglected or too vigorously treated, it may become eczematized, particularly in the skin folds.

Subjective symptoms. Pruritus and burning. If furuncles develop the patient has pain.

Etiology. Contributing factors are excessive heat and humidity, and indulgence in use of alcohol, citrus fruits and soft drinks by those people who have a tendency to hyperhidrosis.

Histopathology. Cystic dilatation of sweat ducts because of occlusion of the orifices, with the presence of an acute inflammatory reaction in the upper cutis about the sweat glands.

Diagnostic aids. The clinical appearance is characteristic.

Relation to systemic disease. The condition is common in obesity, alcoholism and in those individuals suffering from debilitating diseases.

Differential diagnosis. Folliculitis, contact dermatitis, atopic dermatitis, steroid acne.

Therapy. Avoid exposure to excessive heat and wear light clothing. Infants should be kept in a well-ventilated or air conditioned room and wear a minimum of clothing. Cold compresses of Burow's solution (1:32) are of great value. Bland dusting powders used between apposing surfaces also give relief.

CHAPTER 21

Nail Lesions

Anonychia

Synonym. Congenital absence of nails.
Sites of predilection. Fingernails, toenails.
Objective signs. There is usually total absence of all nails on the upper and lower extremities. The nail folds are absent and the dorsal surfaces of the distal phalanges are thin and red.
Subjective symptoms. None usually.
Etiology. Congenital.
Histopathology. Absence of nail fold and absence of eponychium.
Diagnostic aids. Clinical appearance is characteristic.
Relation to systemic disease. Other congenital ectodermal deformities may be present.
Differential diagnosis. Clinical appearance is characteristic.
Therapy. None effective.

Atrophy of the Nail

Synonym. Atrophia unguium.
Sites of predilection. Fingernails, toenails.
Objective signs. Partial or complete atrophy of the nail plates. The condition most commonly occurs on the fingers, and the plates appear lusterless, friable and distorted.
Subjective symptoms. None.
Etiology. Acquired or congenital. May be caused by radiation therapy.
Histopathology. Nonspecific.
Diagnostic aids. Clinical appearance is characteristic.
Relation to systemic disease. None.
Differential diagnosis. Fungus infections.
Therapy. None effective.

Dystrophy, Median Nail

Synonym. Median nail raphe, dystrophia unguium mediana canaliformis.
Sites of predilection. Thumb nails.
Objective signs. A split may develop as the nail emerges from the cuticle. It may be in the center or slightly to one side. As the nail grows, fine cracks develop in the plate on either side of the groove. The canal-like defect extends on the longitudinal axis partially or completely down the plate to the free edge. After a period of a few months to several years the plates return to normal. The condition may be recurrent.
Subjective symptoms. None.

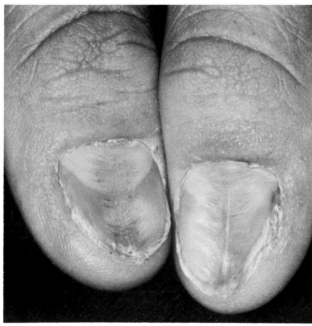

Median nail dystrophy

Etiology. Unknown.
Histopathology. Nonspecific.
Diagnostic aids. None.
Therapy. Condition is self-limited.

Eczematous Eruption of Periungual Tissues

Synonym. None.
Sites of predilection. Fingernails and surrounding tissue.
Objective signs. There is usually an ill-defined, confluent, infiltrated or edematous, scaling and exudative eruption involving the nail folds. After the eruption has been present for a month or longer, changes appear in the nail plates. The nails are discolored, distorted, friable, transversely ridged and frequently shortened at the free edge.
Subjective symptoms. Pruritus.
Etiology. This condition usually develops as a result of

sensitization or primary irritation to some contacted substance. Household detergents, nail polish, paint remover, acids or alkalies, or photographic materials may be causative agents.
Histopathology. Nonspecific.
Diagnostic aids. Culture to rule out fungus infections.
Relation to systemic disease. None.
Differential diagnosis. Onychomycosis, psoriasis of the nails.
Therapy. In chronic cases the nail defect may be permanent. In acute cases remove the patient from exposure to the irritating substance and apply one of the topical corticosteroid preparations.

Hang Nail

Synonym. Agnail.
Sites of predilection. Nail folds of the fingers.
Objective signs. Small tags of skin, attached at the proximal end and free at the distal end, occur in the lateral, medial and proximal nail folds. If these filaments are pulled back they tend to tear into the tissue and become a site of pyogenic infection.
Subjective symptoms. Pruritus or pain.
Etiology. The condition may develop as a result of too frequent use of household detergents or solvents. Biting of the fingernails is a predisposing factor.
Histopathology. Nonspecific.
Diagnostic aids. Clinical appearance is characteristic.
Relation to systemic disease. None.
Differential diagnosis. Clinical appearance is characteristic.
Therapy. Clip the tags of the skin with sharp scissors.

Ingrown Nail

Synonym. Unguis incarnatus.
Sites of predilection. Toenails; most commonly the great toenail.
Objective signs. This condition most commonly involves the great toenail. The involved nail fold becomes swollen, red and exudes serum or pus. A pyogenic granuloma frequently appears in the

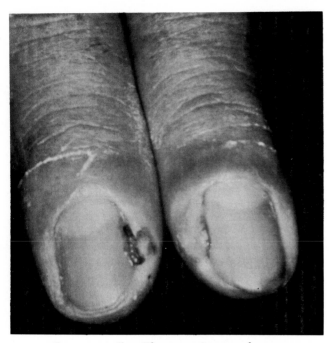

Ingrown nails with pyogenic granulomas

fold and grows across the nail plate. The sharp sides of the nail plate cut into the nail grooves, opening avenues for entrance of infection. Cellulitis and lymphangitis may develop.

Subjective symptoms. Severe pain.

Etiology. Faulty trimming of the nails.

Histopathology. Nonspecific.

Diagnostic aids. Clinical picture is characteristic, culture of the exudate may be necessary.

Relation to systemic disease. None usually.

Differential diagnosis. Onychomycosis, pyogenic granuloma, cellulitis and other tumors.

Therapy. Eradicate secondary infection by the use of hot soaks and the application of an appropriate antibiotic. Remove the portion of the nail which is cutting into the tissue. It may be necessary to fulgurate the pyogenic granuloma. Pack the nail fold with cotton so that when the nail regrows it will find the nail groove. Institute proper nail hygiene.

Wear properly fitting shoes. Surgical removal of part of the nail may be necessary in severe cases.

Leukonychia

Synonym. White nails.

Sites of predilection. Any or all nails may be involved.

Objective signs. The nails become white.

Subjective symptoms. None.

Etiology. Leukonychia may be produced by trauma or associated with many chronic illnesses. It may also be a congenital defect.

Histopathology. Cellular remnants in the nail plate are believed to cause the white color. The cellular material results from abnormal keratinization induced by the underlying disorder.

Diagnostic aids. Nail culture to rule out fungal infections.

Relation to systemic disease. Chronic anemia, renal or hepatic diseases can cause leukonychia.

Differential diagnosis. Tinea infection and trauma have to be carefully eliminated as diagnostic possibilities.

Therapy. No effective specific therapy.

Leukonychia

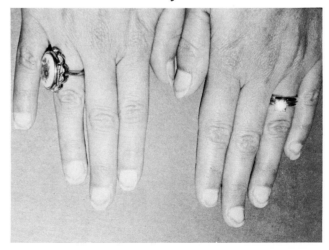

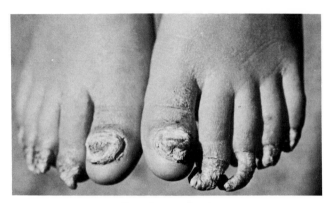

Onychogryphosis

Onychogryphosis

Synonym. Claw nail, talon nail.
Sites of predilection. Toenails.
Objective signs. This condition, which may be acquired or congenital, and involve one or more nails, is characterized by a hypertrophic overgrowth of the nail plate. It may appear as a complication of chronic scaling dermatoses or in association with keratoderma palmaris et plantaris. The nail plates are brittle and friable. In cases of extreme hypertrophy, the nail plates may become greatly elongated and claw-like. Simple hypertrophy of the nail is known as onychauxis.
Subjective symptoms. None usually.
Etiology. Acquired or congenital.
Histopathology. Marked thickening of the nail plate.
Diagnostic aids. Culture to rule out fungus infections, history and physical examination.
Relation to systemic disease. This condition may develop in obese individuals, arthritic patients and in the aged.
Differential diagnosis. Fungus infection of the nail bed.
Therapy. Mechanical removal of the nail plate by the use of clippers or electric drill. Surgical removal may be necessary.

Onycholysis

Synonym. None.
Sites of predilection. Fingernails.
Objective signs. This condition, characterized by separation of the nail plate from the nail bed, usually begins with the development of a brownish arc or brownish spot at the distal edge of the nail. The condition is slowly progressive and may extend from the free edge of the nail to the lanula, or may involve only a portion of the nail. The nail plates are lusterless.
Subjective symptoms. None.
Etiology. The separation may be caused by overzealous cleansing under the nails or constant immersion in household detergents. Nail separation may also be associated with systemic diseases or other dermatoses. Dirt and other detritus may collect in the space between the nail plate and the bed. It is rarely due to pathogenic fungi. Organisms cultured from this area are usually opportunistic. In other instances this lysis may be a reaction to light in a patient receiving a photoactive drug such as tetracycline.
Histopathology. Nonspecific.
Diagnostic aids. Clinical appearance is characteristic; thorough physical examination and history.
Relation to systemic disease. It may be associated with hypothyroidism, pellagra or psoriasis.
Differential diagnosis. Fungus infection, psoriasis of the nails.
Therapy. Avoid immersion in soapy water, detergents or solvents. Avoid overzealous cleansing of the nails. A useful local application is 4% thymol in 95% alcohol applied three times daily. Keep the uninvolved fingers dry.

Onychomadesis

Synonym. Nail shedding.
Sites of predilection. Fingernails, toenails.
Objective signs. One, several or all nails may be involved. The nail separation becomes evident just as it emerges from the cuticle. If only one or two

nails are involved due to trauma, the new nail growth begins before the old nail completely separates. If nail shedding occurs as part of an exfoliative dermatitis syndrome or a bullous drug eruption, next nail growth will not become evident until 6-8 weeks after the acute systemic illness subsides. If the condition is due to poorly fitting foot gear it will be recurrent. If the nail shedding is due to epidermolysis bullosum, the nail beds become scarred and new nail growth does not occur.

Subjective symptoms. Usually none.

Etiology. Trauma, poorly fitting shoes, tight panty hose, exfoliative dermatitis, bullous drug eruption, congenital defect, epidermolysis bullosum, other systemic illnesses.

Histopathology. The histopathologic picture may or may not be specific depending on the basic cause of the problem.

Diagnostic aids. Biopsy of the nail bed.

Relation to systemic disease. May be part of the clinical picture of epidermolysis bullosum, bullous drug eruption, vascular insufficiency, or a prolonged febrile illness.

Differential diagnosis. Lichen planus or psoriasis involvement of nails, yellow nail syndrome, Beau's lines.

Therapy. Treat the underlying cause.

Onychomycosis

Synonym. Ringworm of the nails.

Sites of predilection. Fingernails, toenails.

Objective signs. The involved nail plate is dark, thickened, friable, distorted and usually shortened at the free edge. The nail plate is separated from the nail bed by a dense, hyperkeratotic or caseous substance. In some instances almost the entire nail may be destroyed by the disease process. The condition may involve all of the nails on both upper and lower extremities or only one or two nails may be involved. The condition is frequently limited to one or both of the great toenails.

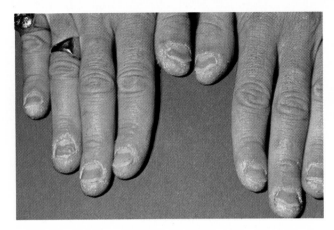

Onychomycosis

Subjective symptoms. Usually none except embarrassment because of the cosmetic defect.

Etiology. Superficial dermatophytes or *Candida albicans*.

Histopathology. By special staining techniques, filaments of the fungi may be seen in the nail bed.

Diagnostic aids. Recognition of fungi by use of the potassium hydroxide preparation, culture on Sabouraud's medium to determine the offending organism.

Relation to systemic disease. None.

Differential diagnosis. Psoriasis of the nails, traumatic onychia.

Therapy. Griseofulvin is effective on systemic administration in the treatment of dermatophyte infections. Favus nails and those caused by *C albicans* have a very poor prognosis. For therapy of *Candida* nail infections, see Candidial Paronychia.

Onychophagia

Synonym. Nail biting.

Sites of predilection. Fingernails.

Objective signs. The nail plates are greatly shortened and irregular at the free edge. The degree of deformity is variable. Some patients even bite the nail plate back to the midportion of the nail bed. In such individuals the distal ends of the fingers become bulbous and extend over the position usually occupied by the free edge of the nail.

Subjective symptoms. Those usually associated with emotional stress.

Etiology. Emotional imbalance.

Histopathology. Nonspecific.

Diagnostic aids. Clinical appearance is characteristic; thorough history and physical examination.

Relation to systemic disease. Associated with tension states.

Differential diagnosis. The clinical appearance is characteristic.

Therapy. Sedation, psychotherapy.

Onychorrhexis

Synonym. Brittleness of the nails.

Sites of predilection. Fingernails.

Objective signs. The nail plates are lusterless and thin. There is frequently sagittal splitting or peeling of the nail plates. Plates are shortened at the free edge.

Subjective symptoms. None.

Etiology. The condition may be caused by nail polish, polish removers, self-inflicted trauma, aging or disorders associated with poor manufacturing of the nail plate.

Histopathology. Nonspecific.

Diagnostic aids. Clinical appearance is characteristic.

Relation to systemic disease. This condition is occasionally observed in emotional tension, hypothyroidism and in protein deficiency diseases or the aged.

Differential diagnosis. Clinical appearance is characteristic.

Therapy. Avoid the use of nail polish and polish remover. The nails should be kept short and the patient should be encouraged to wear gloves while at work. A file or an emery board should be used to keep the nail plates short. Treat any underlying systemic disease.

Onychotillomania

Synonym. None.

Sites of predilection. Any nail.

Objective signs. One or many nails are evulsed.

Subjective symptoms. Variable, usually none.

Etiology. The patient is mentally ill.

Histopathology. Nonspecific.

Diagnostic aids. None.

Relation to systemic disease. None.

Differential diagnosis. Trauma can be ruled out clinically.

Therapy. Psychotherapy.

Paronychia, Candidal

Synonym. None.

Sites of predilection. Proximal nail folds and nail plates.

Objective signs. There is swelling of the proximal nail fold and the medial and lateral folds. Thick, white, caseous material may be expressed in acute cases. Manipulation of the nail fold is not usually painful. The nail plates have a greenish-brown color, particularly on the sides and at the proximal portions. There is occasionally some sealing of the nail plate and distortion of the most proximal portion. In chronic cases the entire nail plate is distorted.

Subjective symptoms. Pruritus or slight pain.

Etiology. Candida albicans. The condition is common in housewives. Immersion in detergents or alkaline solutions destroys the protective pterygium of the proximal nail fold and allows easy access to bacteria and fungi.

Histopathology. Nonspecific.

Diagnostic aids. Culture on Sabouraud's medium for yeast.

Relation to systemic disease. None usually. Administration of broad spectrum antibiotics may cause the condition or aggravate previously existing disease. Patients with debilitating diseases or those who are immunosuppressed may be more prone to acquire this disorder.

Differential diagnosis. Paronychia caused by pyogenic bacteria.

Therapy. Avoid immersion in soapy solutions, detergent solutions, solvents or other irritating substances. Application to the involved areas of nystatin or clotrimazole creams.

Paronychia, Purulent

Synonym. None.

Sites of predilection. Periungual tissues of the fingers and toes.

Objective signs. The condition has an acute onset. The skin of the nail fold is edematous and erythematous. Pustules or vesicles may appear on slight pressure; pus may be expressed from the nail fold. This condition causes temporary or permanent distortion of the nail plate. One or more fingers or toes may be involved.

Subjective symptoms. Pain.

Etiology. Introduction of pyogenic bacteria into the nail folds by trauma. Forcible removal of a hangnail may precipitate the condition.

Histopathology. Nonspecific.

Diagnostic aids. Culture of the pyogenic bacteria on blood agar. Sensitivity tests should be done for antibiotic selection.

Relation to systemic disease. None.

Differential diagnosis. Candidal paronychia, other fungus infections.

Therapy. Hot soaks. Incision and drainage may be necessary. Systemic antibiotic administration is necessary based on results of culture. If neglected, osteomyelitis may develop in the bone of the distal phalanx.

Onycholysis, Photo

Synonym. None.

Sites of predilection. Nails.

Objective signs. Whitish or tan discoloration of the nail plate. Later the nail plate lifts off the bed. Rarely the patient notices any bullous formation.

Subjective symptoms. None to slight pain.

Etiology. The action of light upon the nail bed of a photosensitized patient to produce loss of nail plate adhesion.

Histopathology. Nonspecific destruction of the nail plate. Acute inflammatory changes are present in the nail bed.

Diagnostic aids. None.

Relation to systemic disease. None.

Differential diagnosis. Tinea of the nails, candidiasis.

Therapy. Remove any responsible photosensitizing drug such as tetracyclines, thiazides, sulfonamides, phenothiazines or furocoumarins.

Psoriasis of the Nails

Synonym. None.

Sites of predilection. Nails and other areas. See Psoriasis in Chapter 15: Papular Eruptions.

Objective signs. All or only one or two nails may be affected. Presenting symptoms may be limited to the formation of pits scattered over one or more of the nail plates, or the nail or nails may be pitted, friable, shortened, ridged and discolored. In some instances the nail plates are thickened and elevated from the nail bed by thickly packed, whitish, hyperkeratotic material.

The thickened nail plates, shortened at the face edge may closely resemble onychomycosis.

Subjective symptoms. None except the embarrassment produced by the cosmetic defect.

Psoriasis with pitted nails

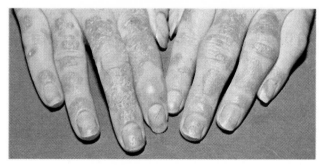

Etiology. Unknown.

Histopathology. See Chapter 15.

Diagnostic aids. Biopsy, history and physical examination, culture to rule out fungus infection.

Relation to systemic disease. May appear in conjunction with psoriatic arthropathy.

Differential diagnosis. Onychomycosis, eczema of the nails, onychia.

Therapy. None specific or effectual. See Chapter 15.

Pterygium

Synonym. None.

Sites of predilection. Fingernails.

Objective signs. There is an abnormal extension of the skin of the proximal nail fold over the lanula at the proximal portion of the nail plate.

Subjective symptoms. None.

Etiology. Unknown.

Histopathology. Nonspecific.

Diagnostic aids. The clinical appearance is characteristic.

Relation to systemic disease. None.

Differential diagnosis. The clinical appearance is characteristic.

Therapy. Removal of the pterygium by surgery, or by the use of 5-10% salicylic acid in 95% alcohol.

Spoon Nails

Synonym. Koilonychia.

Sites of predilection. Fingernails.

Objective signs. The nail plates are thin. In each nail there is a central concavity and the free edge of the plate is everted.

Subjective symtoms. None.

Etiology. Congenital or acquired.

Histopathology. Nonspecific.

Diagnostic aids. Clinical appearance is characteristic.

Therapy. None effective. Treat any associated disease.

Transverse Furrows or Bands

Synonym. Beau's lines.

Sites of predilection. Fingernails.

Objective signs. Transverse furrows appear on the nail plates, beginning in the proximal portion and progressing distally as the nail grows. Usually all of the nails are involved. Transverse arcuate furrows may be preceded by thin whitish bands.

Subjective symptoms. None.

Etiology. This condition, caused by a sudden change in the growth zone, is associated with systemic illness.

Histopathology. A defect in the normal matrix cells of the nails and a break in the continuity of the nail plate.

Diagnostic aids. Clinical appearance is characteristic.

Relation to systemic disease. The condition indicates some previously existing systemic disease such as scarlatina, pneumonia or other febrile illness. The defect in the plate becomes obvious as the nail plate grows out from the proximal fold. It usually appears 4-6 weeks after the onset of the illness.

Differential diagnosis. Clinical appearance is characteristic.

Therapy. Prognosis for the regrowth of the nails to their normal state is good.

Yellow Nail Syndrome

Synonym. None.

Sites of predilection. Fingers, toes.

Objective signs. All of the nails have a decreased growth rate, lose their cuticles and become thickened. Onycholysis may develop. The nail plates assume a yellowish or greenish-yellow color. Edema develops in the lower extremities and occasionally becomes universal.

Subjective symptoms. None produced by the nail change.

Etiology. Unknown.

Histopathology. Thickened nail plate.

Diagnostic aids. None of value.

Relation to systemic disease. Recurrent pleural effusions have been reported in some cases.

Therapy. None effective. The nail changes may spontaneously revert to normal.

CHAPTER 22

Tropical Diseases

In tropical or subtropical regions many common dermatoses are modified by conditions of climate to assume bizarre forms and more extensive involvement. These eruptions include fungus infections, acneform eruptions, eczematous conditions and the pyodermas. Conditions indigenous to the tropical zones include tinea imbricata, yaws, pinta, filariasis, mycetoma, tropical ulcer, ainhum and leishmaniasis.

Ainhum

Synonym. Spontaneous loss of little toe.
Countries. Africa and India.
Sites of predilection. Fifth metatarsophalangeal joint.
Objective signs. Begins as an area of marked hyperkeratosis on the plantar surface of the fifth metatarsophalangeal joint, across which runs a transverse groove or fissure. This groove deepens and extends until it surrounds the toe. The lesion may swell, ulcerate and discharge. Eventually, the constricting band causes spontaneous amputation of the digit. This disease occurs only in blacks.
Subjective symptoms. Usually painless.
Etiology. Unknown. Some cases may be related to trauma.
Histopathology. Nonspecific.

Diagnostic aids. Clinical appearance.
Relation to systemic disease. None.
Differential diagnosis. Congenital constricting bands.
Therapy. Surgical amputation.

Amoebiasis Cutis

This is relatively rare. Ragged ulcers occur in the perianal area, extending on to the rectal mucosa. Occasionally, following operation on an infected bowel, the patient may develop ragged ulcers at the site of the wound in the abdominal wall. The organism may be recovered from the margins of the ulcer. This condition responds readily to injections of emetine hydrochloride.

Urticaria frequently accompanies an attack of intestinal amoebiasis.

Dhobie Mark Dermatitis

Synonym. Dhobie itch, washerman's mark dermatitis, contact dermatitis to litchi nut.
Countries. India.
Sites of predilection. Areas exposed to dhobie mark, such as the back of the neck, the waist and the heels.
Objective signs. The first symptoms are well-defined, localized areas of erythema which develop a few

hours after exposure. These rapidly become edematous and, within a few hours, are recovered with numerous, small, discrete and confluent, closely aggregated, tense vesicles. The original lesions spread to involve larger areas in the same vicinity. Secondary pyogenic infection may occur.

Subjective symptoms. Intense pruritus.
Etiology. Juice of the litchi nut used for laundry marks.
Histopathology. That of contact dermatitis.
Diagnostic aids. Patch tests.
Relation to systemic disease. None.
Therapy. Topical corticosteroids are of value.

Dengue

Synonym. Break-bone fever.

This mosquito-borne disease is characterized by a severe febrile course, retrobulbar pain and intense pain in the bones and joints. Several days after the onset, the patient develops an ill-defined, pinkish, macular eruption over the trunk. Purpura and petechaie occur over the distal portions of the extremities. Axillary lymphadenopathy is a frequent finding. The condition is self-limited. Complications are rare.

Diphtheria

The *Corynebacterium diphtheriae* can be a secondary invader in eczematous eruptions, tinea pedis and traumatized areas and tropical ulcers. An adherent membrane develops. When an attempt is made to detach this, bleeding occurs. In all cases of long-standing cutaneous lesions which are resistant to therapeutic measures and show no tendency to heal, smears and cultures should be made to determine the presence of this organism. Neuritis, cardiac involvement and other toxic manifestations develop as a result of cutaneous diphtheria.

Etiology. C diphtheriae.
Diagnostic aids. Culture diphtheria bacteria.
Treatment. Administration of antitoxin. Penicillin should be given concurrently.

Diphyllobothriasis

Synonym. Tape worm.

Occasionally the parasite invades the skin and produces pseudotumors on the lower extremities. Elephantiasis may develop, with a pruritic, acneform eruption on the overlying skin.

Dracunculiasis

Synonym. Guinea worm infestation.
Countries. India, northern Africa, northern Egypt.
Sites of predilection. Legs.
Objective signs. A small rounded nodule appears on the foot near the ankle. Extending upward from this is a tortuous, cord-like mass. Occasionally, a small ulcer forms at the site of the worm's head at the time the embryos are released. Urticaria and asthma may accompany attacks.
Subjective symptoms. Pruritus and pain.
Etiology. *Dracunculus medinensis* (a worm).
Therapy. Inject tumor with 1:1000 bichloride of mercury and extract the worm. Natives extract the worm by rolling it on a stick and removing a few inches each day. These worms may be several feet in length.

Filariasis

Synonym. Elephantiasis.
Sites of predilection. Legs, scrotum, breasts, forearms.
Objective signs. Onset may be marked with fever and severe systemic symptoms. The affected part becomes edematous and inflamed and may drain a milky fluid. This symptom complex recurs frequently and increases in severity with each attack until the affected part is permanently enlarged. The overlying skin becomes markedly thickened, thrown into folds and verrucoid in appearance.
Subjective symptoms. Severe pain with attack, accompanied by fever and systemic symptoms.
Etiology. *Wuchereria bancrofti.*
Histopathology. Edema, fibrosis and lymphatic stasis.

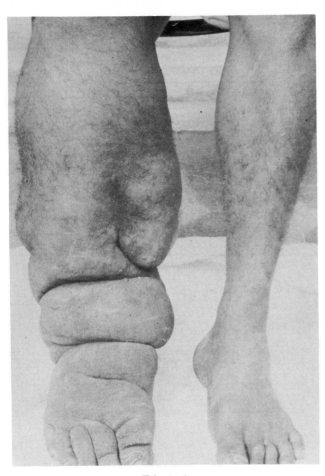

Filariasis

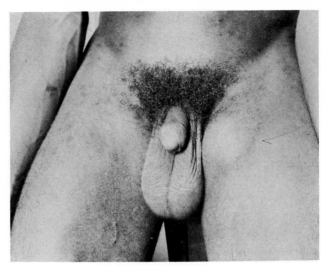

Filariasis, scrotal lesion

The epidermis is acanthotic and verrucoid.

Diagnostic aids. Demonstration of the filaria in blood smears, biopsy.

Relation to systemic disease. Filariasis is a systemic disease.

Differential diagnosis. Other conditions which cause lymphatic obstruction.

Therapy. Remove the patient from the tropics if possible; pressure bandage the involved areas; avoid surgery on the extremities. A plastic operation is the only satisfactory means of treatment for extensive breast and scrotal lesions. Systemic diethylcarbamazine is used to counteract the microfilaria in the blood stream.

Leishmaniasis, Cutaneous and Mucocutaneous

Synonym. Espundia (mucous form), uta (cutaneous form), leishmaniasis of the Brazilian forests.

Countries. Mexico, South America.

Sites of predilection. Exposed parts of the body, cartilage and bones of the nasopharynx.

Objective signs. A primary stage and a late stage form the two distinct phases of the disease. The primary stage occurs after an incubation period of 1-3 months and is marked by the appearance on the lips, face, neck, palms, soles, penis, female genitalia or scalp, of a crusted ulcer (espundic chancre) which heals after a period of months or years with a characteristic, star-shaped scar. The late stage occurs after a period of 1-20 years, with the formation of granulomatous ulcers and destruction of bone and cartilage in the nasopharynx. The tongue is almost invariably spared. Verrucous enlargements of the nose and face may occur. Marked lymphangitis is present in both the early and late phases.

Subjective symptoms. Slight pruritus to intense pain, depending on the type of involvement.

Etiology. *Leishmania brasiliensis.*

Diagnostic aids. Biopsy, culture for leptomonad form of parasite on NNN media.

Relation to systemic disease. Leishmaniasis is a systemic disease.

Differential diagnosis. Other granulomas.

Therapy. Antimony salts by parenteral administration.

Leishmaniasis, Tropical

Synonym. Oriental sore, oriental boil, Biskra button, Aleppo boil, desert sore.

Countries. India, Africa and Mediterranean Coast.

Sites of predilection. Ears, face, legs, arms.

Objective signs. After an incubation period of weeks to years, a small papule develops on the infected site. This gradually enlarges, softens in the center, and breaks down to form an ulcer from one to several centimeters in diameter.

Subjective symptoms. None to slight pain.

Etiology. *Leishmania tropica.*

Diagnostic aids. Demonstration of organism by biopsy or culture. (See Leishmaniasis.)

Therapy. Parenteral use of pentavalent antimony preparations. The disease is self-limited but scarring will occur.

Lepothrix

Synonym. Trichomycosis nodosa; trichomycosis axillaris flava, nigra and rubra.

Sites of predilection. Axillary hair.

Objective signs. Numerous firm yellowish, brownish or blackish concretions surrounding the hair shafts. These masses, which are actually chains and clumps of microorganisms, are bound to the hair shafts by a cement-like substance. Occasionally the hairs are fractured. The surrounding skin may be pinkish in color because of an inflammatory process.

Subjective symptoms. Usually none; may have slight pruritus.

Etiology. Variety of microorganisms.

Histopathology. The concretions on the hair shafts are formed of masses of microorganisms in a homogeneous substance resembling chitin.

Diagnostic aids. Microscopic examination of the involved hair.

Relation to systemic disease. None.

Differential diagnosis. Pediculosis, fungus infections.

Therapy. Shave the axillae and cleanse the skin with mild antiseptics.

Leprosy

Synonym. Lepra, elephantiasis graecorum.

Countries. Asia, Africa, Pacific Islands, Japan, Great Britain and sporadic cases in the United States.

Sites of predilection. See Leprosy in Chapters 14 and 15: Macular and Papular Eruptions.

Loaiasis

Synonym. Calabar swelling, Loa loa.

Countries. Africa.

Sites of predilection. Face, trunk, extremities.

Objective signs. Large, painless swellings resembling giant hives. Urticaria and eosinophilia are present.

Subjective symptoms. Pruritus and malaise.

Etiology. *Loa loa.*

Therapy. Surgical removal of the worm, parenteral use of antimony compounds or diethylcarbamazine.

Mycetoma

Synonym. Madura foot, podelkoma, mossy foot, fungus foot of India.

Countries. India, North Africa, Brazil and the southern part of the United States.

Sites of predilection. See Mycetoma in Chapter 6: Mycology.

Onchocerciasis

Synonym. Craw-craw.

Countries. Central America, Africa.

Sites of predilection. Trunk, extremities, face.

Objective signs. The eruption begins with the formation of follicular papules topped with hyperkeratotic plugs, usually on the extremities and trunk but not on the face and scalp. Pustules and ulcerating plaques heal with scar formation. Urticaria and systemic symptoms occur, and tumor-like lesions may develop on the head. If these lesions develop on the eye, permanent blindness occurs.

Subjective symptoms. Fever, malaise, gastric upsets, pruritus; pain with tumor lesions.

Etiology. Onchocerca volvulus.

Therapy. Preventive by destroying flies, *etc.* Excise tumors as they appear. (See Filariasis.)

Paracoccidioidal Granuloma

Synonym. South American blastomycosis, Almeida's disease.

Countries. Northern part of South America, Central America.

Sites of predilection. Buccal mucosa, pharnyx, skin.

Objective signs. Lesions may begin on the tongue, tonsils or buccal mucosa as papillary vegetations similar to condylomata acuminata. These lesions spread to the lips, nose and the surrounding skin. The fungus may enter through an abrasion on the skin and a primary lesion will develop at the site of inoculation, becoming a precursor of generalized cutaneous involvement. The cutaneous lesions also resemble condylomata acuminata and are granulomatous. Pus which accumulates between the verrucae produces crusting. No constitutional symptoms are produced until later.

The disease usually has a fatal termination.

Subjective symptoms. Discomfort caused by obstruction of the nasopharynx. Late in the course of the disease the general systemic symptoms are pronounced.

Etiology. Blastomyces brasiliensis.

Diagnostic aids. Biopsy and culture on Sabouraud's medium and blood agar.

Relation to systemic disease. Paracoccidioidal granuloma is a systemic disease.

Differential diagnosis. Other deep fungus infections, other granulomas.

Therapy. Amphotericin B.

Pinta

Synonym. Carate, mal del pinto, spotted disease.

Countries. Mexico, Central America.

Sites of predilection. Entire body; more marked on head and extremities.

Objective signs. The onset is marked by mild fever which lasts for a few days and is followed by an eruption of variously sized macules, which may be white, red, yellowish, brownish or violaceous. The lesions are sharply defined and may be covered with a furfuraceous or lamellated scale. In the later stage hyperkeratosis may become very marked. When the lesions undergo involution, permanent depigmentation remains. Unlike syphilis and yaws, pinta does not cause visceral involvement.

Subjective symptoms. Onset of the eruption may be marked with mild malaise and slight pruritus.

Etiology. Treponema carateum.

Diagnostic aids. Demonstration of the treponema by darkfield examination. The lesions must first be scarified in order to obtain the serum. Blood serologic tests.

Relation to systemic disease. Pinta is a systemic disease.

Differential diagnosis. Vitiligo, fungus infections.

Therapy. The treatment is the same as the treatment for syphilis. Penicillin is the drug of choice.

Strongyloidosis

This disease is caused by the *Strongyloides stercoralis* and primarily involves the intestinal tract. At the time of invasion, it produces severe pruritus and localized urticaria.

Schistosomiasis

Synonym. Synonyms for specific schistosome disorders include swimmer's itch, Katayama fever and schistome dermatitis.

Sites of predilection. The extremities exposed to the contaminated water are the sites of swimmer's itch. In visceral schistosomiasis (Katayama fever) there is a generalized eruption and the granulomatous lesions are more commonly observed around the genitalia.

Objective signs. The cutaneous reaction to the schistosomes depends upon the stage of the disease. Swimmer's itch is a pruritic papular eruption which is a reaction to the penetration of schistosome cercariae into the skin. Avian (nonhuman) schistosomes are most commonly involved in the production of this disorder in the United States. Massive infections of *Schistosoma mansoni* or *Schistosoma haematobium* can also produce this eruption. The eruption starts as 1-2 mm macules at the penetration site. Diffuse erythema or urticaria may appear at this time. Ten to fifteen hours later papules with erythematous haloes appear. These lesions may coalesce or form vesicles a few days later. Resolution requires 7-10 days and may be followed by hyperpigmentation.

Katayama fever signifies the egg-laying activity of the adult worm and is characterized by fever, eosinophilia, hepatosplenomegaly, lymphadenopathy, diarrhea and urticaria.

Cutaneous granulomatous lesions with or without fistulas occur as a result of ectopic egg deposition. These lesions consist of flesh-colored, slowly enlarging nodules which may subsequently ulcerate, fissure or form fistulous tracts.

Subjective symptoms. Cercarial entry into the skin may be noted as a prickling or burning when the water evaporates. Other symptoms include pruritus and pain.

Etiology. Swimmer's itch is a result of the entry of cercariae (usually avian) into human skin. Katayama fever is thought to be an immune complex disease coinciding with the entry of eggs into the blood and the cutaneous granulomas are a hypersensitivity reaction against the substance released into the nearby tissues by the egg.

All schistosomes have the same life cycle beginning with the passage of the eggs from the primary host. Three species infect man. *S haematobium*, *S mansoni* and *Schistosoma japonicum*. The eggs from the first species are usually passed from the urine whereas those of the latter two species are excreted in the stool. The eggs develop into a swimming miracidium if they come in contact with water. These structures penetrate the integument of certain snails, migrate to the digestive gland and mature into fork-tailed cercariae. These larval forms leave the snail when mature and search for the primary host. They then penetrate the skin, migrate via the blood stream to the lungs, climb up the trachea and enter the gut where they penetrate the intestine to reside in the venous plexi around the urinary bladder or intestine (depending upon their species). When eggs are laid they repenetrate the viscera and are excreted.

Histopathology. In swimmer's itch only nonspecific inflammatory changes are evident on biopsy. Ectopic schistosome eggs are centered in a granuloma which in turn is replaced by fibrosis. The eggs of some species can be best seen with PAS stains.

Diagnostic aids. History of immersion in epidermic areas. Biopsy of ectopic egg granulomas, blood smear for eosinophilia.

Relation to systemic disease. Visceral schistosomiasis is a generalized disease. Swimmer's itch has no systemic sequellae.

Differential diagnosis. Swimmer's itch may be confused with insect bites or stings from various marine animals. Katayama fever can mimic many systemic diseases. Ectopic egg granulomas may be initially diagnosed as tumors or resolving nodular pyodermas.

Therapy. Therapy for swimmer's itch is mostly symptomatic with antihistamines and antipruritic lotions. Visceral schistosomiasis is usually treated with trivalent antimonials, lucanthone or niridazole (ambilhar).

Tinea Imbricata

Synonym. Tokelau ringworm, Burmese ringworm.

Countries. Fiji Islands, Solomon Islands, India. Occurs only in the natives.

Sites of predilection. Trunk, extremities.

Objective signs. Begins as a pinkish or reddish macule, eventually covered with an adherent whitish scale which peels toward the margin of the lesion. Scaling continues to form in the central portion and, as the lesion spreads peripherally, concentric and polycyclic figures are formed. Annular lesions occur. The disease is persistent.

Subjective symptoms. Varying degrees of pruritus.

Etiology. *Trichophyton concentricum.*

Histopathology. The fungi may be seen in the stratum corneum by use of the PAS stain.

Diagnostic aids. Microscopic examination of scales treated with potassium hydroxide.

Relation to systemic disease. None.

Differential diagnosis. Other fungus infections, pityriasis rosea, seborrheic dermatitis.

Therapy. Systemic griseofulvin.

Tsutsugamushi

Synonym. Japanese river fever.

This disease is characterized by the appearance of the necrotic ulcer at the site of inoculation, and the development of a petechial eruption involving the palms, soles, face, trunk and forearms. It is caused by a rickettsia and has a high mortality rate.

Ulcer, Tropical

Synonym. Tropical phagedenic ulcer, Aden ulcer, Malabar ulcer, Naga sore, desert sore.

Countries. Common in all tropical countries.

Sites of predilection. Legs, usually the lower third.

Objective signs. The lesions begin as small papules or vesicles. These undergo necrosis to form ulcers, which spread peripherally to involve large areas, sometimes encircling the leg. The ulcers have precipitous margins and dirty, greenish-gray bases, and frequently become complicated with cutaneous diphtheria.

Subjective symptoms. Pain at the site of the lesion.

Etiology. Filth. Varieties of microorganisms have been found including staphylococci and streptococci.

Histopathology. Nonspecific.

Tinea imbricata

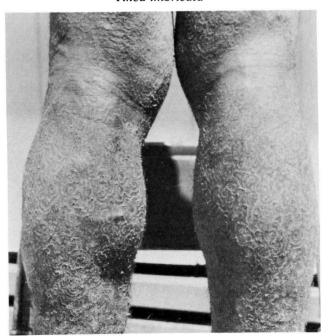

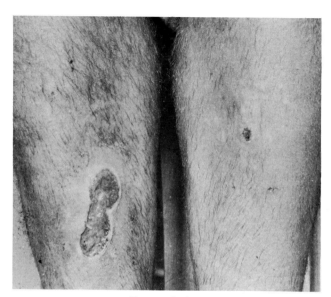

Tropical ulcer

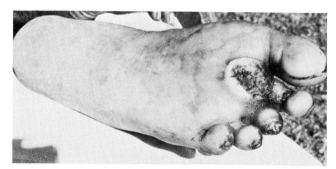

Yaws, primary

Crab yaws

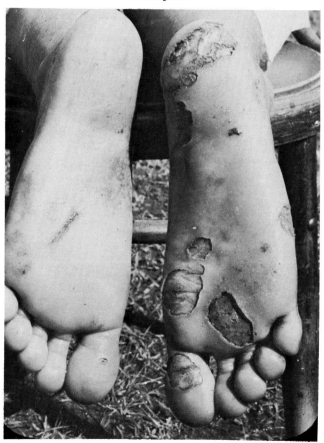

Diagnostic aids. Clinical appearance of the lesion, history and physical examination, cultures of the lesion on blood agar. Serologic tests for streptococci.

Relation to systemic disease. None.

Differential diagnosis. Gumma, tuberculosis, other granulomas.

Therapy. Good hygiene. Administer the proper antibiotic. Surgical repair with grafting may be necessary.

Uncinariasis

Synonym. Hookworm disease.

Frequently the early symptoms are ignored or misdiagnosed as epidermophytosis. At the site of inoculation of the parasite, one may find a vesicular eruption on the soles which resembles a fungus infection.

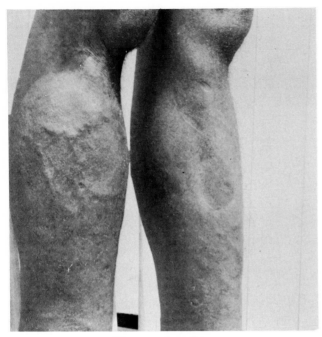

Yaws, saber shins

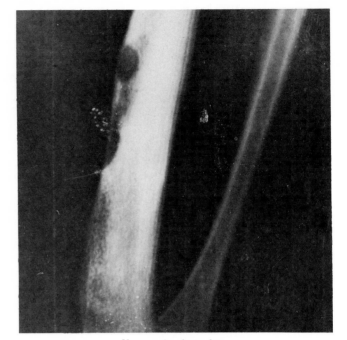

X ray of saber shins

Yaws

Synonym. Frambesia, pian, treponematosis.

Countries. Central and South Pacific Islands, North Africa, West Indies, Asia. Occurs only in natives.

Sites of predilection. In the early stages only the skin is involved; later, destructive lesions appear in the bone and soft tissue.

Objective signs. The primary lesion or "mother yaw" usually occurs on the feet or legs, and begins as a papule or small nodule, which breaks down to form a granulomatous mass, usually topped with a serosanguinous crust. The margins of this lesion are folded back like petals. In 1-4 weeks, secondary lesions develop, and vary in appearance from dull reddish papules to crusted ulcers. The crusts covering the ulcers have a piled-up appearance ("oyster shell crust"). Tertiary of late yaws appears in 1-3 years, forming destructive, gum-matous lesions in bone or skin.

Subjective symptoms. Variable degrees of pruritus and occasionally, transient fever with early yaws. Pain with late lesions.

Etiology. *Treponema pertenue.* This is not a sexually transmitted disease but is carried by insect vectors (*eg,* flies).

Histopathology. Histopathologic picture is similar to that observed in syphilis.

Diagnostic aids. Demonstration of the *T pertenue* by darkfield examination from early lesions; blood serologic tests.

Relation to systemic disease. Yaws is a systemic disease.

Differential diagnosis. Syphilis, tuberculosis, deep fungus infections, other granulomas.

Therapy. The same as the therapy for syphilis. Penicillin is the drug of choice.

CHAPTER 23

Peripheral Vascular Diseases

Angiokeratoma

See Angiokeratoma in Chapter 15: Papular Eruptions.

Angioneurotic Edema

See Angioneurotic Edema in Chapter 15: Papular Eruptions.

Arteriosclerosis

Synonym. Hardening of the arteries.

Sites of predilection. Cutaneous symptoms are usually noted on the distal portions of the lower extremities.

Objective signs. Occlusion or extreme narrowing of the lumen of an artery may result in anoxia of the distal portion of the extremity, causing dry atrophy of the digits, which become black and undergo spontaneous amputation.

Subjective symptoms. Moderate to severe pain in the affected extremity. Intermittent claudication is a frequent symptom.

Etiology. Thickening of the arterial intima with resultant narrowing of the lumen.

Histopathology. Loss of elastic tissue and calcification of artery wall. Intimal thickening and rupturing or erosion of the endothelium.

Relation to systemic disease. Arteriosclerosis is a disseminated disease with cerebral and cardiac symptoms.

Diagnostic aids. History and physical examination.

Differential diagnosis. Raynaud's disease, Buerger's disease.

Therapy. None effective.

Cutis Marmorata

See Cutis Marmorata in Chapter 14: Macular Eruptions.

Dermatomyositis

See Dermatomyositis in Chapter 14: Macular Eruptions.

Erythema ab Igne

See Erythema ab Igne in Chapter 14: Macular Eruptions.

Frostbite

Synonym. Dermatitis congelationis, trench foot, im-

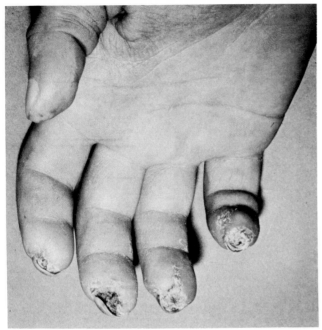

Frostbite

mersion foot, pernio.

Sites of predilection. Nose, ears, cheeks, fingers, toes.

Objective signs. The symptoms vary from a mild, transitory erythema to a deep-seated inflammatory process which involves nerves and blood vessels and frequently results in gangrene.

The milder degrees of frostbite are evidenced by initial vasoconstriction then subsequent erythema and edema and, occasionally, vesiculation. In the more severe forms, gangrene may occur without vesicle formation. Pulses may be absent. Bones may be involved. The condition tends to recur on reexposure to cold.

Subjective symptoms. Vary from mild paresthesias to severe pain.

Etiology. Usually associated with prolonged exposure to below freezing temperatures or contact with cold metals which are good heat conductors. Symptoms may follow immersion in cold water,

wearing wet clothing, or standing on cold ground for long periods (as soldiers in combat). Ingestion of alcohol causes vasodilatation and increases susceptibility to cold.

Histopathology. Occlusion of superficial blood vessels with resultant cutaneous changes.

Diagnostic aids. History and physical examination.

Relation to systemic disease. None usually.

Differential diagnosis. Raynaud's disease.

Therapy. Prophylaxis is the best treatment. Layers of warm, clean, dry clothing should be worn and changed frequently. Rapid rewarming of the affected part with controlled heat slightly over 37.7°C is indicated. If gangrenous changes are present, surgical intervention is usually necessary.

Glomus Tumor

See Glomus Tumor in Chapter 15: Papular Eruptions.

Hemangioma

See Hemangioma in Chapter 15: Papular Eruptions.

Telangiectasia, Hereditary Hemorrhagic

Synonym. Rendu-Osler-Weber syndrome.

Sites of predilection. Face, tongue, buccal surfaces, nasal septum, viscera.

Objective signs. Multiple purpuric lesions are present on the fingertips, tongue, palpebral conjunctivae and buccal mucosae. Visceral telangiectasias rupture and cause intestinal bleeding which may reach major proportions.

Subjective symptoms. There may be abdominal discomfort associated with hemorrhage, plus the psychic trauma associated with the cosmetic defect.

Histopathology. The histopathologic picture is that of a nonspecific telangiectasia.

Diagnostic aids. History and physical examination.

Relation to systemic disease. The disease is systemic.

Differential diagnosis. Multiple benign telangiectasias, senile angioma, purpura, "spiders."

Therapy. None effective. Transfusions may be necessary.

Lupus Erythematosus

See Lupus Erythematosus in Chapter 14: Macular Eruptions.

Nevus Araneus

Synonym. Spider nevus.

See Nevus Araneus in Chapter 14: Macular Eruptions.

Nevus Flammeus

Synonym. Port wine stain.

See Nevus Flammeus in Chapter 14: Macular Eruptions.

Periarteritis Nodosa

See Periarteritis Nodosa in Chapter 14: Macular Eruptions.

Peripheral Vascular Diseases

The objective symptoms of many peripheral vascular diseases are primarily cutaneous. These are described in detail in the following outline.

I. Intrinsic diseases of the peripheral blood vessels
  A. Congenital anomalies
    1. Arteriovenous aneurysm
  B. Nevi
    1. Port wine stain (nevus flammeus)
    2. Hemangiomas
      a. Superficial (strawberry mark, hemangioma simplex)
      b. Deep (cavernous)
      c. Nevus araneus (spider nevus)
  C. Tumors
    1. Glomus tumor
    2. Angiosarcoma
    3. Angioendothelioma
    4. Senile angiomas and angiokeratomas
    5. Multiple idiopathic hemorrhagic sarcoma (Kaposi's)
  D. Traumatic
    1. Arteriovenous aneurysm
    2. Erythema ab igne
    3. Frostbite
    4. Varix of the lips and other isolated varices
    5. Cutis marmorata
    6. Radiodermatitis
II. Inflammatory and obstructive lesions of the peripheral vessels, associated with systemic disease
  A. Capillaries
    1. Idiopathic telangiectasia
    2. Hereditary telangiectasia
    3. Hemosideroses
      a. Purpura annularis telangiectodes
      b. Progressive pigmentary dermatosis
      c. Pigmented purpuric lichenoid dermatitis
    4. Necrobiosis lipoidica
  B. Veins
    1. Varicose veins
    2. External thrombosed hemorrhoids
    3. Thrombophlebitis and phlebothrombosis
  C. Arteries
    1. Arteriosclerosis
    2. Periarteritis nodosa
    3. Buerger's disease (thromboangiitis obliterans)
    4. Diabetes mellitus (arteriosclerosis)
    5. Erythromelalgia
    6. Syphilis
III. Functional disturbances of the peripheral vessels, associated with systemic disease
  A. Psychosomatic responses
    1. Angioneurotic edema
    2. Flush or blush
    3. Red, sweaty palms
    4. Acrocyanosis
  B. Organic lesions (connective tissue or autoimmune)
    1. Raynaud's disease

2. Scleroderma
3. Dermatomyositis
4. Lupus erythematosus
5. Periarteritis nodosa

Purpuric Pigmented Eruption of the Lower Extremities

Synonym. Purpura annularis telangiectodes, Schamberg's disease, pigmented purpuric lichenoid dermatitis. These are probably variants of the same condition.

See these conditions in Chapter 14: Macular Eruptions.

Raynaud's Disease

See Raynaud's Disease in Chapter 14: Macular Eruptions.

Scleroderma

See Scleroderma in Chapter 14: Macular Eruptions.

Telangiectasia

Synonym. None.

Sites of predilection. Face, trunk and other areas.

Objective signs. Tortuous, dilated, small blood vessels develop on the nose and contiguous portions of the cheeks. Other areas of the body may be affected. The condition is not inflammatory.

Subjective symptoms. Vary with the severity of the condition and the underlying disease.

Etiology. The variety of causes includes X-ray damage, actinic rays, alcoholism, drug reactions, liver disease, blood dyscrasias, *etc.* Telangiectasia may be associated with rosacea, or may occur following prolonged, repeated exposure to sun, wind or excessive heat.

Histopathology. Dilated vessels; usually little or no inflammation is present.

Diagnostic aids. History and physical examination, hemograms and other laboratory studies for a suspicious underlying cause.

Relation to systemic disease. Cirrhosis of the liver, blood dyscrasias, rosacea, allergic reactions and malignancies are among those conditions which produce telangiectasia.

Differential diagnosis. None usually necessary.

Therapy. If the cosmetic defect is annoying, the vessels may be treated with electrolysis (occlusion by the galvanic or high frequency current). Treat the underlying disease.

Thromboangiitis Obliterans

Synonym. Buerger's disease.

Sites of predilection. Extremities.

Objective signs. This condition may be unilateral or bilateral. Scattered areas of obliterative endovasculitis of arteries and veins cause symptoms which include gangrene of toes, ulcers and other dystrophies. Arterial pulsations may be absent.

Subjective symptoms. None to severe pain.

Etiology. Buerger's disease has been associated with the use of tobacco. The condition occurs most frequently in men.

Histopathology. Vasculitis with thrombus formation at intervals along the course of arteries and veins.

Diagnostic aids. Biopsy, history and physical examination.

Relation to systemic disease. This is a disease of peripheral blood vessels.

Differential diagnosis. Thrombophlebitis, Raynaud's disease, arteriosclerosis.

Therapy. Of little value. Avoid use of tobacco. Amputation of part or all of the affected extremity may be necessary.

Varicose Veins

Synonym. None.

Sites of predilection. Lower extremities, scrotum, occasionally trunk.

Objective signs. Dilated, tortuous, superficial and deep veins, occasionally forming large cutaneous masses. Palpable thrombus formation may occur. Inflammatory reaction in the vein walls may predispose to clot formation (phlebothrombosis). If these thrombi become infected, intense pain may result (thrombophlebitis). Ulceration may occur, caused by slight trauma or spontaneous rupture of a dilated vein.

Subjective symptoms. None to intense pain in the extremities.

Etiology. Weakening of the valves in the intercommunicating veins.

Histopathology. Dilated vessels. If inflammatory reaction is present, there may be an infiltration of polymorphonuclear cells or thrombus formation.

Diagnostic aids. History and physical examination.

Relation to systemic disease. None usually, although an abdominal mass productive of increased venous pressure predisposes to varicosities.

Differential diagnosis. The condition is characteristic.

Therapy. Varicose vein stripping may be necessary in selected cases.

Varix of the Lip

Synonym. None.

Sites of predilection. Usually the lower lip.

Objective signs. The lesions are small, purplish, soft masses, measuring 1-2 mm in diameter. They are easily compressed free of blood, unless an organized thrombus is present.

Subjective symptoms. The cosmetic defect causes some concern.

Etiology. May be caused by trauma.

Histopathology. Dilated vein containing a clot.

Diagnostic aids. Biopsy, history and physical examination.

Relation to systemic disease. None.

Differential diagnosis. Hemangioma, nevi.

Therapy. Obliteration of lesion by electrodesiccation.

Vasculitis

This is a symptom complex covering a spectrum of disorders of unknown etiology.

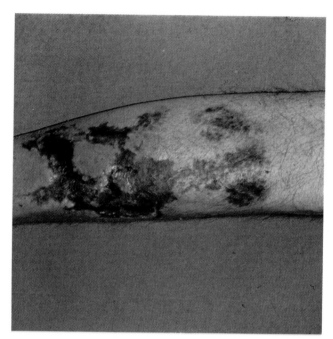

Necrotizing vasculitis

Synonym. Toxic vasculitis, nodular vasculitis, necrotizing vasculitis.

Sites of predilection. The extremities.

Objective signs. Lesions of vasculitis range from

Necrotizing angiitis

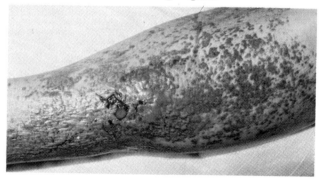

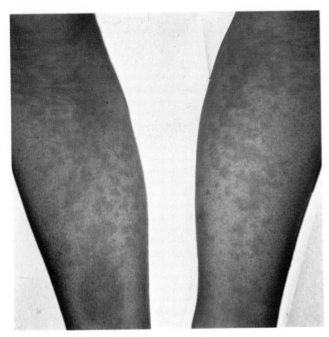

Toxic vasculitis

small, purpuric macules to necrotic ulcers of variable sizes. The lesions are usually discrete and violaceous with some surrounding telangiectasia. Tenderness may be present. Red or bluish, tender nodules may occur along the arterioles and occasional hemorrhagic vesicles or bullae may be seen.

Subjective symptoms. Pain.

Etiology. This symptom complex is currently regarded as an idiopathic hypersensitivity phenomenon, which possibly develops in response to allergens such as food additives, drugs or infection.

Histopathology. There is a polymorphonuclear leukocytic infiltration of the vessel walls and the vascular tissue. The damaged vessels become surrounded by mononuclear cells and may later thrombose.

Diagnostic aids. Biopsy, serum complement, sedimentation rate.

Relation to systemic disease. This condition may develop as a symptom of serum sickness, drug sensitivity or reaction to infection.

Differential diagnosis. Purpura, erythema nodosum, periarteritis nodosa.

Therapy. Search for and eliminate any possible allergen. Systemic therapy with corticosteroids may be necessary.

CHAPTER 24

Some Syndromes of Dermatologic Significance

Achard-Thiers Syndrome
syn: *Diabetic bearded women syndrome*
Diabetes mellitus
Facial hirsutism and other signs of masculinization in
women
Obesity
Hypertension

Acrodermatitis Enteropathica
Cutaneous lesions on extremities and in perioral area
Gastrointestinal disturbances
Alopecia

Acute Defibrination Syndrome
Ecchymoses into the skin
Areas of gangrene
Absence of plasma fibrinogen

Addisonian Syndrome
syn: *Adrenocortical insufficiency syndrome*
Mental, muscular and cardiovascular asthenia
Diarrhea and digestive disturbances
Bronze-like pigmentation of the skin and mucous
membranes
Progressive anemia

Adrenogenital Syndrome
syn: *Adrenal virilism syndrome*
Increased production of androgens
Masculinization in the female
Sexual precocity in the male

Albright's Syndrome
syn: *Albright-McCune-Sternberg syndrome, Wright's
syndrome*
Melanotic pigmentation of the skin
Osteitis fibrosa cystica
Precocious puberty in the female

Aldrich's Syndrome
Thrombocytopenic purpura
Chronic eczema
Recurrent purulent infections

Allergic Dermal-Respiratory Syndrome
Urticaria or eczema
Asthma, hay fever or perennial rhinitis

Allergic Granulomatosis Syndrome
See Churg-Strauss syndrome

Angioendotheliomatosis Proliferans Systemisata Syndrome
Chills and fever
Nodules of various sizes on the trunk and extremities
Diffuse malignant proliferation of vascular endothelium

Angiomatosis Retinae et Cerebelli Syndrome
See von Hippel-Lindau syndrome

Ascher's Syndrome
Edema of the upper eyelids
Blepharochalasis
Hyperplastic labial glands
Acquired double lip

Ataxia-Telangiectasia Syndrome
syn: Louis-Bar syndrome, cephalo-oculocutaneous-telangiectasia syndrome
Progressive cerebellar ataxia
Oculocutaneous telangiectasia
Peculiar eye movements
Frequent sinopulmonary infections

Auriculotemporal Syndrome
syn: Frey's syndrome
Pain, vasodilatation and hyperhidrosis of the cheek while eating

Basal Cell Nevus Syndrome
Multiple basal cell nevi
Dyskeratosis of the palms and soles
Multiple dental follicular cysts of the jaws
Skeletal changes: spina bifida, bifid ribs, *etc.*
Hypertelorism

Behcet's Syndrome
syn: Triple symptom complex
Recurrent ulceration of the genitals
Intermittent aphthous lesions of the mouth
Uveitis or iridocyclitis followed by hypopyon

Bloch-Sulzberger Syndrome

syn: Incontinentia pigmenti syndrome; Siemens' syndrome
Irregular pigmentation often preceded by bullous or verrucous phases
Neurologic, mental, bony, ocular, and dental defects

Bloom's Syndrome
Primordial dwarfs
Telangiectatic erythematous areas resembling lupus erythematosus on face
Crusted bullous lesions on lips
Sun sensitivity
Café au lait spots

Blue Rubber-Bleb Nevus Syndrome
Bluish bladder-like hemangiomas of the skin
Spontaneous nocturnal pain
Supralesional sweating
Bleeding from intestinal hemangiomas

Brunsting's Syndrome
Chronic herpetiform plaques about the head and neck
Atrophic scarring of affected sites
Severe burning and pruritus
Mostly middle-aged or older men

Brushfield-Wyatt Syndrome
Extensive port-wine staining of the skin
Hemiplegia
Mental retardation
Various stigmata of degeneration

Bürger-Grütz Syndrome
syn: Idiopathic familial hyperlipemia syndrome
Xanthomas of skin and mucous membranes
Hepatosplenomegaly
Lipemia retinalis
Recurrent attacks of abdominal pain

Buschke-Ollendorff Syndrome
Multiple cutaneous fibromas
Osteopoikilosis

Carcinoid Syndrome

syn: Thorson-Biörck syndrome
Peripheral vasomotor phenomena, notably peculiar flushing and episodic cyanosis
Asthma
Refractory diarrhea
Cardiac symptoms
Pellagroid dermatitis
Scleroderma-like changes of the lower extremities

Cat Scratch Syndrome

Red, tender papule at the site of a cat scratch
Regional lymphadenopathy
Irregular fever
Systemic manifestations

Chédiak-Higashi Syndrome

Anomalous leukocytic inclusions
Photophobia, pale ocular fundi and decreased lacrimation
Hyperhidrosis
Pigmentary disturbances: partial albinism and excessive pigmentation of areas exposed to sunlight
Hepatosplenomegaly and lymphadenopathy

Chlorpromazine Pigmentation Syndrome

Light brown, slate-gray, or violaceous discoloration of the exposed parts
Deposition of fine particulate matter in the cornea and lens
Star-shaped opacities in the anterior portion of the lens

Chondrodystrophia Congenita Punctata Syndrome

See Conradi's syndrome

Chondroectodermal Dysplasia Syndrome

See Ellis-van Creveld syndrome

Chronic Familial Neutropenia Syndrome

Constant depression of neutrophil count
Marked periodontal lesions

Churg-Strauss Syndrome

syn: Allergic granulomatosis syndrome
Debilitation
Attacks of fever
Eosinophilia
Asthma, ulcerative colitis or organic disease of the heart and spleen
Erythematous papules or nodules on the extensor surfaces of the extremities and scalp

Clouston's Syndrome

syn: Hidrotic ectodermal dysplasia syndrome
Generalized hypotrichosis
Dystrophy of the nails
Hyperkeratosis of the palms and soles
Pigmentation

Cockayne's Syndrome

Lupus erythematosus-like dermatitis
Atrophy of subcutaneous fat
Defective mental and physical development
Various ocular manifestations
Progressive loss of hearing

Conradi's Syndrome

syn: Chondrodystrophia congenita punctata syndrome
Stippled foci of calcification within hyaline cartilage
Dwarfing
Stiff contracted joints
Congenital cataracts
Diffuse dry, scaly, rough, thick, red or pigmented skin
Few and rudimentary hairs, eyebrows and eyelashes

Cornelia de Lange's Syndrome

Primordial growth failure
Various skeletal abnormalities
Mental retardation
Characteristic cry
Hirsutism
Cutis marmorata and facial "cyanosis"

Crigler-Najjar Syndrome

syn: Familial nonhemolytic jaundice with kernicterus
syndrome, kernicterus syndrome
Marked retention icterus
Severe neurologic disease

Cronkhite-Canada Syndrome
Gastrointestinal polyposis
Generalized alopecia
Diffuse and spotty pigmentation
Atrophy of the nails
Diarrhea

CRST Syndrome
Subcutaneous calcinosis
Raynaud's phenomenon
Sclerodactyly
Multiple telangiectasia

Cushing's Syndrome
Hirsutism
Acne
Abdominal striae
Moon face
"Buffalo type" obesity
Insulin-resistant diabetes
Arterial hypertension

Degos' Syndrome
syn: Cutaneointestinal syndrome
Crops of crusted umbilicated papules
Depressed atrophic scars
Acute abdominal symptoms
Fatal fulminating peritonitis

Dennie-Marfan Syndrome
Congenital syphilis
Spastic paralysis
Mental retardation

Dercum's Syndrome
Multiple, painful, symmetric lipomas
Obesity

Neuritis
Mental depression and deterioration

DeSanctis-Cacchione Syndrome
Xeroderma pigmentosum
Mental deficiency
Stunted growth
Occasional gonadal immaturity

Down's Syndrome
syn: Mongolism, Trisomy 21 anomaly
Mental retardation
Brachycephaly
Acromicria
Characteristic changes in skin, mucosae, hair and eyes

Dubin-Johnson Syndrome
Chronic idiopathic icterus (direct bilirubin)
Greenish-black discoloration of liver

Dyskeratosis Congenita Syndrome
Atrophy and pigmentation of skin
Dystrophy of nails and teeth
Oral leukoplakia and sometimes bullae
Various ocular manifestations

Dysplasia Oculodentodigitalis Syndrome
Microphthalmos, bilateral medial epicanthus, high
    myopia, glaucoma
Enamel defect, microdontia, missing teeth
Camptodactylia of the fifth fingers, variable syndactyly,
    missing middle phalanges of the toes
Hypotrichosis of the scalp, eyebrows, eyelashes;
    cutaneous atrophy
Small alae nasi with anteverted nostrils

Ectodermosis Erosiva Pluriorificialis Syndrome
See Klauder's syndrome

Ehlers-Danlos Syndrome
syn: Cutis hyperelastica syndrome
Hyperextensibility of joints

Hyperelasticity and friability of the skin
Fragility of blood vessels
Papyraceous scars
Pseudotumors
Spherules

Elastoidosis Syndrome
Numerous small cutaneous cysts, nodules and comedones
Abnormal folds and wrinkles on face, neck, ears

Ellis-van Creveld Syndrome
syn: Chondroectodermal dysplasia syndrome
Ectodermal dysplasia affecting the nails, hair and teeth
Chondrodysplasia
Polydactyly
Congenital cardiac defect

Encephalotrigeminal Angiomatosis Syndrome
See Sturge-Weber syndrome

Erythema Multiforme Exudativum Major Syndrome
See Stevens-Johnson syndrome

Erythema Nodosum-Hilar Adenopathy Syndrome
Erythema nodosum
Bilateral hilar lymphadenopathy

Familial Idiopathic Dysproteinemia Syndrome
Familial edema of legs
Leg ulcers in males
Functional vascular changes in females

Familial Nonhemolytic Jaundice with Kernicterus Syndrome
syn: Familial Mediterranean fever syndrome
Short recurrent bouts of fever
Pain in abdomen and/or chest and/or joints
Erysipelas-like erythema

Familial Ulceration of the Extremities Syndrome
See Thévenard's syndrome

Fanconi Syndrome
Severe progressive refractory hypoplastic anemia
Generalized brown pigmentation of skin
Various congenital defects

Felty's Syndrome
Chronic deforming arthritis
Splenomegaly and lymphadenopathy
Leukopenia
Nodules and pigmentation of skin

Focal Dermal Hypoplasia Syndrome
Linear areas of pigmentation and thinning of the skin with herniation of adipose tissue
Papillomatosis of the mucous membranes and skin
Dystrophy of the nails
Defects of the eyes, bones, teeth, heart, central nervous system

Gardner-Diamond Syndrome
Painful ecchymoses at the sites of trauma followed by progressive erythema and edema
Limited to women
Possible autosensitization by the patients to their own extravasated red blood cells

Gardner's Syndrome
Multiple polyposis of colon
Bony exostoses
Soft tissue tumors

Gaucher's Syndrome
Hepatosplenomegaly
Brown pigmentation of skin
Mucocutaneous hemorrhage
Cuneiform thickenings of ocular conjunctiva

Gianotti-Crosti Syndrome
syn: Infantile acrodermatitis papulosa syndrome
Erythematopapular lesions on face, neck and extremities of children
Respiratory or gastrointestinal symptoms

Lymphadenopathy
Fever and malaise

Glomangiomatous-osseous Malformation Syndrome
Multiple glomus tumors
Hypoplasia and osteoporosis of the bones of the affected forearm

Gopalan's Syndrome
Malnutrition
Burning and prickling sensation in extremities
Hyperhidrosis

Gorlin-Chaudhry-Moss Syndrome
Craniofacial dysostosis
Patent ductus arteriosus
Hypertrichosis
Hypoplasia of the labia majora
Dental and ocular abnormalities

Gougerot Trisymptomatic Syndrome
Papuloerythematous rash resembling erythema multiforme
Purpuric macules
Discrete dermal or hypodermal nodules

Graham-Little Syndrome
syn: *Feldman's syndrome*
Lichen planus
Acuminate follicular papules
Cicatricial alopecia

Grönblad-Strandberg Syndrome
Pseudoxanthoma elasticum
Angioid streaks of retina

H Disease
See Hartnup syndrome

Hallermann-Streiff Syndrome
syn: *François syndrome*

Malformation of the skull
Proportionate nanism
Hypotrichosis
Atrophy of skin
Congenital cataracts

Hand-Foot Syndrome
Painful symmetrical swelling of hands or feet or both
Sickle cell disease
Periosteal elevation or lytic areas or both in the metacarpals, metatarsals, and phalanges

Hand-Schüller-Christian Syndrome
Defects in the membranous bones
Exophthalmos
Diabetes insipidus
Cutaneous xanthoma
Stomatitis and gingivitis

Hanot-Chauffard Syndrome
syn: *Bronze diabetes syndrome, hemochromatosis*
Diabetes mellitus
Hypertrophic cirrhosis of liver
Dark brown pigmentation of skin

Harada's Syndrome
syn: *Uveomeningitis syndrome*
Bilateral posterior uveitis
Retinochoroidal detachment
Signs of meningeal irritation with pleocytosis
Alopecia, vitiligo and poliosis may be temporarily associated

Hart Syndrome
See Hartnup syndrome

Hartnup Syndrome
syn: *Hart syndrome, H disease*
Pellagra-like skin rash
Intermittent cerebellar ataxia
Psychiatric manifestations
Constant aminoaciduria

Sensitive to sunlight

Hemangioma-Thrombocytopenia Syndrome
Giant vascular tumor
Thrombocytopenic purpura

Hereditary Anhidrotic Ectodermal Dysplasia Syndrome
See Siemens' syndrome

Hereditary Benign Intraepithelial Dyskeratosis Syndrome
Soft, white asymptomatic thickenings of oral mucosa
Bulbar conjunctivitis

Hereditary Hemorrhagic Telangiectasia Syndrome
See Rendu-Osler-Weber syndrome

Hereditary Onycho-osteodysplasia Syndrome
See nail-patella syndrome

Herpes Zoster-Hemiplegia Syndrome
Herpes zoster ophthalmicus
Contralateral hemiplegia developing about 4 weeks later

Herricks's Syndrome
See Sickle cell disease

Hidrotic Ectodermal Dysplasia Syndrome
See Clouston's syndrome

Hines-Bannick Syndrome
Intermittent attacks of low temperature and disabling sweating

Horner's Syndrome
Enophthalmos
Ptosis of upper eyelid
Miosis
Absence of sweating on the ipsilateral side of face and neck

Increased secretion of tears
Facial hemiatrophy

Hunterian Glossitis Syndrome
Atrophic glossitis
Achylia gastrica
Primary macrocytic anemia

Hunt's Syndrome
syn: *Ramsay Hunt syndrome*
Herpes zoster oticus
Facial palsy

Hurler-Pfaundler Syndrome
See Hurler's syndrome

Hurler's Syndrome
syn: *Gargoylism, Hurler-Pfaundler syndrome*
Dwarfism with bizarre skeletal deformities
Hepatosplenomegaly
Clouding of cornea in autosomal recessive form
Mental retardation
Deafness
Various cutaneous manifestations
    a. Specific papular and nodular lesions
    b. Thickening of skin of hands
    c. Hypertrichosis

Hutchinson-Gilford Syndrome
syn: *Progeria syndrome, premature senility syndrome*
Infantilism with dwarfism
Alopecia: head, eyebrows, eyelashes
Premature aging

Hutchinson's Syndrome
syn: *Hutchinson's triad*
Interstitial keratitis
Eighth nerve deafness
Characteristic incisors and molars

Hutchinson's Triad
See Hutchinson's syndrome

Hydantoin Syndrome
Morbilliform, scarlatiniform, urticarial or exfoliative
  eruptions
Fever
Lymphadenopathy, particularly cervical nodes
Splenic or hepatic enlargement
Eosinophilia

Hydralazine Syndrome
Simulates systemic lupus erythematosus

Hypertrophied Frenuli Syndrome
syn: Orofaciodigital syndrome
Abnormally developed frenuli
Pseudoclefts in upper lip, tongue and palate
Mental retardation
Familial trembling
Syndactyly

Idiopathic Familial Hyperlipemia Syndrome
See Bürger-Grütz syndrome

Incontinentia Pigmenti Syndrome
See Bloch-Sulzberger syndrome

Infantile Acrodermatitis Papulosa Syndrome
See Gianotti-Crosti Syndrome

Intestinal Lipodystrophy Syndrome
See Whipple's Disease

Jacquet's Syndrome
Hypotrichosis of scalp
Congenital absence of nails
Dental anomalies

Jadassohn-Lewandowsky Syndrome
See pachyonychia congenita syndrome

Joliffe's Syndrome
Nicotinic acid deficiency

Kernicterus Syndrome
See Crigler-Najjar syndrome

Klauder's Syndrome
*syn: Ectodermosis erosiva pluriorificialis syndrome,
  erythema multiforme bullosum*
Fever and constitutional symptoms
Erythema multiforme with involvement of orificial
  mucous membranes

Klippel-Feil Syndrome
Shortness of neck
Limitation of head movements
Growth of hair low down on neck

Klippel-Trenaunay-Weber Syndrome
Congenital angiomatosis of an extremity
Developmental hypertrophy of underlying bone and
  soft structures

Kwashiorkor Syndrome
Edema
Depigmentation of hair and skin
Failure of growth
Various dermatoses

Lawford's Syndrome
Facial nevi
Chronic simple glaucoma
May be unilateral or bilateral

Leschke Syndrome
General weakness
Numerous brownish macules
Hyperglycemia

Letterer-Siwe Disease
Cutaneous changes
      a. Hemorrhagic manifestations
      b. Maculopapular or papular lesions
      c. Typical seborrheic dermatitis
      d. Moist erosions and ulcers

Hepatosplenomegaly
Generalized lymphadenopathy

Lindau's Disease
See von Hippel-Lindau disease

Lipoatrophic Diabetes Syndrome
Generalized and marked wasting of subcutaneous fat
Diabetes mellitus
"Acromegaloid" overgrowth
Hepatosplenomegaly
Generalized muscular hypertrophy
Hypertrichosis
Hyperpigmentation
Hypertension
Corneal opacities

Lipomelanotic Reticulosis Syndrome
See Pautrier-Woringer Syndrome

Lobstein's Syndrome
Fragility of bones and laxity of ligaments
Blue sclerae and often precocious arcus senilis
Otosclerosis
Defects in dental enamel
Unusual fineness of hair

Lorain-Lévi Syndrome
syn: Pituitary nanism syndrome
Dwarfism
Infantilism
Absence of pubic and axillary hair
Premature aging of skin

Maffucci's Syndrome
syn: Dyschondroplasia with hemangiomas syndrome
Multiple hemangiomas of the skin, mucosae and internal organs
Bone lesions
Dyschondroplasia
Phleboliths

Malignant Granulomatous Syndrome of Childhood
Eczematoid dermatitis of central part of face
Chronic suppurative lymphadenitis
Hepatosplenomegaly
Infiltration of pulmonary tissue

Marchesani's Syndrome
Short stocky well-developed stature
Thick skin and hair
Spade-like hands with short stubby fingers
Various ocular abnormalities

Marfan's Syndrome
syn: Arachnodactyly
Skeletal abnormalities, notably arachnodactyly
Ocular lesions
Cardiovascular disease
Striae atrophicae

Margolis Syndrome
Sex-linked deaf-mutism
Total albinism

Mastocytosis
Urticaria pigmentosa
Hepatosplenomegaly
Generalized lymphadenopathy
Osteolytic or sclerotic changes in the bones
Symptoms resembling those of carcinoid syndrome

McCarthy-Shklar Syndrome
Pyostomatitis vegetans
Ulcerative colitis

Melkersson-Rosenthal Syndrome
Recurring facial paralysis or paresis
Edema and granuloma formation of lips
Scrotal tongue

Metastasizing Lipase-Forming Pancreatic Adenoma Syndrome
Polyarthritis

Nonsuppurating panniculitis
Eosinophilia

Mikulicz's Syndrome
Bilateral painless enlargement of salivary and lacrimal
glands
Xerostomia
Decrease in or absence of lacrimation

Milian's Syndrome
Fever and systemic manifestations
Ninth-day erythema after the first injection of an
arsphenamine

Monilethrix Syndrome
Spindle hair formation
Keratosis pilaris
Koilonychia

Morgagni's Syndrome
Almost entirely in women
Symmetric benign thickening of the inner table of the
frontal bone of the skull
Obesity
Hirsutism and other signs of virilism
Neuropsychiatric symptoms
Progressive visual failure

Morvan's Syndrome
Recurrent painless whitlows
Syringomyelia or occasionally leprosy

Moynahan's Syndrome
Multiple symmetrical mottling with moles
Genital hypoplasia
Stunted growth
Psychic infantilism despite normal intelligence
Congenital mitral stenosis

Muckle-Wells Syndrome
Recurrent urticaria
Deafness

Nephritis

Mucocutaneous Ocular Syndrome
See Stevens-Johnson Syndrome

Mucosal Respiratory syndrome
Influenza-like symptoms or pneumonia
Manifestations of Stevens-Johnson syndrome

Myotonia Dystrophica Syndrome
syn: Steinert's Disease
Tonic spasm of muscle
Atrophy of skin, panniculus, musculature
Hypogonadism
Hypotrichosis
Cataracts
Premature aging

Naegeli's Syndrome
syn: Melanophoric nevus syndrome
Reticular pigmentation of skin
Yellowish spots on enamel of teeth
Hypohidrosis
Keratosis palmaris et plantaris

Nail-Patella Syndrome
*syn: Hereditary onycho-osteodysplasia syndrome,
congenital iliac horns syndrome, Fong's syn-
drome*
Onychatrophia
Absent or rudimentary patellae
Congenital dislocation of head of radius
Iliac horns

Netherton's Syndrome
Congenital ichthyosiform erythroderma
Bamboo hairs
Atopy

Niemann-Pick Disease
Malnutrition and retarded development
Hepatosplenomegaly

Occasional cutaneous xanthomas
Pigmentation of skin

Oculo-oro-genital Syndrome
Stomatitis with ulcers on buccal mucosa
Conjunctivitis and keratitis
Exfoliative dermatitis of scrotum
Diarrhea
Inadequate rice diet

Oid-Oid Disease
See Sulzberger-Garbe syndrome

Orofaciodigital Syndrome
See hypertrophied frenuli syndrome

Pachyonychia Congenita
syn: *Jadassohn-Lewandowsky syndrome*
Thickening of nails
Plantar and palmar bullae and keratoses
Follicular papules on buttocks and extremities
Leukoplakia oris
Corneal dyskeratoses and cataracts

Papillon-Lefèvre Syndrome
Palmar and plantar hyperkeratosis
Periodontosis with loss of teeth

Parotitis-herpangina-Coxsackie Virus Syndrome
Inflammation of parotid glands
Vesicular and ulcerative lesions in the faucial area
Presence of Coxsackie virus

Pautrier-Woringer Syndrome
syn: *Lipomelanotic reticulosis syndrome*
Generalized superficial lymphadenopathy
Chronic nonspecific pruritic skin disorder

Pemphigus Erythematosus
See Senear-Usher syndrome

Petges-Clégat Syndrome

syn: *Poikilodermatomyositis*
Poikiloderma
Dermatomyositis

Peutz-Jeghers Syndrome
Melanin pigmentation in and about body orifices and
    on digits
Generalized intestinal polyposis

PHC Syndrome
Premolar aplasia
Hyperhidrosis
Canities prematura

Pierre Robin Syndrome
Micrognathia
Microglossia
Glossoptosis
Cleft palate

Plummer-Vinson Syndrome
Atrophy of mucosa of mouth, tongue, pharynx and
    esophagus
Dysphagia
Thinning of lips and angular cheilitis
Koilonychia
Microcytic hypochromic anemia
Middle-aged women

Premature Senility
See Hutchinson-Gilford syndrome

Pretibial Fever Syndrome
Erythematous rash in pretibial area
Mild respiratory symptoms
Febrile illness of five days' duration

Pringle's Syndrome
syn: *Bourneville's disease, epiloia*
Adenoma sebaceum
Epilepsy
Mental deficiency

Refsum's Syndrome
Ichthyosis simplex
Chronic polyneuritis
Retinitis pigmentosa
Progressive nerve deafness
Cerebrospinal fluid shows albuminocytologic dissociation

Reiter's Syndrome
Polyarthritis
Conjunctivitis
Nonspecific urethritis
Cutaneous lesions resembling erythema multiforme or keratosis blenorrhagica

Rendu-Osler-Weber Syndrome
syn: *Hereditary hemorrhagic telangiectasia, Osler's disease*
Numerous telangiectases on skin and mucous membranes
Frequent or severe hemorrhage from the mucous membranes

Riley-Day Syndrome
syn: *Familial autonomic dysfunction, dysautonomia*
Intermittent erythematous patches while eating or during excitement
Excessive perspiration
Drooling persisting beyond infancy
Absence of lacrimation

Riley-Smith Syndrome
Macrocephaly without hydrocephalus
Multiple subcutaneous hemangiomas
Pseudopapilledema

Rosenthal-Kloepfer Syndrome
Corneal leukomata
Acromegaloid appearance
Cutis verticis gyrata

Rothmann-Makai Syndrome

Spontaneous circumscribed panniculitis

Rothmund-Thomson Syndrome
syn: *Poikiloderma congenitale*
Poikiloderma
Juvenile cataracts
Congenital bone defects
Disturbances of hair growth
Sensitivity to sunlight
Defective development of teeth and nails
Hypogonadism

Rud's Syndrome
Ichthyosis simplex
Mental deficiency
Epilepsy
Infantilism

Savill's Syndrome
syn: *Epidemic exfoliative dermatitis*
Dry or moist exfoliative dermatitis of face, scalp and upper limbs
Appears as epidemics in institutions

Scalded Skin Syndrome
syn: *Toxic epidermal necrolysis, Lyell's disease*
Premonitory symptoms such as vomiting, diarrhea and sore throat
Initial widespread erythema and edema
Extensive loosening of the skin with or without bullae
Denudation with raw red oozing surfaces sometimes involving practically the entire body
Extreme toxicity, frequent death

Schäfer's Syndrome
Pachyonychia congenita
Retardation of development with oligophrenia and hypogenitalism

Schönlein-Henoch Syndrome
Nontraumatic hemorrhage in skin, subcutaneous tissue and joints

Gastrointestinal pain and hemorrhage
Painful swelling of joints
Localized edema of backs of hands, face or elsewhere

Senear-Usher Syndrome
syn: Pemphigus erythematosus
Lupus erythematosus-like lesions on face
Changes related to seborrheic eczema
Positive Nikolsky's sign

Sézary Reticulosis Syndrome
See Sézary syndrome

Sézary Syndrome
syn: Sézary reticulosis syndrome
Generalized exfoliative erythroderma
Intense pruritus
Pigmentation
Benign lymphadenopathy
Monocytosis
Alopecia

Sickle Cell Anemia
syn: Dresbach's syndrome, Herrick's anemia
Chronic leg ulcers
Green sclerae
Pain in bones and joints
Weakness and dyspnea
Attacks of acute abdominal pain
Recurrent swelling of hands and feet in children

Siemens' Syndrome
syn: Hereditary anhidrotic ectodermal dysplasia
Absence or paucity of sweat, sebaceous and mucous
   glands
Hypotrichosis
Anodontia

Sjögren-Larssen Syndrome
Congenital ichthyosiform erythroderma
Mental deficiency
Cerebral spastic diplegia

Frequently degenerative retinitis

Sjögren's Syndrome
*syn: Sicca syndrome, Gougerot-Houwer-Sjögren syn-
   drome*
Dryness of all the mucous membranes and skin
Rheumatoid arthritis
Anemia
Sometimes scleroderma-like changes, alopecia or tel-
   angiectasia

Speransky-Richen-Siegmund Syndrome
Necrosis and sloughing in the oral cavity leading to
   perforation of the hard palate into the maxillary
   sinus and detachment of the alveolar processes

Stein-Leventhal Syndrome
Bilateral polycystic ovaries
Amenorrhea or oligomenorrhea
Obesity
Sterility
Hirsutism

Stevens-Johnson Syndrome
*syn: Erythema multiforme exudativum major syn-
   drome, mucocutaneous ocular syndrome*
Fever and severe constitutional symptoms
Extensive stomatitis
Conjunctivitis, keratitis, uveitis and even panophthal-
   mitis
Ulcerative lesions on mucosa of nose, penis, vagina
   and around the anus
Vesicobullous or petechial and hemorrhagic eruption
   of face, hands and feet

Stewart-Treves Syndrome
Edematous upper extremity after radical breast surgery
Lymphangiosarcoma

Still-Chauffard Syndrome
Arthritis of cervical spine
Anemia and leukemia

Splenomegaly and lymphadenopathy
Cutaneous pigmentation especially on cheeks

Stryker-Halbeisen Syndrome
Scaly and vesicular patches of erythroderma on face, neck and upper chest
Intense pruritus
Macrocytic anemia

Sturge-Weber Syndrome
syn: Encephalotrigeminal angiomatosis
Angiomas of the choroid and pia mater
Ipsilateral port-wine stain along the course of the superior and middle branches of the trigeminal nerve
Convulsions
Paralysis
Mental retardation
Visual disturbances

Sudeck's Disease
Acute pain
Atrophy of skin, subcutaneous tissue and bone
These manifestations occur at site of minor injury

Sulzberger-Garbe Syndrome
syn: Oid-oid disease
Chronic exudative discoid and lichenoid dermatitis
Severe nocturnal pruritus
Chiefly middle-aged men

Sweat Retention Syndrome
syn: Tropical anhidrotic asthenia
Anhidrosis
Miliaria
Attacks of pruritus
Severe systemic symptoms
Collapse

Thévenard's Syndrome
syn: Familial ulceration of the extremities, familial mutilating ulcerous acropathy

Trophic ulcers of soles
Hypoesthesia to pain and temperature on soles
Osteodystrophies of the feet and spine

Thibierge-Weissenbach Syndrome
syn: Scleroderma-calcinosis syndrome
Scleroderma
Small areas of periarticular and subcutaneous calcification

Thorson-Biörck Syndrome
See carcinoid syndrome

Thyrohypophyseal Syndrome
Euthyroidism
Ocular manifestations suggestive of hyperthyroidism
Facial, temporal and pretibial edema

Thyroid Acropachy Syndrome
Hyperthyroidism with exophthalmos
Pretibial myxedema
Clubbing and/or hypertrophic osteoarthropathy

Tietze Syndrome
Albinism
Deaf-mutism
Hypoplasia of the eyebrows

Touraine-Solente-Golé Syndrome
Cutis verticis gyrata of scalp, forehead, face and extremities
Periosteal lesions and hypertrophy of long bones
Clubbing of fingers and toes

Toxic Epidermal Necrolysis
See scalded skin syndrome

Triparanol Syndrome (Mer-29 syndrome)
Alopecia
Depigmentation of hair
Ichthyosis
Cataracts

Trisomy 18 Syndrome
Loose folds of skin with typical dermal patterns
Horizontal palmar creases and downy hair
Poor subcutaneous tissue
Multiple congenital anomalies

Trisomy 21 Syndrome
See Down's syndrome

Troisier's Syndrome
Bronzed cachexia
Diabetes

Tropical Anhidrotic Asthenia
See sweat retention syndrome

Turner's Syndrome
syn: Bonnevie-Ullrich syndrome
Webbed neck
Lymphangiectatic edema of hands and feet
Cutis laxa and hyperelastica
Mental and physical retardation
Variable multiple congenital abnormalities
Forty-five chromosomes (XO)

Uveomeningitis
See Harada's syndrome

van der Hoeve's Syndrome
Blue sclerae
Brittle bones
Deafness
Frequently abnormalities of nails, hair and dental
    enamel

Vogt-Koyanagi Syndrome
Severe bilateral anterior uveitis with iritis and glaucoma
Vitiligo
Alopecia
Poliosis
Dysacusis
Deafness may occur

von Hippel-Lindau Disease
syn: Lindau's disease, angiomatosis retinae et cerebelli
    syndrome
Angiomatosis of retinae and cerebellum
Tumors and cysts of various organs
Rarely, vascular nevi of face

Waardenburg's Syndrome
Pigmentary disturbances including partial albinism,
    white forelock and partial or complete hetero-
    chromia iridis
Congenital deafness
Fused thick eyebrows, broad nasal root and laterally
    displaced inner canthi

Waldenström's Syndrome
Relapsing nonthrombocytopenic purpura
Xerostomia and xerophthalmia
Hepatosplenomegaly and lymphadenopathy
Mild anemia
High erythrocyte sedimentation rate
Marked increase in serum gamma globulin
Rarely, infiltrated cutaneous and mucosal nodules and
    plaques

Waterhouse-Friderichsen Syndrome
Cyanosis
Purpuric macules
Meningococcal septicemia

Weber-Christian Syndrome
syn: Relapsing febrile nodular nonsuppurative pan-
    niculitis
Recurrent attacks of malaise and fever
Localized inflammatory subcutaneous nodules
Subcutaneous atrophy at the sites of nodules

Wegener's Syndrome
syn: Wegener's granulomatosis
Severe sinopulmonary inflammation
Generalized necrotizing angiitis
Symmetrical papulonecrotic lesions of extremities

Widespread vesicular or urticarial lesions
Pyoderma gangrenosum
Terminal renal insufficiency

Werner's Syndrome
syn: Progeria of the adult
Premature graying and loss of hair
Atrophy of the skin and subcutaneous tissue
Precocious cataracts
Endocrine disturbances

Whipple's Disease
syn: Intestinal lipodystrophy
Arthritis
Abdominal symptoms
Diarrhea with evidence of steatorrhea
Cough
Loss of weight

Asthenia
Patchy brown pigmentaton of the skin
Purpura

Willan-Plumbe Syndrome
Psoriasis

Wilson's Syndrome
syn: Hepatolenticular degeneration
Kayser-Fleischer rings
Azure lunulae of nails
Behavior disorders frequent
Disturbance in copper metabolism

Yellow Nail Syndrome
Slow-growing discolored nails
Edema, usually of the ankles

INDEX

Page numbers in boldface indicate main discussion of disease entity.